Bio-mathematics, Statistics, and Nano-Technologies

Finding effective methods for mosquito control remains one of the great global challenges facing this generation. ***Bio-mathematics, Statistics and Nano-Technologies: Mosquito Control Strategies*** brings together experts from a large array of disciplines in order to provide a comprehensive overview of cutting-edge techniques to model, analyse and combat mosquito-transmitted vector-borne diseases.

Features

- Includes multiple case studies
- Suitable for scientists and professionals working on methods for mosquito control and epidemiology
- Provides a much-needed focal point for interdisciplinary discussion

Bio-mathematics, Statistics, and Nano-Technologies

Mosquito Control Strategies

Edited by
Peyman Ghaffari
Chair of IMAAC & CIDMA, University of Aveiro, Portugal

CRC Press
Taylor & Francis Group
Boca Raton London New York

CRC Press is an imprint of the
Taylor & Francis Group, an **informa** business
A CHAPMAN & HALL BOOK

First edition published 2023
by CRC Press
6000 Broken Sound Parkway NW, Suite 300, Boca Raton, FL 33487-2742

and by CRC Press
4 Park Square, Milton Park, Abingdon, Oxon, OX14 4RN

CRC Press is an imprint of Taylor & Francis Group, LLC

Library of Congress Cataloging-in-Publication Data

Names: Ghaffari, Peyman, editor.
Title: Bio-mathematics, statistics and nano-technologies : mosquito control strategies / edited by Peyman Ghaffari, CIDMA, University of Aveiro, Portugal.
Other titles: Mosquito control strategies
Description: First edition. | Boca Raton : C&H/CRC Press, 2023. | Includes bibliographical references.
Identifiers: LCCN 2022061381 (print) | LCCN 2022061382 (ebook) | ISBN 9780367477004 (hardback) | ISBN 9781032524764 (paperback) | ISBN 9781003035992 (ebook)
Subjects: LCSH: Mosquitoes--Control. | Mosquitoes as carriers of disease. | Mosquitoes--Control--Mathematical models. | Mosquitoes as carriers of disease--Mathematical models.
Classification: LCC RA640 .B536 2023 (print) | LCC RA640 (ebook) | DDC 614.4/323--dc23/eng/20230419
LC record available at https://lccn.loc.gov/2022061381
LC ebook record available at https://lccn.loc.gov/2022061382

ISBN: 978-0-367-47700-4 (hbk)
ISBN: 978-1-032-52476-4 (pbk)
ISBN: 978-1-003-03599-2 (ebk)

DOI: 10.1201/9781003035992

Typeset in Nimbus Roman
by KnowledgeWorks Global Ltd.

Publisher's note: This book has been prepared from camera-ready copy provided by the authors

In Memory of Rajesh Madhukar Pai
My Friend and First Member of IMAAC

Contents

Foreword xix

Contributors xxi

CHAPTER 1 ▪ Introduction and Overview 1

PEYMAN GHAFFARI

SECTION I **Control of Mosquitoes and Their World: An Overview**

CHAPTER 2 ▪ Practical Control Methods and New Techniques for Mosquito Control 9

RUI-DE XUE, STEVE PEPER, AND GUNTER C. MULLER

2.1 INTRODUCTION 10
2.2 PERSONAL AND COMMUNITY PROTECTION 10
2.2.1 Repellent 10
2.2.2 Community Protection and Participate 11
2.3 SPACE SPRAYING 11
2.3.1 ULV 11
2.3.2 Thermal Fogging 11
2.3.3 Barrier Spray 12
2.4 INDOOR RESIDUAL SPRAYING (IRS) 12
2.5 INSECTICIDE-TREATED BED NETS (ITN) 12
2.6 NEW CONTROL TECHNIQUES 13
2.6.1 Genetic Control, Gene Drive, and GMO 13
2.6.2 Incompatible Insect Technique (IIT) 14
2.6.3 Sterile Insect Technique (SIT) 14
2.6.4 Adult Mosquito Control Traps 14
2.6.5 Lethal Ovitrap and Autocidal Gravid Ovitrap (AGO) 15
2.6.6 Larvicide Traps 15
2.6.7 Auto-dissemination Method 15
2.6.8 Endectocides 16

2.6.9 Attractive Toxic Sugar Bait (ATSB) 16

2.6.10 Vaccine 16

2.6.11 Challenges and Conclusions 16

CHAPTER 3 ▪ Concepts of the Best Management Practices for Integrated Pest, Mosquito, and Vector Management 19

RUI-DE XUE AND TONG-YAN ZHAO

3.1 INTRODUCTION 19

3.2 CONTROL METHODS/TOOLS 20

3.2.1 Immature Stage Control 20

3.2.2 Adult Control 21

3.3 INTEGRATED PEST MANAGEMENT (IPM) 21

3.4 INTEGRATED MOSQUITO MANAGEMENT (IMM) 22

3.5 INTEGRATED VECTOR MANAGEMENT (IVM) 24

3.6 BEST MANAGEMENT PRACTICE (BMP) 25

3.7 SUMMARY 25

CHAPTER 4 ▪ Overview of Personal Protection Measures Through the Innovative Use of Repellent-Textiles 27

ASGHAR TALBALAGHI, SAHAR HASSANDOUST, AND CHINAZOM ENUKOHA

4.1 INTRODUCTION 28

4.2 INNOVATIVE VECTOR CONTROL 29

4.3 INSECT REPELLENT MODE OF ACTION 31

4.4 TEXTILE AND PERSONAL PROTECTION 32

4.5 IMPREGNATION OF TEXTILE 33

4.6 EVALUATION OF REPELLENTS 33

4.7 MEASURING THE ENTOMOLOGICAL PERFORMANCE OF TEXTILES 35

4.7.1 Open field, Italian Mosquito Control Association Alessandria Italy, 2019 35

4.7.2 Laboratory test at Anastasia Mosquito Control District St. Augustine, Florida, USA 2020 36

4.7.2.1 Measuring the efficacy of textile samples already treated for arm test 37

4.7.2.2 Measuring the efficacy of textile samples treated with 2 types of micro spraying treatment before the test 38

4.7.2.3 Measuring the efficacy of textile samples already treated for glove test (Figures 4.7 and 4.8) 39

4.7.2.4 Evaluation of lotions of botanical-based repellents 39
4.7.3 Measuring the efficacy of repellent by use of olfactometer 39
4.7.3.1 Measuring the efficacy of Ultrasound devices 40
4.8 DISCUSSION ON LAB TEST 40
4.9 RESULTS 42
4.10 FUTURE PERSPECTIVE AND OUTLOOK 43
4.11 CONCLUSION NOTE 44

CHAPTER 5 ▪ Biology, Surveillance and Control of Mosquito Vectors 47

ELTON ROGOZI

5.1 INTRODUCTION ON THE MOSQUITO BIOLOGY 48
5.2 BIOLOGY OF MOSQUITOES (*CULICIDAE*) 49
5.3 LIFE STAGES OF MOSQUITOES 49
5.3.1 Eggs stage of mosquitoes 50
5.3.2 Larval stage of mosquitoes 51
5.3.3 Pupal stage of mosquitoes 51
5.3.4 Adults stage of mosquitoes 52
5.4 MOSQUITOES CONCERNS FROM THE PUBLIC HEALTH OVERVIEW 53
5.5 ROLE OF MOSQUITOES IN DISEASE TRANSMISSION 54
5.6 MOSQUITOES AS VECTOR OF DISEASES 55
5.7 VECTORIAL CAPACITY AND COMPETENCE OF MOSQUITOES 55
5.8 PATHOGENS THAT CAN BE TRANSMITTED BY MOSQUITOES 55
5.8.1 Parasites 55
5.8.2 Viruses 56
5.8.3 Bacteria and other pathogens 56
5.9 BITING ACTIVITY OF MOSQUITOES 56
5.10 MOSQUITO AS NUISANCE 57
5.11 SURVEILLANCE AND ENTOMOLOGICAL STUDIES OF MOSQUITO VECTOR 57
5.12 MOSQUITO SURVEILLANCE AND COLLECTION 58
5.12.1 Light traps 58
5.12.1.1 CDC light traps 59
5.12.2 Human landing catch (collection) 60
5.12.2.1 Resting catch 60
5.13 OTHER TECHNIQUES USED FOR MOSQUITO COLLECTION 61
5.13.1 Adult sampling 61

5.13.2 Gravid Trap Box 62
5.13.3 The ovitraps 62
5.13.4 The Fay Prince trap 62
5.13.5 Precaution during human landing catch 63
5.14 MOSQUITO PRESERVATION, LABELING AND TRANSPORTATION 63
5.14.1 Preservation 63
5.14.2 Labeling 64
5.14.3 Mosquito identification 64
5.14.4 Dynamic and density of mosquito population 64
5.15 DATA PROCESSING AND FIELD EVALUATION OF MOSQUITO BITES VIA HLC METHOD FOR TESTING REPELLENT TREATED TEXTILES 64
5.15.1 Calculation for the efficacy 64
5.16 MOSQUITO LANDING RATES FOR THE EVALUATION OF REPELLENT IMPREGNATED TEXTILES EFFICACY! 65
5.16.1 Mosquito biting activity 65
5.16.2 Main objectives 65
5.16.3 Study site 66
5.16.4 Technique used to measure the mosquito landing bites rates 66
5.16.4.1 Results from Divjake study site 67
5.16.4.2 Results from Durres study site 68
5.16.4.3 Results from the Darzeze, Fier study site 69
5.17 CONCLUSION 70
5.18 PROSPECTIVE FOR FUTURE STUDY 71
5.18.1 The protocol used to test the repellent treated t-shirts 71

SECTION II **Mathematical Modelling of Immunity: An Overview based on Malaria**

CHAPTER 6 ▪ Models of Acquired Immunity to Malaria: A Review 75

MIRACLE AMADI, GERRY KILLEEN, AND HEIKKI HAARIO

6.1 INTRODUCTION 76
6.2 COMPLEX FACTORS OF ACQUIRED IMMUNITY AND THEIR MODELING APPROACHES 79
6.2.1 Misleading binary view on malaria immunity 80
6.2.2 Functional immunity/clinical immunity 84
6.2.3 Unfounded assumptions about what protective efficacy of immunity constitutes 85

6.2.3.1 Transmission-blocking immunity (TBI) 85
6.2.3.2 Increase in recovery rate/Decrease in infection duration 86
6.2.4 Age and acquired immunity 87
6.2.5 Duration of acquired immunity to malaria 90
6.2.6 Malaria parasite variants 92
6.2.7 Acquired variant-specific and variant-transcending immunity 94
6.2.8 Superinfection/ Reinfection and acquired immunity 96
6.2.9 Other factors influencing the acquisition of immunity 97
6.2.9.1 Effect of intervention measures on immunity acquisition and malaria prevalence 97
6.2.9.2 Climatic driving effect on immunity acquisition 98
6.2.9.3 Effect of population dynamics on immunity acquisition 99
6.2.10 Summary of modelling approaches 100
6.3 DISCUSSION 102

Appendices 105

6.A METHODS FOR LITERATURE SEARCH 107
6.A.1 Literature search strategy and selection criteria 107
6.A.2 Outcome of literature search 107
6.B DETAILED MODEL DESCRIPTIONS 109

SECTION III **Mathematical Epidemiology including Mosquito Dynamics and Control Theory**

CHAPTER 7 ▪ Multi-strain Host-vector Dengue Modelling: Dynamics and Control 117

PETER RASHKOV, EZIO VENTURINO, AND BOB W. KOOI

7.1 INTRODUCTION 118
7.2 DESCRIPTION OF THE MODELS 119
7.2.1 Equilibria and basic reproduction number $\mathcal{R}_0$ 121
7.2.2 Time scale separation 122
7.2.3 Example: SIR-UV model 124
7.3 TWO-STRAIN DENGUE MODELS 125
7.3.1 Host-only models 125
7.3.2 Host-vector models 128
7.4 COMPARISON OF HOST-ONLY AND HOST-VECTOR MODEL 130
7.4.1 Results for autonomous systems 130

7.4.2 Results for seasonally-forced systems 131

7.5 MODELING AND ANALYSIS OF CONTROL MEASURES FOR DENGUE FEVER 132

7.5.1 Description of a model with vaccination 132

7.5.1.1 Analysis of the SIRvUV model 133

7.5.1.2 Sensitivity analysis of the SIRvUV model 136

7.5.2 Model with vector control 137

7.5.2.1 Analysis of the SIRqVM model 139

7.5.2.2 Sensitivity analysis of the SIRqVM model 140

7.5.3 Viability analysis of vector control 141

7.6 CONCLUSIONS 142

Appendices 145

7.A TIME SCALE SEPARATION, EXAMPLE: SIR-UV MODEL 147

7.B PARAMETER VALUES 148

Chapter 8 ▪ Mathematical Models and Optimal Control in Mosquito Transmitted Diseases 149

Peyman Ghaffari, Cristiana J. Silva, and Delfim F. M. Torres

8.1 INTRODUCTION 149

8.2 CONTROLLED MODEL 151

8.3 OPTIMAL CONTROL PROBLEM 153

8.4 NUMERICAL RESULTS AND DISCUSSION 154

Appendices 159

8.A UNIQUE OPTIMAL SOLUTION 161

Section IV **Topological Studies: Topology Meets Mosquito Control**

Chapter 9 ▪ On the Shape and Design of Mosquito Abatement Districts 165

James R. Bozeman

9.1 INTRODUCTION 165

9.2 DESIGNS OF CURRENT MOSQUITO ABATEMENT REGIONS 166

9.2.1 Rhode Island, USA [3] 166

9.2.1.1 Mosquito Control Measures: 2019 Pesticide Applications 166

9.2.1.2 Mosquito Control Measures: 2019 Pesticide Applications 167
9.2.2 Winnipeg, Canada [4] 168
9.3 FLIGHT DISTANCES, PATTERNS AND TIMES OF VARIED MOSQUITOES AND DISEASE AGENTS 168
9.4 CREATION OF DISTRICTS 169
9.5 ANALYSIS AND CONCLUSIONS 171

SECTION V **Chemometric and Mathematical Approach for Modelling and Designing Mosquito Repellents**

CHAPTER 10 ■ A Multiplatform Chemometric Approach to Molecular and Mathematical Modeling of Mosquito Repellents 177

MILICA Z. KARADZIC BANJAC, STRAHINJA Z. KOVACEVIC, AND SANJA O. PODUNAVAC-KUZMANOVIC

10.1 INTRODUCTION 178
10.2 REPELLING COMPOUNDS IN THE SPOTLIGHT 179
10.3 THE IMPORTANCE OF CHEMOMETRIC MODELING IN DESIGN, CLASSIFICATION AND SELECTION OF REPELLING COMPOUNDS 182
10.3.1 QSAR platform for modeling of repellent activity 182
10.3.2 Linear chemometric regression modeling of repellence index 182
10.3.3 Non-linear chemometric regression modeling of repellence index 184
10.3.4 Mathematical validation of QSAR models 186
10.3.5 Chemometric classification methods as a platform for repellents selection 187
10.3.5.1 Cluster analysis 187
10.3.5.2 Principal component analysis 188
10.3.5.3 Sum of ranking differences 189
10.4 CONCLUDING REMARKS AND FURTHER RESEARCH 191

SECTION VI **Pharmacy Meets Mosquito Control: Using Pharmacological Tools Combating Mosquito Transmitted VBDs**

CHAPTER 11 ■ Pharmacological Approach to Combat Mosquito Transmitted Malaria 195

ELLEN KALESI GONDWE MHANGO, BAXTER HEPBURN KACHINGWE, PETER E. OLUMESE, PRECIOUS NGWALERO KATUNDU, KAMUNKHWALA GAUSI, AND SVEINBJORN GIZURARSON

11.1 INTRODUCTION 196
11.2 PHARMACOLOGICAL TREATMENT OF MALARIA 197

11.3 RESISTANCE TO ANTIMALARIAL TREATMENT, A GLOBAL THREAT 198
11.4 CLINICAL PHARMACOKINETICS OF ANTIMALARIAL DRUGS 200
11.5 TREATMENT OF PREGNANT WOMEN 203
11.6 TREATMENT OF INFANTS AND YOUNG CHILDREN 205
11.7 CONCLUSION 209

SECTION VII **Using Natural Oils Combatting Mosquitoes: An Overview**

CHAPTER 12 ▪ Plant Based Repellents: Green Mosquito Control 213

KIRIL LISICHKOV, KATERINA ATKOVSKA, ERHAN MUSTAFA, STEFAN KUVENDZIEV, AND MIRKO MARINKOVSKI

12.1 INTRODUCTION 214
12.2 PLANT ESSENTIAL OILS - COMPOSITION AND EXTRACTION 215
12.3 EFFICACY OF DIFFERENT ESSENTIAL OILS AS MOSQUITO REPELLENTS 216
12.3.1 Lemon eucalyptus oil 216
12.3.2 Immortelle oil 216
12.3.3 Lavender oil 216
12.3.4 Citronella oil 217
12.3.5 Basil oil 217
12.3.6 Thyme oil 217
12.3.7 Neem oil 218
12.3.8 Rosemary oil 218
12.4 IMPROVING THE REPELLENT EFFICIENCY OF ESSENTIAL OILS 218
12.5 CONCLUSION 219

CHAPTER 13 ▪ Microencapsulation of Essential Oils for Antimicrobial Function and Mosquito Repellency 221

KATIE LAIR, ANITA SOROH, AND JINSONG SHEN

13.1 INTRODUCTION 222
13.2 MICROENCAPSULATION TECHNOLOGY 223
13.2.1 Complex coacervation 223
13.2.2 Ionic-Gelation 225
13.2.3 Freeze-Drying 225
13.2.4 Spray-Drying 225
13.2.5 Emulsification 226
13.3 CHARACTERIZATION OF MICROCAPSULES 226

13.3.1 Particle size and size distribution 226
13.3.2 Surface charge 226
13.3.3 Release of the core material 227
13.4 ANTIMICROBIAL ACTIVITY AND MOSQUITO REPELLENCY OF ENCAPSULATED ESSENTIAL OILS 227
13.5 CONCLUSION 229

SECTION VIII **Textiles and Paints as Mosquito Control Tools**

CHAPTER 14 ▪ Mosquito Repellent against *Anopheles SPP.* and *Aedes Aegypti* on Cotton Fabric 233

ANA MARIJA GRANCARIC, LEA BOTTERI, PEYMAN GHAFFARI, JOSE HERIBERTO OLIVEIRA DO NASCIMENTO, RENATA ANTONACI GAMA, RIVALDO LEONN BEZERRA CABRAL, AND RENATO CESAR DE MELO FREIRE

14.1 INTRODUCTION 234
14.2 MATERIAL AND METHODS 236
14.3 RESULTS 237
14.4 CONCLUSION 239

CHAPTER 15 ▪ Silica-Based Organic-Inorganic Hybrid Treatments as Anti-Mosquito Textile Finishing 243

VERONICA MIGANI, ANA MARIJA GRANCARIC, MARIA ROSARIA PLUTINO, VALENTINA TROVATO, AND GIUSEPPE ROSACE

15.1 INTRODUCTION 244
15.2 ENCAPSULATION TECHNIQUES AND SOL-GEL CHEMISTRY 245
15.3 ANTI-MOSQUITO FINISHING BY SOL-GEL TECHNIQUE 247
15.4 CONCLUSIONS 249

CHAPTER 16 ▪ Cotton and Polyester Fabrics Plasma Coated with Hydrogenated Amorphous Carbon Films 251

MELANIE FRITZ, ANA MARIJA GRANCARIC, LEA BOTTERI, AND CHRISTIAN B. FISCHER

16.1 INTRODUCTION 252
16.2 COATING PROCESS AND ANALYTICS 253
16.3 RESULTS 254
16.4 CONCLUSION 256

SECTION IX **Testing Methods for Treated Textiles with Mosquito-Repellents: An Overview**

CHAPTER 17 ▪ Testing Methods for Mosquito-Repellent Treated Textiles 261

HITOSHI KAWADA AND RUI-DE XUE

17.1 INTRODUCTION 261
17.2 ACTIVE INGREDIENT 262
17.3 TREATED METHOD 262
17.4 LABORATORY TESTING 262
17.5 FIELD TESTING 269
17.6 INFLUENCING FACTORS 270
17.7 CHALLENGES AND CONCLUSIONS: TOWARDS AN INTERNATIONAL STANDARD 271

SECTION X **Case Studies: Putting the Knowledge into Action**

CHAPTER 18 ▪ A Case Study: How the Rephaiah Project Combats Malaria in Young Children 275

SVEINBJORN GIZURARSON, PRECIOUS NGWALERO KATUNDU, EMMANUEL MWATHUNGA, GUDLAUG MARIA SVEINBJORNSDOTTIR, URDUR NJARDVIK, TITHA DZOWELA, WILFRED DODOLI, AND KRISTIN LINDA RAGNARSDOTTIR

18.1 INTRODUCTION 276
18.2 MOSQUITO TRANSMITTED MALARIA IN MALAWI 278
18.3 GEOGRAPHICAL STRUCTURE AND DEMOGRAPHY OF THE COUNTRY 278
18.4 WHO OPERATION AND MOSQUITO CONTROL IN MALAWI 281
18.5 SUCCESSES AND FAILURES IN MOSQUITO CONTROL IN MALAWI 282
18.5.1 Successes 282
18.5.2 Failures 283
18.6 CONSEQUENCES OF CEREBRAL MALARIA IN YOUNG CHILDREN 283
18.7 SUPPORTING THE PROJECT 284
18.8 CONCLUSION 285

CHAPTER 19 ▪ Strengthening the control of mosquito vectors in Cabo Verde; New Approaches to Improve Intervention Strategies 289

LARA FERRERO GOMEZ, DERCILIANO LOPES DA CRUZ, MORGANA DO NASCIMENTO XAVIER, DEINILSON CONSELHEIRO MENDES, ROSANGELA MARIA RODRIGUES BARBOSA, AND HELIO DANIEL RIBEIRO ROCHA

19.1 INTRODUCTION 290
19.2 STUDY AREA 291
19.3 PILOT STUDY I 292
19.3.1 Assessment of the use of substances with attractive power in ovi-traps 292
19.3.2 Material and Methods 292
19.3.3 Results 294
19.3.4 Discussion 295
19.3.5 Conclusion 295
19.4 PILOT STUDY II 295
19.4.1 Sticky BR-OVT evaluation 295
19.4.2 Material and Methods 297
19.4.3 Results 298
19.4.4 Discussion 299
19.4.5 Conclusion 299
19.5 PILOT STUDY III 299
19.5.1 Evaluation of the effectiveness of insecticide paints 299
19.5.2 Material and method 299
19.5.3 Results and discussion 300
19.5.4 Conclusion 301

Bibliography 303

Foreword

Prevention is often better than treatment, and this is certainly true for a number of insect-borne diseases such as malaria, dengue, and visceral leishmaniasis. The push for malaria elimination over the last decade, with the rapid scale-up of the use of long-lasting insecticide impregnated bed nets and the increased use of indoor residual spraying, supported by the US Presidents' malaria initiative, combined with better combination anti-malaria drug treatment and prophylaxis has dramatically reduced infant mortality. The surprise for many malariologists was the extent to which insect control was responsible for this reduction, with around 67% of the reduction coming from the two vector control interventions. It took the availability of large-scale data sets and cutting-edge spatial and mathematical modelling to demonstrate this. The poorly informed consensus prior to this work being published was that the gains were driven by access to combination drug treatment with vector control playing a more minor support role. Key lessons here are the importance of different disciplines engaging in the development, deployment, and assessment of global infectious disease control efforts and understanding properly what is working and why.

If we are to fully realize the benefits in global health from vector control, we need to add to the arsenal of proven technologies and establish exactly how these control tools can be effectively integrated. For too long the field has been dominated by insect control specialists often using small-scale field experimental approaches in different formats that do not have the power to provide a solid evidence base for policy changes at scale. It is obvious that the field would benefit from a disruptive multi-disciplinary approach to assessing and validating different vector control approaches, building on the strengths that mathematical and theoretical modelers could bring to the subject.

This book is a welcome start to this journey, bringing together a multidisciplinary team from many countries to look at a range of well-embedded and more experimental vector control approaches. Their thought provoking and novel approaches provide an engaging platform for more traditional vector control specialists at all stages of their career. I am delighted to see the outputs of this European Union funded collaborative effort in this engaging book format, that is well-targeted for both entomology students and vector control practitioners and demonstrates to those across a range of other disciplines how they might engage productively in the debate on how we evolve insect control over the next decades.

Professor Janet Hemingway , CBE, FRS, AcadMedSci, FRCP, NAS USA

October 2022

About Professor Janet Hemingway:

Professor of Tropical Medicine, Liverpool School of Tropical Medicine Janet Hemingway has 40 years' experience of working in multiple disease control programs across Africa and Asia. Established the IVCC in 2005 to work with industry to generate new public health insecticides and vector control tools, bringing a range of new vector control tools to the market over the last decade. She was the Director of LSTM from 2000 to 2019 and currently heads the £200 M Infection Innovation Consortium (iiCON).

Contributors

** The List of Contributors in Alphabetic Order:*

Miracle Amadi
LUT School of Engineering Science,
Lappeenranta University of Technology,
Lappeenranta, Finland

Katerina Atkovska
Faculty of Technology and Metallurgy,
University Ss. Cyril and Methodius,
Skopje, North Macedonia

Lea Botteri
University of Zagreb,
Faculty of Textile Technology (TTF),
Zagreb, Croatia

James R. Bozeman
Department of Mathematics,
American University of Malta (AUM),
Bormla, Malta

Deinilson Conselheiro Mendes
Unidade de Ciências da Natureza,
da Vida e do Ambiente,
Universidade Jean Piaget de Cabo Verde,
Praia, Cabo Verde

Wilfred Dodoli
Malaria Programme,
World Health Organization (WHO),
Lilongwe, Malawi

Titha Dzowela
UNC Project,
Fleming Fund Country Grant Malawi,
Lilongwe, Malawi

Chinazom Enukoha
Department of Epidemiology and
Medical Statistics,
University of Ibadan, Nigeria

Christian B. Fischer
Department of Physics,
University Koblenz-Landau,
Koblenz, Germany **&**
Materials Science, Energy and
Nano-Engineering Department,
Mohammed VI Polytechnic University,
Ben Guerir, Morocco

Melanie Fritz
Department of Physics,
University Koblenz-Landau,
Koblenz, Germany

Renata Antonaci Gama
Laboratory of Entomology,
Department of Microbiology and Parasitology,
Universidade Federal do Rio Grande do Norte,
Natal, Rio Grande do Norte, Brazil

Kamunkhwala Gausi
Division of Clinical Pharmacology,
University of Cape Town,
Cape Town, South Africa

Peyman Ghaffari
Chair of IMAAC
(COST Action CA 16227) **&**
Center for Research
and Development in Mathematics
and Applications (CIDMA),
University of Aveiro,
Aveiro, Portugal

Sveinbjorn Gizurarson
Faculty of Pharmaceutical Sciences, School of Health Sciences, University of Iceland, Reykjavik, Iceland &
Department of Pharmacy, College of Medicine, University of Malawi, Blantyre, Malawi &
Hananja plc, Reykjavik, Iceland

Lara Ferrero Gomez
Unidade de Ciências da Natureza, da Vida e do Ambiente, Universidade Jean Piaget de Cabo Verde, Praia, Cabo Verde

Ana Marija Grancaric
Co-chair of IMAAC (COST Action CA 16227) &
University of Zagreb, Faculty of Textile Technology (TTF), Zagreb, Croatia

Heikki Haario
LUT School of Engineering Science, Lappeenranta University of Technology, Lappeenranta, Finland

Sahar Hassandoust
Italian Mosquito Control Association (IMCA), San Lazzaro di Savena (BO), Italy

Baxter Hepburn Kachingwe
Department of Pharmacy, College of Medicine, University of Malawi, Blantyre, Malawi

Ellen Kalesi Gondwe Mhango
Faculty of Pharmaceutical Sciences, School of Health Sciences, University of Iceland Reykjavik, Iceland &
Department of Pharmacy, College of Medicine, University of Malawi, Blantyre, Malawi

Milica Z. Karadzic Banjac
University of Novi Sad, Faculty of Technology Novi Sad, Department of Applied and Engineering & Chemistry, Novi Sad, Serbia

Hitoshi Kawada
Department of Vector Ecology & Environment, Institute of Tropical Medicine, Nagasaki University, Nagasaki, Japan

Gerry Killeen
AXA Research Chair in Applied Pathogen, Ecology at the Environmental Research Institute and School of Biological Earth & Environmental Sciences, University College Cork, Cork, Ireland

Bob W. Kooi
Faculty of Science, VU University Amsterdam, HV Amsterdam, The Netherlands

Strahinja Z. Kovacevic
University of Novi Sad, Faculty of Technology Novi Sad, Department of Applied and Engineering & Chemistry, Novi Sad, Serbia

Stefan Kuvendziev
Faculty of Technology and Metallurgy, University Ss. Cyril and Methodius, Skopje, North Macedonia

Katie Lair
Leicester School of Pharmacy, Infectious Disease Research Group, De Montfort University, Leicester, United Kingdom

Kiril Lisichkov
Faculty of Technology and Metallurgy, Skopje, University Ss. Cyril and Methodius, North Macedonia

Derciliano Lopes da Cruz
Departamento de Entomologia, Instituto Aggeu Magalhães, Fundação Oswaldo Cruz-PE, Recife, Pernambuco, Brazil

Mirko Marinkovski
Faculty of Technology and Metallurgy, University Ss. Cyril and Methodius, Skopje, North Macedonia

Renato Cesar de Melo Freire
Laboratory of Entomology,
Department of Microbiology and Parasitology,
Universidade Federal do Rio Grande do Norte,
Natal, Rio Grande do Norte, Brazil

Veronica Migani
University of Bergamo, Department of
Engineering and Applied Sciences,
Dalmine, Bergamo, Italy

Gunter C. Muller
Malaria Research & Training Centre,
Faculty of Medicine, University of Sciences,
Techniques, and Technology of Bamako,
Bamako, Mali

Erhan Mustafa
Faculty of Technology and Metallurgy,
University Ss. Cyril and Methodius,
Skopje, North Macedonia

Emmanuel Mwathunga
Ministry of Natural Resources,
Energy and Mining,
Lilongwe, Malawi

Morgana do Nascimento Xavier
Secretaria Estadual de Saúde de
Pernambuco, Recife, Brazil

Precious Ngwalero Katundu
Department of Pharmacy, College of Medicine,
University of Malawi, Blantyre, Malawi &
Division of Clinical Pharmacology, University
of Cape Town, Cape Town, South Africa

Urdur Njardvik
Faculty of Psychology, School of Health
Sciences, University of Iceland,
Reykjavik, Iceland

Jose Heriberto Oliveira do Nascimento
Departamento de Engenharia Têxtil,
Universidade Federal do
Rio Grande do Norte UFRN,
Centro de Tecnologia,
Campus Universitário Lagoa Nova,
Lagoa Nova Natal/RN, Brazil

Peter E. Olumese
Diagnosis Medicines and Resistance,
Global Malaria Programme,
World Health Organization (WHO),
Geneve, Switzerland

Steve Peper
Anastasia Mosquito Control District
of St. Johns County,
St. Augustine, Florida, USA

Maria Rosaria Plutino
Institute for the Study of Nanostructured
Materials, ISMN – CNR, O.U. Palermo
c/o Department of ChiBioFarAm,
University of Messina, Vill. S. Agata,
Messina, Italy

Sanja O. Podunavac-Kuzmanovic
University of Novi Sad,
Faculty of Technology Novi Sad,
Department of Applied and Engineering &
Chemistry, Novi Sad, Serbia

Kristin Linda Ragnarsdottir
Hananja plc,
Reykjavik,
Iceland

Peter Rashkov
Institute of Mathematics and Informatics,
Bulgarian Academy of Sciences,
Sofia, Bulgaria

Helio Daniel Ribeiro Rocha
Unidade de Ciências da Natureza,
da Vida e do Ambiente,
Universidade Jean Piaget de Cabo Verde,
Praia, Cabo Verde

Rivaldo Leonn Bezerra Cabral
Universidade Federal do Rio Grande
do Norte Centro de Tecnologia
Departamento de Engenharia Têxtil –
DET Nanociências e Têxteis Funcionais
Lagoa Nova Natal/RN, Brazil

Rosangela Maria Rodrigues Barbosa
Departamento de Entomologia,
Instituto Aggeu Magalhães,
Fundação Oswaldo Cruz-PE,
Recife, Pernambuco, Brazil

Elton Rogozi
Vectors' and
Rodent's Control Unit (VRCU),
Control of Infectious Diseases
Department (CIDD),
Institute of Public Health (IPH),
Tirana, Albania

Giuseppe Rosace
University of Bergamo, Department of
Engineering and Applied Sciences,
Dalmine, Bergamo, Italy

Cristiana J. Silva
Center for Research and Development
in Mathematics and Applications (CIDMA),
University of Aveiro, Aveiro, Portugal

Jinsong Shen
School of Fashion and Textiles,
Textile Engineering and Materials (TEAM)
Research Group,
De Montfort University,
Leicester, United Kingdom

Anita Soroh
School of Fashion and Textiles,
Textile Engineering and Materials (TEAM)
Research Group,
De Montfort University,
Leicester, United Kingdom

Gudlaug Maria Sveinbjornsdottir
Faculty of Psychology, School of Health
Sciences, University of Iceland,
Reykjavik, Iceland

Asghar Talbalaghi
Italian Mosquito Control Association
(IMCA),
San Lazzaro di Savena (BO), Italy

Delfim F. M. Torres
Center for Research and Development
in Mathematics and Applications (CIDMA),
University of Aveiro, Aveiro, Portugal

Valentina Trovato
University of Bergamo, Department of
Engineering and Applied Sciences,
Dalmine, Bergamo, Italy

Ezio Venturino
Dipartimento di Matematica "Giuseppe Peano",
Università di Torino,
Torino, Italy

Rui-De Xue
Anastasia Mosquito Control District
of St. Johns County,
St. Augustine, Florida, USA

Tong-Yan Zhao
Department of Vector Biology and Control,
Institute of microbiology and Epidemiology,
Fengtai, Beijing, China

CHAPTER 1

Introduction and Overview

Peyman Ghaffari

CONTENTS

This editorial book is the result of the cooperation starting from September 2017 between different scientific disciplines within the framework of IMAAC (`www.imaac.eu`) related to the COST Action CA 16227 (Investigation & Mathematical Analysis of Avant-garde Disease Control via Mosquito Nano-Tech-Repellents, `https://www.cost.eu/actions/CA16227/`), supported by COST Association (European Cooperation in Science and Technology). The European Action consisted of almost 100 members from nearly 35 countries, scientists, health experts, and professionals, aimed to develop new techniques in combatting mosquito-transmitted Vector-borne Diseases (VBDs) using nano- and micro-particles attached to textiles and paints to reduce the danger of mosquito bites. It was necessary to develop new methods to measure the efficacy of such techniques. Unfortunately, it was impossible to perform field studies during the Action, which needed huge funding and was out of the scope of the Grant and Action.

Mosquito-transmitted diseases are among the most dangerous problems in many countries. Experts estimated that VBDs account for around 17% of all infectious diseases, causing more than 700,000 deaths annually (See Section I). Controlling the mosquito population in living areas is difficult and often has side effects. Zika, dengue, chikungunya, and yellow fever are vector-borne diseases transmitted by daytime active mosquitoes. These diseases have a significant health risk and a negative economic factor in 128 countries, mainly in tropical and subtropical regions of Asia, Africa, and Latin America. In recent years, however, VBDs and, specifically, dengue fever has been occurring in Europe. Some reasons for this are the worldwide flow of trade and traveling tourism. Increasing urbanization and regional warming due to global climate change have amplified the spread of mosquitoes like *Aedes albopictus*, even in Europe.

One of the biggest challenges of IMAAC was bringing together many experts from different disciplines, i.e., mathematics, biology, epidemiology, entomology, physics, chemistry, textile engineering, and even social sciences, to discuss various topics and find a common language. This book aims to give a brief overview and understanding of the different disciplines involved in researching this exciting topic without going too in-depth. Some chapters, for instance, in mathematical epidemiology, are difficult to understand by non-mathematicians but fulfill the purpose of clarifying how mathematics can contribute to research.

DOI: 10.1201/9781003035992-1

This editorial book is divided into ten parts or sections. All authors of the chapters within a section are listed in alphabetic order at the beginning. The sections are as follows:

(I) Control of Mosquitoes and Their World: An Overview

(II) Mathematical Modeling Of Immunity: An Overview

(III) Mathematical Epidemiology including Mosquito Dynamics and Control Theory

(IV) Topological Studies: Topology meets Mosquito Control

(V) Chemometric and Mathematical Approach for Modeling and Designing Mosquito Repellents

(VI) Pharmacy Meets Mosquito Control: Using Pharmacological Tools Combating Mosquito Transmitted VBDs

(VII) Using Natural Oils and Micro-encapsulation Combatting Mosquitoes: An Overview

(VIII) Textiles and Paints as Mosquito Control Tools

(IX) Testing Methods for Treated Textiles with Mosquito-Repellents: An Overview

(X) Case Studies: Putting Knowledge into Action

In the **first section**, the authors try to give a brief overview of the life of mosquitoes and mosquito control. Mosquitoes are semi-aquatic insects of which approximately more than 3,200 species worldwide have been described. As known, mosquito vector control is one of the most effective and successful strategies and methods for controlling mosquito-transmitted vector-borne diseases (WHO 2008), such as malaria, Zika, dengue fever, chikungunya, and yellow fever. Mosquitoes evolve in four life stages: egg, larva, pupa, and adult. Besides causing diseases for humans, mosquitoes can also transmit diseases to animals since they feed from the blood of animals such as frogs, toads, birds, etc., and transmit infectious diseases from animals to humans.

The **second section** reviews malaria and the naturally acquired immunity (NAI) related to this disease. The consequences of NAI in a population are of immense interest, and the interaction with a possible malaria vaccine is important for the efficacy of the vaccine. This section also aims to develop mathematical models that can be used and translated for other mosquito-transmitted diseases.

The **third section** is mathematically challenging for researchers unfamiliar with mathematical epidemiology but can highlight the importance of mathematics in mosquito-transmitted diseases. The chapters give a brief overview of the inclusion of mosquito dynamics in the epidemiological models expanding the famous SIR (susceptible, infected, and recovered population) model to SIRUV model (inclusion of infected and healthy mosquitoes). One chapter is dedicated especially to the implications of Optimal Control Theory. Interventions usually include vector control through insecticide-treated nets

(ITNs) and Human behavior change interventions, including information, education, and communication (IEC) campaigns. Mathematical models can be introduced mimicking ITN and IEC interventions using Optimal Control Theory. Resulting equations can be solved to minimize the number of infectious humans while keeping costs low. At the end of the chapter, numerical results are provided, showing the effectiveness of the optimal control interventions. In the final chapter of this section or part, a deterministic model based on SIRUV is used and analyzed by complexity reduction using time scale separation and singular perturbation analysis. This method allows the representation of host-only models connected to vector-borne disease dynamics without including the mosquito population.

The **fourth section** is dedicated to topological concepts applied to mosquito control. This field is relatively unexplored. For instance, developing a solid theory connecting the topological characteristics of an area under mosquito control with mathematical models using Optimal Control Theory needs to be better understood mathematically and developed. Many considerations must be taken into account when designing the regions for spraying, fogging, or ground placement of insecticides. These include the type of mosquito being eradicated, their flight ranges, flight patterns of vectors, population density, and already used control measures in the region. Also of concern is the region's demographics to be sprayed, including vulnerable populations and its topography. Political issues must often be considered, e.g., public opposition to spraying, which is very similar to the matters of interest when designing voting districts, which is the mathematical expertise of the author.

The **fifth section** aims to design and model efficient mosquito repellents. Most repellents, insecticides, and pesticides contain biological and natural chemical compounds. Discoveries and developments in novel biologically active compounds are largely potentiated by computational and numerical methods using tools like chemometrics, mathematical modeling, and molecular docking. Since mosquitoes rapidly develop resistance to repelling compounds, it is necessary to involve various chemometric techniques to shorten the time for laboratory experiments and save resources in searching for new effective repellents. Multiple linear regression (MLR), principal component regression (PCR), partial least squares (PLS), and artificial neural networks (ANN), together with pattern recognition techniques such as principal component analysis (PCA) and hierarchical cluster analysis (HCA), as well as molecular docking approach, can be used for screening of many compounds with potential repelling or different physicochemical properties. Ideas about the development of effective vaccines are also briefly discussed.

The **sixth section** is focused on the pharmacological treatment of malaria with the quick and complete removal of the Plasmodium parasites from a patient's circulation to prevent uncomplicated malaria from progressing to a severe infection or mortality. It is well known that effective malaria management also decreases disease transmission to other population members by decreasing the disease reservoir and preventing the emergence and spread of resistance to antimalarial drugs.

The **seventh section** is dedicated to repellents and insecticides from plant extracts or natural essential oils. Natural products are effective, environmentally friendly, biodegradable, inexpensive, and vastly available and are an alternative to conventional synthetic repellents and insecticides. Many plant-essential-oils extracted from different families can be applied as green repellents against mosquito vectors, such as citronella, peppermint, clove, eucalyptus, catnip, immortelle, basil, thyme, lavender, rosemary, and others. These oils are considered safe by the Environmental Protection Agency (EPA) at low concentrations but provide a limited duration of protection against mosquitoes, less than usually three hours. Therefore, Essential Oils cannot achieve their full potential because of the chemical volatility and instability characteristics exposed to environmental factors such as oxygen, heat, light, and moisture. Microencapsulation has been used as a viable technique to preserve the oils' essential biological and functional characteristics and achieve the required full potential. Microencapsulation can prevent the loss of volatile oil compounds while allowing for the controlled and sustained release of essential oils, enhancing bioavailability and efficacy against pathogens.

The **eighth section** deals with mosquito repellents applied on cotton fabric to protect people against *Anopheles spp* and *Aedes aegypti*. For this purpose, the bleached cotton fabric was scoured and treated with natural immortelle essential oil and ingredients, such as water glass and Vibro-activated zeolites, and analyzed. In general, to apply repellents on textiles, finishing is necessary. Various attempts have been made to replace environmentally hazardous products and to use new procedures in preparing functional coatings for medical applications, which allow combining the entrapment of bioactive compounds with their controlled release. The sol-gel process has demonstrated its exceptional potential among the different methods proposed. In one of the chapters within this section, the new trends in textile engineering toward green finishing processes, such as plasma technology, are discussed. It has been shown that cold plasmas were found suitable for surface modification of temperature-sensitive textile materials.

The **ninth section** evaluates and tests mosquito-repellent-treated textile products. The use of insecticide or repellent-treated bed nets, head nets, jackets, uniforms, and curtains is increasing, and objective, standardized testing methods for the efficacy of the products are crucial. This chapter briefly reviews repellents, treated methods, and several bioassay methods in the laboratory and field for anti-mosquito textiles and proposes advisable standard methods.

The **tenth and final section** discuss specific case studies in two African countries, namely Republic of Malawi and Republic of Cabo Verde. One chapter focuses on the Rephaiah project in Malawi. As is well known, if malaria is not treated, it can quickly become life-threatening, affecting children under five very hard with severe or cerebral malaria. The Rephaiah project is based on the need for pediatric dosage forms to treat children under five years with the simple dosage form. This project focuses on providing health to these children by establishing a not-for-profit pharmaceutical manufacturing entity in Malawi. The other chapter is about the national program in Cabo Verde combatting mosquito-transmitted VBDs. These control activities as national efforts include using larvivores fish, physical control of solid waste cleaning, communication campaigns during outbreaks, and periods of greater risk. To help the health authorities implement more proactive vector control strategies, the Tropical Diseases Research Group at the Jean Piaget University of Cabo Verde – GIDTPiaget conducts applied research on control methodologies and interventions for vector mosquitoes in the country. In this context, three pilot studies are discussed.

We hope that this editorial book could initiate a dialogue between the different science disciplines in understanding controlling mosquito-transmitted infectious diseases and contribute to bridging this barrier, which is, in the opinion of the author, needing to improve significantly and make progress in this crucial field difficult. The editor thanks all authors involved in the book for their kind engagement and support. He also thanks the COST Association for making networking through the Grant IMAAC (CA 16227) possible and always supported this exciting project. Special thanks also go to Professor Grancaric for co-chairing IMAAC and Professor Hemingway for writing the foreword to this book. The editor also thanks Karin for her great help and patience while preparing this book.

Finally, it is worth mentioning that the editor of this book has no responsibility for the contents of the chapters not authored or co-authored. In case of readers' comments or suggestions regarding chapter's contents, the responsible contributors (mentioned in alphabetic order by the editor) should be contacted directly.

Dr Peyman Ghaffari, Dipl. -Phys., DIC, Ph.D.

Chair of IMAAC (COST Action CA 16227) **&**
Center for Research and Development in Mathematics
and Applications (CIDMA),
University of Aveiro, Aveiro, Portugal

Lisbon, July 2022

About Dr Peyman Ghaffari*:

Dr Ghaffari received his Ph.D. in Mathematical-Physics (Non-linear Dynamics and Complex Systems) at Imperial College London (UK) in 1997. He also received his German Diploma in Physics (Dipl. -Phys.) 1993 in Theoretical Plasma Physics at Heinrich Heine University Düsseldorf (Germany). After completing his Ph.D. at Imperial College London, he worked as an industrial consultant for years focusing on establishing Joint-Ventures between International companies wanting to penetrate the European and Middle Eastern markets. In 2006 Dr Ghaffari returned to academia as a visiting/associate scientist at Imperial College London, parallel to his consultancy. In 2007 he co-founded the "Complexity and Interdisciplinary Research Centre (CIRC)" at Imperial College London providing a platform to transmit the ideas of "Complexity Research" into Industry. Since March 2010 until Dec 2018, he has worked at the University of Lisbon in the Biomathematics and Statistics Group and has participated in several scientific projects resulting in scientific articles. Since 2020 he is continuing his research as an associate researcher at CIDMA ("Center for Research and Development in Mathematics and Applications", University of Aveiro, Portugal). In June 2017 he won the prestigious EU - COST Grant (CA16227) as proposal writer (estimates for 4.5 years circa 570.000 Euro). Since September 2017 he has been the Chair of this Action with the acronym IMAAC ("Investigation and Mathematical Analysis of Avant-garde Disease Control via Mosquito Nano-Tech-Repellents", `www.imaac.eu`) with around 100 members from about 35 countries involved. He also founded 2018 a yearly Training School ("International Training School on Optimal Control Theory and Mosquito Control Strategies") and a conference in 2019 on "Political Decision Making and Vector-Borne Diseases" aiming to bring political decision makers and scientists together. Dr Ghaffari is working now on application of Optimal Control Theory on deterministic and stochastic epidemiological models. Other scientific interests include Complex Systems, Self-Organization, Fractional Derivatives, Neuronal Networks and Industrial Mathematics.

* e-mail: pgsaid@fc.ul.pt

I

Control of Mosquitoes and Their World: An Overview

CHAPTER 2

Practical Control Methods and New Techniques for Mosquito Control

Rui-De Xue*
Anastasia Mosquito Control District, EOC Drive, St. Augustine, Florida, USA
** corresponding author, e-mail: rxue@amcdfl.org*

Steve Peper
Anastasia Mosquito Control District, EOC Drive, St. Augustine, Florida, USA

Gunter C. Muller
Malaria Research & Training Centre, Faculty of Medicine, University of Sciences, Techniques, and Technology of Bamako, Bamako, Mali

CONTENTS

2.1 Introduction 10
2.2 Personal and Community Protection 10
2.2.1 Repellent 10
2.2.2 Community Protection and Participate 11
2.3 Space Spraying 11
2.3.1 ULV 11
2.3.2 Thermal Fogging 11
2.3.3 Barrier Spray 12
2.4 Indoor Residual Spraying (IRS) 12
2.5 Insecticide-Treated Bed Nets (ITN) 12
2.6 New Control Techniques 13
2.6.1 Genetic Control, Gene Drive, and GMO 13
2.6.2 Incompatible Insect Technique (IIT) 14
2.6.3 Sterile Insect Technique (SIT) 14
2.6.4 Adult Mosquito Control Traps 14
2.6.5 Lethal Ovitrap and Autocidal Gravid Ovitrap (AGO) 15
2.6.6 Larvicide Traps 15
2.6.7 Auto-dissemination Method 15
2.6.8 Endectocides 16
2.6.9 Attractive Toxic Sugar Bait (ATSB) 16

DOI: 10.1201/9781003035992-2

2.6.10 Vaccine 16
2.6.11 Challenges and Conclusions 16

2.1 INTRODUCTION

Vector control is one of the most effective and successful strategies and methods for control of vector-borne diseases (WHO 2008), such as malaria, dengue, west nile, zika, and so on. Typical methods for mosquito control include source reduction, personal protection, and prevention through the elimination or limitation of contact opportunities between adult mosquitoes and people, and directly or indirectly killing of larval and adult mosquitoes. Many traditional control methods, for example, space spraying, indoor residual spraying (IRS), bed nets, and long-last insecticide-treated bed nets (LLIN), are practical and useful for the control of major vector mosquitoes and mosquito-borne diseases, like malaria (WHO 2006, 2019). Due to recent new emerging, resurgent, and outbreak of several mosquito-borne diseases, and spread and invasion of several species of important vector mosquitoes, several traditional practical control methods and new control techniques have been brought more attention and developed. In this chapter, we will give an overview of the most practical control methods and new control techniques for the control of vector mosquitoes.

2.2 PERSONAL AND COMMUNITY PROTECTION

Elimination and limitation of the contact opportunity between vector mosquitoes and people, eradication of vector mosquitoes, and mass administration of drugs (MAD) or vaccination to sensitive people are the three major elements in a successful control program for mosquito-borne diseases. Traditional personal protection methods, such as wearing long sleeves, long pants, using bed nets, and insect repellents, are the most practical methods. The old prevention strategies, such as avoiding outdoor activity during dusk and dawn when mosquitoes are most active, reducing breeding resources by dumping and eliminating standing water, fixing screening doors and windows are the most simple and effective methods.

2.2.1 Repellent

Currently, there are numerous commercial insect-repellent products available on the market (Xue et al. 2015). However, the most effective and reliable repellent products all included one of the following active ingredients: DEET, Picaridin, para-menthane-3,8-diol (PMD), and IR 3535 (Barnard & Xue 2004). Botanical resource repellents have received more attention recently, but only a few products included the active ingredients of lemongrass, geranium, coconut, and soy bean oils, which each provide different effective protection time (Xue et al. 2015). Also, there are many spatial repellent products and devices, such as coils, torches, candles, different bands and patches, Clip-on, ThermaCell, and so on, on the market for personal and community protection. However, the products that include the active ingredients of metofluthrin, transfuthion, d-cis/trans allethrin, and other pyrethroid insecticides showed different effective functions against adult mosquitoes by killing and repelling (Bibbs & Kaufman 2017). Also, several products with active ingredients from botanical resources provide a short protection time.

2.2.2 Community Protection and Participate

Community and family protection is most effective as all community members participate in the education and community prevention program. Community members can participate in such programs by emptying containers and eliminating standing water for source reduction, fixing screen doors and windows for family protection, wearing long sleeve shirts and long pants, avoiding outdoor activity during dawn and dusk, and using effective repellents for personal protection. When available, all residents should participate in the mass drug administration (MDA) and vaccination for prevention and control of mosquito-borne diseases in epidemic or hot spot areas. Although there are not many vaccine products currently available for preventing mosquito-borne diseases, the mass vaccination against yellow fever and Japanese type B encephalitis in several countries showed the successful control against the outbreak of these diseases.

2.3 SPACE SPRAYING

Space spraying is one of the delivery methods of insecticides for control of adult and larval mosquitoes. The traditional application methods are applied by hand and backpack sprayers, aerosol spraying, and ultra-low-volume (ULV) spraying by ground and aerial application (Bonds 2012). By law, the application of any kind of insecticides requires following the labels of the insecticide and operation instruction. The equipment, especially the nozzles, should be matched with the requirement of insecticide formulations and the droplet of insecticides needs to be calibrated before use.

2.3.1 ULV

The ULV is an ultra-low-volume of insecticide formulation and sprayed out by a high-pressure machine or equipment and provides effective and quick control of mosquitoes (Bonds 2012). The ULV application is usually conducted by a truck-mounted ULV machine (Mount 1998) or an aircraft equipped with the ULV spraying system (Mount et al. 1996). Also, there are small hand-held and backpack ULV machines available on the market. The ULV method is more effectively used for the treatment of larger areas, and the insecticides with small droplet size result in a quicker knockdown and effective killing of adult mosquitoes. Several pyrethroid insecticides, permethrin, deltamethrin, alpha-cypermethrin, bifenthrin, sumithrin, and pyrethethin, and organophosphates insecticides, malathrin, and naled (for aerial application only in the USA) are available on the market for mosquito control.

2.3.2 Thermal Fogging

Thermal fogging is a very old spraying method performed by heating insecticide solution or oil, which becomes a fog and is used to kill adult mosquitoes. Thermal fogging needs to have a specific fogging machine to deliver the insecticides in oil formulation and are mostly used during the day. Thermal fogging machines are available in trucked-mounted, hand-held, or backpack form. The droplets generated by fogging are very small and can be used to treat heavily vegetated areas. Several products included pyrethroid insecticides, permethrin, deltamethrin, and sumithrin are available on the market.

2.3.3 Barrier Spray

This method has been used since the 1960s and recently has been given more attention (Stoops et al. 2018). Barrier spraying uses a long residual formulation of insecticides sprayed on vegetation and materials to control adult mosquitoes when they contact the surface treated by an insecticide. In some instances, the effectiveness of barrier spraying could last for a few weeks. The most popular insecticides used in barrier spraying include bifenthrin, lambda-cyhalothrin, and deltamethrin. The commercial product called Talstar (7% bifenthrin) is currently available on the market.

2.4 INDOOR RESIDUAL SPRAYING (IRS)

Indoor residual spray (IRS) is an application method of insecticide for the control of adult mosquitoes that enter and rest indoors, and requires the use of long residual active ingredients. Adult mosquitoes are killed by contacting the long residual insecticides on the walls and other materials indoors. The IRS has been recommended and used as a successful malaria vector control by the World Health Organization (WHO, 2006) for many years. The most successful insecticide for IRS is DDT, an old and effective organochlorine insecticide, which has been banned in many countries, and currently, is only used for IRS in a handful of countries for malaria mosquito control. Other common insecticides used for IRS are pyrethroids (deltamethrin, alpha-cypermethrin, cyfluthrin, etofenprox, bifenthrin, lambda-cyhalothrin, and permethrin), and organophosphates (malathion and fenitrothion), and carbamates (propoxur and bendiocarb). Detailed instructions for the selection and application of insecticides for IRS have been published by the WHO (2006) and also described and reviewed by Najera & Zaim (2002) and Pluess et al. (2010).

2.5 INSECTICIDE-TREATED BED NETS (ITN)

Insecticide-treated nets (ITNs) and long-last insecticide treated nets (LLINs) use different materials treated by insecticides or a long residual formulations of insecticides. ITNs and LLINs are designed to kill adult mosquitoes as they contact the treated bed nets and materials. ITN and LLIN have been recommended by the WHO (2008, 2019) for control of malaria vector mosquitoes in communities, and the mass application of the LLIN in many countries have aided in successfully reducing the incidence of malaria. The materials used for bed nets are usually cotton and polyesters, and the control efficacy varies based on the specific materials and insecticidal formulations used. The most common insecticides for ITN and LLIN are permethrin, deltamethrin, alpha-cypermethrin, and Lambda-cyhalothrin. Recent reports have shown the development of resistance to these control techniques. This issue is being overcome by mixing active ingredients with the insect growth regulator, pyriproxyfen, and attractive toxic sugar baits, ivermectin and BTi, to overcome the resistance and improve the control efficacy (Furnival-Adam et al. 2020). There are several products available on the market for private/residential purchase and professional mosquito control use. Any application should follow the product labels and instructions to select the ITN and LLIN for specific control program needs. Najera & Zaim (2002) provided detail instructions and guidelines about decision-making criteria and procedures for judicious use of insecticides for malaria vector mosquito control. These guidelines benefit all vector mosquito control. The WHO's Pesticide Evaluation Scheme recommended the following insecticide products for the treatment of mosquito nets: Alpha-cypermethrin 10% suspension concentrate (SC) (active ingredient (a.i.) in 20-40 mg/m² of netting) at 6 mL per net, Cyfluthrin 5% oil in water emulsion (EW) (a.i. in 50 mg/m² of netting) at 15 mL per net, Deltamethrin 1% SC (a.i. in 15-25 mg/m² of netting) at 40 mL per net and 25% WT 25% (water dispersible table at 1 table), Etofenprox 10% EW (a.i. in 200 mg/m² of netting) at 30 mL per net, Lambda-cyhalothrin 2.5% capsule suspension (CS) (capsule suspension) (a.i. in 10-15 mg/m² of netting) at 10 mL per net, and Permethrin 10% emulsifiable oncentrate (EC) (a.i. in 200-500 mg/m² of netting) at 75 ml per net.

2.6 NEW CONTROL TECHNIQUES

2.6.1 Genetic Control, Gene Drive, and GMO

Genetic control of mosquitoes is a form of biological control of mosquitoes, which exploits the mosquitoes-mate-seeking expertise to introduce genetic abnormalities into the eggs of the wild population of mosquitoes (WHO 2019). Genetics provide new, species-specific, and environmentally friendly methods /tools for control of mosquitoes. Genetic control aims either to suppress target populations or to introduce a harm-reducing novel trait and intends to persist indefinitely in the target mosquito population, and may invade other populations (Alphey 2013). A next-generation control tools for mosquito-borne diseases has been designed to eliminate mosquito populations or to replace them with mosquitoes that are less capable of transmitting major pathogens due to recent advances in CRISPR/Cas9-based genome editing, such as pathogen-resistant lines, new genetics-based sexing strain (Bernardini et al. 2018) and methods, driving desirable genetic traits into mosquito populations (Caragata et al. 2020).

Capitalizing on the RNA interference (RNAi) machinery to suppress interest genes of mosquitoes may be a promising direction for mosquito control. The RNAi pathway could be activated via RNA molecule with a double-stranded appearance (RNAi triggers), resulting in silencing of target genes. This approach could provide a new paradigm for mosquito control in the future (Airs & Bartholomay 2018). There are many studies about transgenes and fitness and strain replacement in the laboratory and field trails. Oxitech, a U.K. company, has developed several genetically modified strains of *Aedes aegypti*. Field studies have shown success of strain OX513A, which has been tested in the Cayman Islands, Panama, Malaysia, and Brazil. The OX513A mosquito strain has been produced to alter the female offspring to die in the larval stage, thus preventing adult mosquitoes from emerging. Release of a new strain, OX5034, has been developed and was tested in south Florida in 2021.

2.6.2 Incompatible Insect Technique (IIT)

The incompatible insect technique (IIT) employs the symbiont-associated (e.g., *Wolbachia* bacteria) reproductive **incompatibility** as a biopesticide for the control of insect pests and disease vectors (WHO 2019, Mains et al. 2019). *Wolbachia* bacteria are obligatory intracellular and maternally inherited bacteria that infect and spread through natural arthropod populations by inducing male-killing, feminization, parthenogenesis, and, most commonly, unidirectional and bidirectional cytoplasmic incompatibility (CI). Cytoplasmic incompatibility can be used to control natural populations of mosquitoes, in a way analogous to the Sterile Insect Technique (SIT). For the successful application of IIT (based on a unidirectional CI approach) against a target species of mosquitoes, it is essential that only males are released, as the release of females would lead to fertile mating between the released males and the released females and the establishment of a *Wolbachia*-carrying field population. Release of *Wolbachia* infected male *Aedes* mosquitoes showed a significant reduction in a natural population of mosquitoes (Mains et al. 2019). The combined SIT and IIT also provided more effective control of dengue vector mosquito populations in Thailand (Kittayapong et al. 2019).

2.6.3 Sterile Insect Technique (SIT)

The sterile insect technique (SIT) is a method of biological insect control and requires the release of a large number of sterile insects into the wild. This technique was developed in the 1940s and 1950s and adopted for *Anopheles*, *Culex*, and *Aedes* mosquito control in the early 1970s and is now being utilized and accepted by some mosquito control programs. The released mosquitoes are preferably sterile males that compete with wild males to mate with females of the natural populations. After mating with a sterile male, females produce no offspring, thus reducing the next generation's population. This is an environmentally friendly control method involving mass-rearing and sterilization by radiation and other methods. The release of sterile male mosquitoes requires repeated mass releases over low population densities to control target populations of mosquitoes in certain areas. There are many reports about the successful mass rearing and release of male *Aedes* mosquitoes sterilized by radiation against dengue vector mosquitoes in Malaysia, Brazil, and several other countries. Recently, the International Atomic Energy Agency (IAEA) and WHO (2020) published a comprehensive guideline for the testing and application of SIT for control of *Aedes* mosquitoes and mosquito-borne diseases.

2.6.4 Adult Mosquito Control Traps

Usually mosquito traps, such as New Jersey light trap, CDC light trap, Biogenet (BG) traps, DynaTraps, and other traps baited with different attractants (UV, LED, regular light, CO_2, octenol, lactic acid, naphtha, human and animal odors, or heat) have been used for the surveillance of adult mosquito populations. Several new trap designs, have been developed for control of adult mosquitoes through direct killing by electric wires or collecting adult mosquitoes to be killed (Kline 2006). These traps use UV, LED, and regular light plus different attractants to attract adult mosquitoes to the traps and killed by electric shock, pesticides, sticky pads, and other mechanical methods. The traps usually operated by a suction fan powered by electricity, batteries, or solar-power. There are many commercial mosquito control traps on the market. The selection and application of traps and trapping for adult mosquito control are based on the location, target species, economic, and power supply availability.

2.6.5 Lethal Ovitrap and Autocidal Gravid Ovitrap (AGO)

The Centers for Disease Control and Prevention's (CDC) autocidal gravid ovitraps (AGO) by attract-stick-killing are an inexpensive, simple-to-assemble, and easy-to-maintain trap that targets gravid female mosquitoes looking for a place to lay eggs. The AGO trap has been successfully used by mosquito control programs for the surveillance and control of *Aedes* mosquitoes in several countries. Field trials in which the AGO trap has been installed in most homes in a community have shown it not only reduces mosquito populations but also reduces the rates of virus infection (Barrera et al. 2014).

The fertility of *Ae. aegypti* populations can be reduced by the use of autocidal oviposition cups, sticky pad gravid traps, and insecticide-treated oviposition cups. These techniques prevent the development of mosquitoes inside the trap by mechanical means or larvicides/adulticides, as well as by releasing sterile, transgenic, and para-transgenic mosquitoes. In southern Puerto Rico, significant reductions in the capture of female *Ae. aegypti* (53-70%) in the intervention area were observed. Placing three to four AGO traps per home in 81% of the community prevented outbreaks of *Ae. aegypti*. The documents showed that the AGO traps are useful and inexpensive surveillance and control devices for container-inhabiting mosquitoes (Barrera et al. 2014). Zhu and colleagues (2019) added BG lure and a suction fan to the AGO traps and increased the collection and control of both host-seeking and gravid container-inhabiting mosquitoes.

2.6.6 Larvicide Traps

Usually ovitraps treated with insecticides have been used to kill larvae after egg hatching. Most of these traps are designed for the control of container-inhabiting mosquitoes. There is a new kind of larval trap on the market through the restriction of larvae in the containers after egg hatching to kill new emerged adult mosquitoes (no way to get out from the containers after emerging). This kind of trap and modified by additional sticky paper are a simple and economic tool for the surveillance and control of *Culex* and *Aedes* mosquitoes in residential homes (Talbalaghi et al. 2020).

2.6.7 Auto-dissemination Method

Insect growth regulator (IGR) pyriproxyfen has been studied for the auto-dissemination through gravid female mosquitoes for dispersion to other breeding containers or bodies of water to control mosquitoes at the larval stage. Also, IGRs and other insecticides could be auto-disseminated by male mosquitoes, acting as vehicles for dispersion (Mains et al. 2015, Brelsfoard et al. 2019). Auto-dissemination has also been documented through fecal deposits by adult mosquitoes to control larvae (Scott et al. 2017). Methoprene, another commonly used IGR, has also shown the function for larval control by auto-dissemination in the laboratory (Bibbs et al. 2016). In2Care traps are specifically designed for larval control by auto-dissemination of IGRs (Buckner et al. 2017).

2.6.8 Endectocides

This is a systematic administration with the toxic ivermectin or other related drugs by humans and animals. When people and animals take in ivermectin, the toxin will be circulated into the blood, then the biting mosquitoes and other blood-sucking insects take in the toxin and other drugs to kill mosquitoes and the insects (WHO 2019). Currently, there are only products available for dogs and cats to use by orally administration against mosquitoes and fleas.

2.6.9 Attractive Toxic Sugar Bait (ATSB)

ATSB is a novel control method for adult mosquitoes based on sugar feeding behavior (Xue et al. 2013, Kline et al. 2018). There are several reports about the active ingredients for the ATSB and the most effect ingredient is boric acid (Xue & Barnard 2003) and dinotefuran (Traore et al. 2002). ATSBs can be effectively used as bait stations or sprayed on vegetation as demonstrated by the effective control of malaria vector mosquitoes (Traore et al. 2020). Another benefit of ATSBs is the small impact on non-target organisms (Fiorenzano et al. 2017). There are also several reports about using U.S. Environmental Protection Agency (EPA) 25B exemption of essential oils extracted from botanical resources along with ivermectin, and other insecticides as the active ingredient against mosquitoes. Recently documentations showed that the ATSB could kill the resistant strains of *Culex quinquefasciatus* (Gu et al. 2019) and *Aedes aegypti* (Pearson et al. 2020) and mixed with the insect growth regulator, pyriproxyfen, could control adult and larval mosquitoes (Fulcher et al. 2014, Scott et al. 2017).

2.6.10 Vaccine

There is a plethora of research on vaccines for several mosquito-borne diseases. So far, vaccines for yellow fever and Japanese B encephalitis virus are successful and have been marketed for many years. Vaccines for West Nile and East Equine Encephalitis (EEE) viruses are successful for animals, but not for human beings. The first-generation malaria vaccine (RTS,S/AS01 vaccine (Mosquirix™) was created in 1987 and began pilot implementation in endemic countries in 2019 and demonstrates modest efficacy against malaria illness and holds promise, especially for children (Laurens 2020). However, after several field trials, the vaccines for malaria parasites and dengue fever viruses have not been marketed yet due to complications with multiple species of malaria parasites and various serum types of dengue virus. Vaccines for Zika and other viruses have been explored, without any successful progress reported.

2.6.11 Challenges and Conclusions

Humans are at an increased risk of mosquito-borne diseases in the world and the people in the world, are not adequately prepared to respond to public health threats (CDC

2020) despite malaria cases being dramatically reduced over the past few decades. However, malaria is still the most deadly mosquito-borne virus as it kills about 500,000 per year worldwide. The emergence and spread of yellow fever, zika, chikgunya, West Nile viruses, the lack of vaccines, the shortage of effective insecticides, the increasing resistance to insecticides by target mosquitoes, and increasing of pathogens to drugs are still a big challenge for the effective control of vector mosquitoes and mosquito-borne diseases. The U.S. reported that vector-borne cases have more than double from 2004 to 2018 and are now at an all-time high (Petersen et al. 2019). Based on a CDC report (CDC, 2020), during the last 15 years, the number of vector-borne disease cases has increased dramatically as the ranges of vectors have expanded, and the number of emerging pathogens have multiplied (Petersen et al. 2019). In part, this may be caused by global warming, climate, and environmental changes (Bezirtzoglou et al. 2011), expansion of transportation, migration, and general globalization. Vector mosquito control remains one of the most critical measures for the effective prevention and control of mosquito bites and mosquito-borne diseases.

ACKNOWLEDGMENTS

This chapter is partly based on work performed within the framework of IMAAC (`https://imaac.eu/`) related to COST Action CA16227 (*Investigation & Mathematical Analysis of Avant-garde Disease Control via Mosquito Nano-Tech-Repellents*, `https://cost.eu/actions/CA16227/`), supported by COST Association (European Cooperation in Science and Technology).

CHAPTER 3

Concepts of the Best Management Practices for Integrated Pest, Mosquito, and Vector Management

Rui-De Xue*
Anastasia Mosquito Control District,
St. Augustine, Florida, USA
** corresponding author, e-mail: rxue@amcdfl.org*

Tong-Yan Zhao
Department of Vector Biology and Control,
Institute of microbiology and Epidemiology,
Dongdajie, Fengtai, Beijing, China

CONTENTS

3.1 Introduction 19
3.2 Control Methods/Tools 20
  3.2.1 Immature Stage Control 20
  3.2.2 Adult Control 21
3.3 Integrated Pest Management (IPM) 21
3.4 Integrated Mosquito Management (IMM) 22
3.5 Integrated Vector Management (IVM) 24
3.6 Best Management Practice (BMP) 25
3.7 Summary 25

3.1 INTRODUCTION

Mosquitoes are semi-aquatic insects (family Culicidae, order Diptera) of which approximately 4,000 species from around the world have currently been described. Mosquitoes have four life stages that include egg, larva, pupa, and adult. Eggs, larvae, and pupae are the immature stages and reside in water, unlike adults which have matured and emerged with two wings to live in an air environment. Adult mosquitoes are either male or

DOI: 10.1201/9781003035992-3

female, but it is only the adult females that bite and suck blood, excluding several species of *Toxorhynchites*. Adult mosquitoes are the number one most dangerous animals to kill and detriment the health of humans and other animals because many species act as pathogen vectors and transmit different diseases such as yellow fever, dengue, zika, chikungunya, West Nile, St. Louis encephalitis (SLE), Japanese type B encephalitis, eastern and western equine encephalitis (EEE & WEE), lymphatic filariasis, and malaria (AMCA 2017). Mosquitoes also cause annoying nuisance problems and economic losses due to host-seeking and blood-sucking behaviors. Therefore, control and management of vector and pest mosquito populations are critical for the protection of both public health and the quality of life. This chapter provides a description of concepts, principle, major methods and tools for the control of pest and vector mosquitoes in addition to the terminology and components of Integrated Pest Management (IPM), Integrated Mosquito Management (IMM), Integrated Vector Management (IVM), and Best Management Practices (BMP).

3.2 CONTROL METHODS/TOOLS

3.2.1 Immature Stage Control

Traditional methods to control immature mosquito stages focus on **Source Reduction**. The simple principle is NO WATER AND NO Mosquitoes due to the necessity of water for egg hatching and larval/pupal growth. Prevention of mosquito breeding is one of the most effective and permanent measures to control larvae through techniques of (1) ditching, impounding, and filling to eliminate standing water (Lloyd et al. 2018), (2) emptying water from containers and/or covering up open containers to prevent gravid female mosquitoes from laying eggs, or (3) directly restricting and killing mosquito larvae and emerged adult mosquitoes. For egg control, there are several kinds of **Mechanical or Physical Control** methods , such as commercially available ovitraps or lethal ovitraps (Xue et al., 2021). For larval control, several species of mosquito larvae have siphons that attach to the roots of aquatic weeds and plants to obtain oxygen, and thus the control of these larval stage mosquitoes is directly related to the management of the aquatic plants. However, the most effective method for general larval control is **Chemical Control** via application of larvicides such as organophosphates (temephos), pyrethroid insecticides, biopesticides or microbial larvicides (*Bacillus thuringiensis israelensis* (BTi), *Bacillus sphaericus*, and Spinosad), insect growth regulators (methoprene, pyriproxyfen, and diflubenzuron), or even surface oil and monomolecular surface films for both pupal and larval control. Such insecticides and chemicals can be applied with either ground or aerial application techniques.

Biocontrol and Biorational Control measures instead work to control larval populations by use of natural predators like predatory mosquito fish, *Toxorhynchites* mosquito larvae, or pathogens (protozoan and nematodes). In several countries, there are national or locally established laws and regulations regarding the application and implementation of mosquito control methods; this is so-called **Legal and Regulation Control**. Usually, these measures apply to larval and adult mosquito control or other public health issues directly occurring within urban regions or cities.

3.2.2 Adult Control

The most practical methods for prevention and control of adult mosquitoes are **Prevention and Personal Protection**. This involves personal protective measures of wearing long sleeves shirts and pants, avoiding outdoor activity at peak mosquito activity (usually dawn and dusk), and applying insect repellents such as DEET, Picaridin, or *para*-menthane-3,8-diol (PMD). Another measure is to repair screened windows and doors before the onset of mosquito season in order to prevent adult mosquitoes from entering buildings. The purposes of these methods are to limit or prevent the opportunity for contact between mosquitoes and human beings by targeting mosquito behaviors, biology, and habitats. **Mechanic and Physical Control** measures involve a variety of different trap devices, removal techniques, and bug zappers to attract, collect and/or kill adult mosquitoes. Other routes include the use of specific materials and tools to create a physical barrier between mosquitoes and humans. However, **Chemical Control** provides the most effective and rapid control of adult mosquitoes via insecticide application and implementation techniques like indoor residual spraying (IRS), long last insecticide-treated bed nets (WHO 2006), or space fogging and cold/ thermal spraying, particularly ultra-low-volume (ULV) applications (UCSF 2020, WHO 2006a). Convention insecticides include variants of organophosphates (malathion, chlorpyrifos, and naled (the USA only)) and pyrethroids (permethrin, deltamethrin, cypermethrin, Lambda-cyhalothrin, Cyfluthrin, Bifenthion, D-phenothrin (sumithrin), and Etofenprox). Unfortunately, a downside to chemical control that the long-term use of insecticides and the large quantities applied has resulted in instances of chemical resistance in mosquitoes which leads to major challenges for control efforts. Targeted pest management also takes into consideration that adult mosquitoes are a part of an ecosystem and that there exist many natural and predatory enemies in such systems such as birds, bats, dragonflies, etc., that can impact and adjust the natural mosquito populations. Within **Biocontrol and Biorational Control**, biocontrol involves the release of natural predators to control adult mosquitoes; however, the predator species are not typically mosquito-specific killers and they eat or kill a range of bugs that may include beneficent insect species. Biorational control methods such as sterile insect technology (SIT), *Wolbachia* bacteria-infection (IAEA & WHO/TDR 2019), genetically modified organisms (GMO), and attractive toxic sugar baits (ATSB) have recently showed promise for controlling vector mosquitoes (WHO 2019, 2019a). **Legal and Regulation Control** for adult mosquitoes has mostly been implemented in urban areas using measures of surveillance, like trapping or measuring human landing rate count, and/or awarding cities, town, and villages the title of "mosquito free" to promote public and governmental appreciation of mosquito control in China. These control efforts are directly regulated and overseen by the local government systems.

3.3 INTEGRATED PEST MANAGEMENT (IPM)

Integrated Pest Control (IPC) or **Integrated Pest Management (IPM)** is a broad-based approach that integrates practices to achieve an economically sound control of pests and vectors. IPM aims to suppress pest populations below the level or threshold that is economically justified and consequently minimize the risks to human and environmental health (ESA 2020). The principles for the screening and selection of control methods involves comparing the effectiveness, safety, economics, and simplicity across all available pest control techniques and the subsequent integration of appropriate measures (EPA 2020, WHO 2008). IPM combinations of varying methods and tools are designed to control either a prioritized major species or a multiple species of pests and/or vectors. The first choices for IPM are source reduction and environmental control methods that may be the permanent solution. Importantly, these methods have to be adapted to the local climate, economy, and community in addition to being practical, acceptable, and sustainable. In the United States, IPM was formulated into national policy in 1972 when President Richard Nixon directed federal agencies to take steps to advance the application of IPM in all relevant sectors. In 1979, President Jimmy Carter established an interagency IPM Coordinating Committee to ensure the development and implementation of IPM practices (ESA 2020). The IPM strategy was later extended towards integrated mosquito management (IMM) and integrated vector management (IVM).

3.4 INTEGRATED MOSQUITO MANAGEMENT (IMM)

IMM is a control strategy that manages mosquito populations based on risk thresholds, ecological characteristics of mosquitoes and ecosystems, economic and environmental conditions, community participation, and an overall method selection process (FMCA 2012, CDC 2020a). The traditional IMM methods involve the use of standard traps to first conduct surveillance of mosquito population and consequently define an appropriate action threshold for justifying control methods, insecticide application, and equipment for control action (AMCA 2017) (Figure 3.1). Based on the multitude of known breeding habitats of pest and vector species, the emphasis of mosquito control is divided into the sectors of container-breeding mosquito management, waste water or storm drain mosquito management, floodwater mosquito management, salt marsh mosquito management, and rice field mosquito management (Lu 1986). There is additional emphasis for control practices based on the exact diseases trasmitted by vector mosquitoes, specifically divided into dengue, Yellow fever, Chikungunya, and Zika vector mosquito management sectors. Notably, the principles of container-breeding mosquito management match the practices for managing vector species of Zika and other arboviruses (SLE, WNV, EEE/WEE, Japanese encephalitis), as well as malaria vectors, lymphic filiarisis vectors, and urban mosquito species (Lu 1999).

Typical control methods involve simple mechanical and physical controls such as handpicking, barriers, traps, vacuuming, and tillage disrupt breeding (Lloyd et al. 2018). Additionally, source reduction is performed through environmental management and modifications, which are considered permanent solutions that limit and reduce breeding sites and/or limit and reduce the opportunities for mosquitoes to come into contact with humans or other animals. Chemical control is also implemented through use of registered insecticides in aerial applications or ground application techniques like indoor residual spraying (IRS), long last insecticide-treated bed nets, ULV spraying (WHO 2006, WHO 2006a), and barrier spraying (Najera & Zaim 2002). Biocontrol or biorational control measures are also common in IMM and involve the use of pathogens, parasites, predators, sterile insect

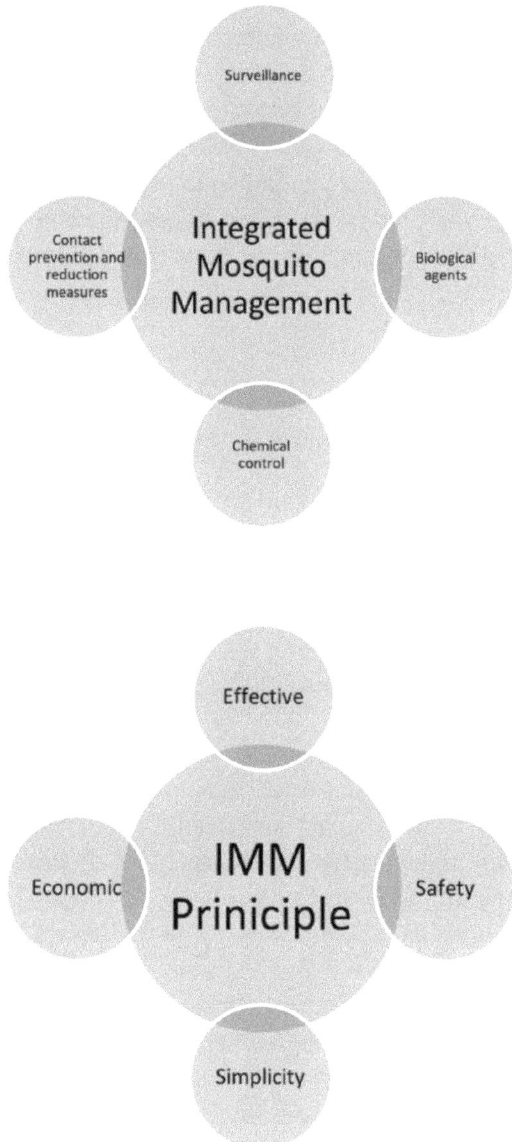

Figure 3.1: Control methods and priniciple of integrated mosquito management (IMM)

technology (SIT), and genetic modifications (IAEA & WHO/TDR 2019). Law and regulation control that is implemented at the local level benefits the community by controlling and reducing both the presence of mosquito breeding sites and the opportunity for disease trasminission. Overall, the selection of single or combination method is based on the target species, threshold regulations, local conditions, funding situation, and the available labor and equipment resources (EPA 2020).

Due to the innovation and application of new technology, the traditional IMM has been updated and improved (Fouet & Kamdem 2019). The increased availability of new technology and novel techniques have played major roles in supplementing the activities of data collection, data management, and data analysis in addition to increasing the effectiveness and speed of control measures. Important innovations include Georgraphic Information Systems (GIS) and mapping software (UCSF 2020), GIS-based vehicles and spraying equipment, new aircrafts and drones, smart traps, species-specific traps, and attractant-based collection devices. Additonally, technological advancements in genetic control tools and techniques allow greater accuracy in the diagnosis and testing for pathogens and insecticide resistance, and thus better guide operational decisions and improve control efforts (WHO 2019).

3.5 INTEGRATED VECTOR MANAGEMENT (IVM)

The term "vector" defines all arthropod species that can carry and transmit pathogens to humans and which thus present a risk to public health. Known vectors include species of mosquitoes, sand flies, black flies, fleas, lice, chagas, and ticks. IVM is a rational decision-making process focused on protecting public health through the environmentally sound management of vector populations and the reduction or interruption of vector-borne pathogen transmission. The ultimate goal of IVM is to prevent and control the transmission of vector-borne diseases such as malaria, Zika, dengue, Japanese encephalitis, leishmaniosis, schistosomiasis, Lyme diseases, and Chagas disease (WHO 2008). IVM attempts an optimal use of resources and the overall principle seeks to improve the efficacy, cost-effectiveness, ecological soundness, and sustainability of disease-vector control efforts via collaboration with many related partners and agencies. Because IVM requires collaboration, the U.S. Centers for Disease Control and Prevention (CDC, 2020) developed a network of partners within the United States. The framework includes: federal government agencies (CDC, NIH, USDA, EPA, and military vector control units) for policing, guidelines, and diagnosis; the State Departments of Health for surveillance, diagnosis, and guidelines; local control agencies for control action; local health providers for treatment of patients and case reporting; academic and industry partners for research into pathogens and control techniques; industry for development of tools and equipment; policy makers to create regulations and make decisions; public health partners to promote the policy; the public for community participation and follow through of preventative behaviors.

To select the most appropriate control methods, IVM strives for informed decisions based on knowledge of ecological characteristics & behaviors of mosquitoes and ecosystems and consideration of the current environmental and economic conditions. This approach attempts to overcome the typical challenges experienced with conventional single-intervention approaches by taking advantage of collaborative opportunities and new technologies and thus promoting multi-sectoral approaches for the protection of humans and animals from infection and disease. The Global Strategic Framework (WHO 2004,WHO 2016) for IVM notes that IVM requires the establishment of principles, decision-making criteria and procedures, timeframes, and target goals, in addition to addressing program suitability and sustainable management. The framework identifies the following five key elements for the successful implementation of IVM: (1) advocacy, social mobilization, and regulatory controls for public health and the empowerment of communities; (2) collaboration within and outside of the health sector for planning, monitoring, decision-making, and achieving an optimal use of resources; (3) integration of non-chemical and chemical control methods plus further integration with other disease control measures; (4) evidence-based decision making guided by operational research in addition to entomological and epidemiological surveillance and evaluation; and (5) development of adequate human resources, training, and career structures at national and local levels to promote capacity building and effective management of IVM programs.

3.6 BEST MANAGEMENT PRACTICE (BMP)

BMP was originally used for water and plant management in the early 1980s but was later expanded to cover IPM, IMM, and IVM. The BMP for IPM, IMM, and IVM represents a practice (or combination of practices) that is promoted as an effective and practicable means (with technological, economic, and institutional considerations) of preventing or reducing the risk of mosquito-borne disease transmission to below threshold levels (Figure 3.2). Major components of BMP are based on surveillance of vector species (distribution, seasonal activity & activity behaviors), GIS mapping, development of regulatory action thresholds for immature and adult stages (FMCA 2012, AMCA 2017), monitoring mosquito resistance, conducting source reduction, biocontrol and biorational controls, proper application of chemical controls like larvicides and adulticides, and using physical or cultural controls to cut and limit the contact opportunities between vectors and people. Additional components include monitoring the efficacy and quality of control efforts and operations, record-keeping, sustainable management practices, public education, citizen science and community outreach, and encouragement of community participation.

3.7 SUMMARY

In summary, the management approaches for mosquito control are quite different from one another and there are benefits and limitations to each other. Integrated Pest Mangement (IPM) is a broad category that applies to many kinds of pests and vectors including a multutide of mosquito species. IPM is broken down into Integrated Vector Management (IVM) and Integrated Mosquito Management (IMM). IVM is the broad subcategory and applies to all kinds of vectors including mosquitoes, ticks, sand flies, black flies, fleas, lice, etc. Comparitively, IMM is a narrowed subcategory that only applies to mosquitoes, primarily pest and vector species but also concerns benefient species like *Toxorhynchites*. Best Management Practices (BMP) is the effective action and implementation of management plans and strategies for the IPM, IMM, and IVM, which results in the interconnectedness of IPM, IMM, IVM, and BMP within the grand scheme of mosquito control.

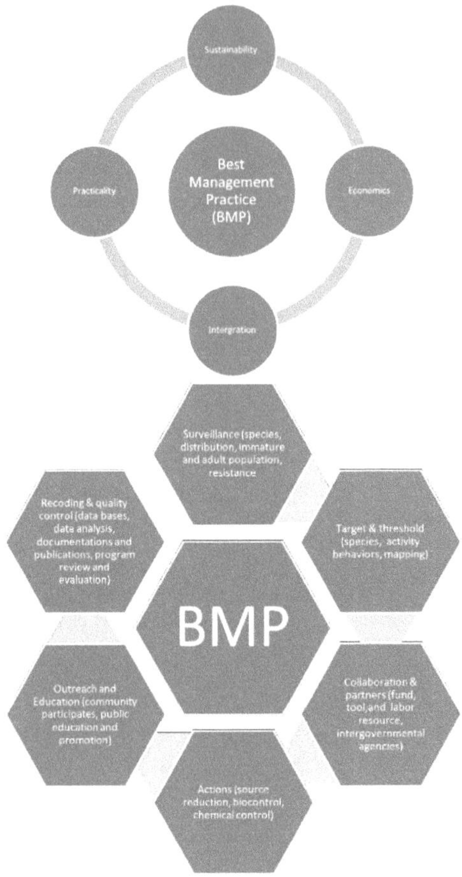

Figure 3.2: Principles and compents of best management practices (BMP) for integrated mosquito management (IMM).

ACKNOWLEDGMENTS

This chapter is partly based on work performed within the framework of IMAAC (`https://imaac.eu/`) related to COST Action CA16227 (*Investigation & Mathematical Analysis of Avant-garde Disease Control via Mosquito Nano-Tech-Repellents*, `https://cost.eu/actions/CA16227/`), supported by COST Association (European Cooperation in Science and Technology).

CHAPTER 4

Overview of Personal Protection Measures Through the Innovative Use of Repellent-Textiles

Asghar Talbalaghi*

Italian Mosquito Control Association, Alessandria, Italy
** corresponding author, e-mail: talbalaghi@libero.it*

Sahar Hassandoust

Italian Mosquito Control Association, Alessandria, Italy

Chinazom Enukoha

Department of Epidemiology and Medical Statistics, University of Ibadan, Nigeria

CONTENTS

4.1 Introduction ... 28
4.2 Innovative Vector control ... 29
4.3 Insect Repellent Mode of Action ... 31
4.4 Textile and Personal Protection ... 32
4.5 Impregnation of Textile ... 33
4.6 Evaluation of Repellents ... 33
4.7 Measuring the entomological performance of textiles ... 35
4.7.1 Open field, Italian Mosquito Control Association Alessandria Italy, 2019 ... 35
4.7.2 Laboratory test at Anastasia Mosquito Control District St. Augustine, Florida, USA 2020 ... 36
4.7.2.1 Measuring the efficacy of textile samples already treated for arm test ... 37
4.7.2.2 Measuring the efficacy of textile samples treated with 2 types of micro spraying treatment before the test ... 38
4.7.2.3 Measuring the efficacy of textile samples already treated for glove test (Figures 4.7 and 4.8) ... 39
4.7.2.4 Evaluation of lotions of botanical-based repellents ... 39
4.7.3 Measuring the efficacy of repellent by use of olfactometer ... 39
4.7.3.1 Measuring the efficacy of Ultrasound devices ... 40

DOI: 10.1201/9781003035992-4

4.8 Discussion on lab test 40
4.9 Results 42
4.10 Future perspective and outlook 43
4.11 Conclusion Note 44

4.1 INTRODUCTION

Mosquitoes are vectors of arboviruses affecting animals and human health (Moutailler et al. 2019). Vector-borne diseases account for more than 17% of all infectious diseases, causing more than 700,000 deaths annually. Diseases such as malaria, Zika, chikungunya, dengue fever, and West Nile fever are major health problems in the world that are transmitted by *Culicidae* mosquitoes (WHO 2017).

Every year, malaria alone, transmitted by the Anopheles mosquito, kills 400,000 people (mainly children) and incapacitates another 200 million for days. Knowing where vector species occur is crucial for the assessment of vector-borne disease risk (European Centre for Disease Prevention and Control and European Food Safety Authority, 2018). The extensive outbreak of Chikungunya in the Indian Ocean between 2005 and 2006 and the subsequent outbreak in the Emilia Romagna region of Italy in August 2007 prompts a number of actions which must be carried out without delay in order to prevent any future recurrence of outbreaks (Talbalaghi 2008).

Climate change and the movement of humans infected with vector borne diseases across the world will increase the risk of new local transmission of diseases. The rapidity of transport systems which facilitates the movement of goods and people from one part of the globe to another also permits the introduction of varieties of exotic insects in every form: eggs, larvae and winged forms into different territories (Talbalaghi 2012). Early surveillance of mosquitoes and the appropriate standard monitoring of adult mosquitoes species is a key step to be established in vector control. The main principle of mosquito research can therefore be summarized in one question: "Where are the mosquitoes coming from?" and not, "Where are they are migrating to" (Talbalaghi 2008 ECDC Report). Within the strategies for lowering the risk of transmission of disease vectored by mosquitoes there is personal protection. Personal protection involves protective clothing and use of repellents. Improper use of repellents may limit the action of the repellent if the repellent does not last long and its persistence is not assured conveniently. The innovative approach, through Mosquito Nano-Tech-Repellents, is however a promising path. Scientific research has shown that through the textiles, it is possible to achieve this goal.

4.2 INNOVATIVE VECTOR CONTROL

Prior to the discovery of modern mosquito repellent devices, people often used natural ingredients and traditional methods to repel mosquitoes. Usually, they utilise scents that repel insects, such as dried orange peels, lemons, and lemongrass stems (Arief, Saratian, Permana, Soelton, and Rohman 2019). However, this method is considered unreliable due to the quick biodegradation of the composites.

Targeting the disease agent is one of the main strategies for the control of vector-borne diseases. These tactics include preventative measures, widespread medicine distribution campaigns, vaccinations, antibiotic medications, and antiviral therapies that specifically target the parasite or inhibit the replication of the arbovirus in the host (Tolle 2009). While extremely successful in the control of certain agents of disease etiology, such as filarial parasites and some strains of Plasmodium, the resistance of parasites to various drugs and the lack of antivirals and vaccines for many disease agents limit the success of this control technique for many vector-borne disease agents (Mok et al. 2015). The second method of control involves the prevention of transmission of the disease agent by the vector. This is accomplished by a variety of means including the abatement of vector populations and the use of biting deterrents or repellents such as insecticide-treated bed nets.

As more of the limited insecticidal classes approved for use against vectors fail in controlling vector populations and with the ever increasing vectorial capacity, the need for novel control strategies becomes ever more necessary. Within the control strategies of bloodsucking arthropods, personal protection is of growing importance and it is an in-equitable solution in some socio-economic and environmental contexts considering the target species to ward off. Personal protection applied by persons against arthropods, is basically an important, simple strategy and economically it is considered cost effective.

Consequently, it is essential to gauge how well repellant-infused nanotechnological materials work. The most effective way to combat Leishmaniosis, which is spread by sand flies,; Chagas disease, spread by triatomine bugs,; and tick-borne diseases, which are spread by numerous ticks, is to implement personal protection methods by using repellents.

In order for an arthropod control strategy to be a valid option, it's implementation should guaranty its sustainability over time, as suggested in Figure 4.1; "Good for mosquito control (A)". Figure 4.2 illustrates "We should work on where the mosquitoes are coming from but not where the mosquitoes are going to", an emphasis on the implementation of source reduction operations, larviciding through the routine application of microbial or chemical insecticides, and operation of breeding sites as opposed to adulticiding intervention through the application of pesticides (chemical) to kill adult mosquitoes, which may have a possible immediate effect but often with an impact on the environment over a long period of time.

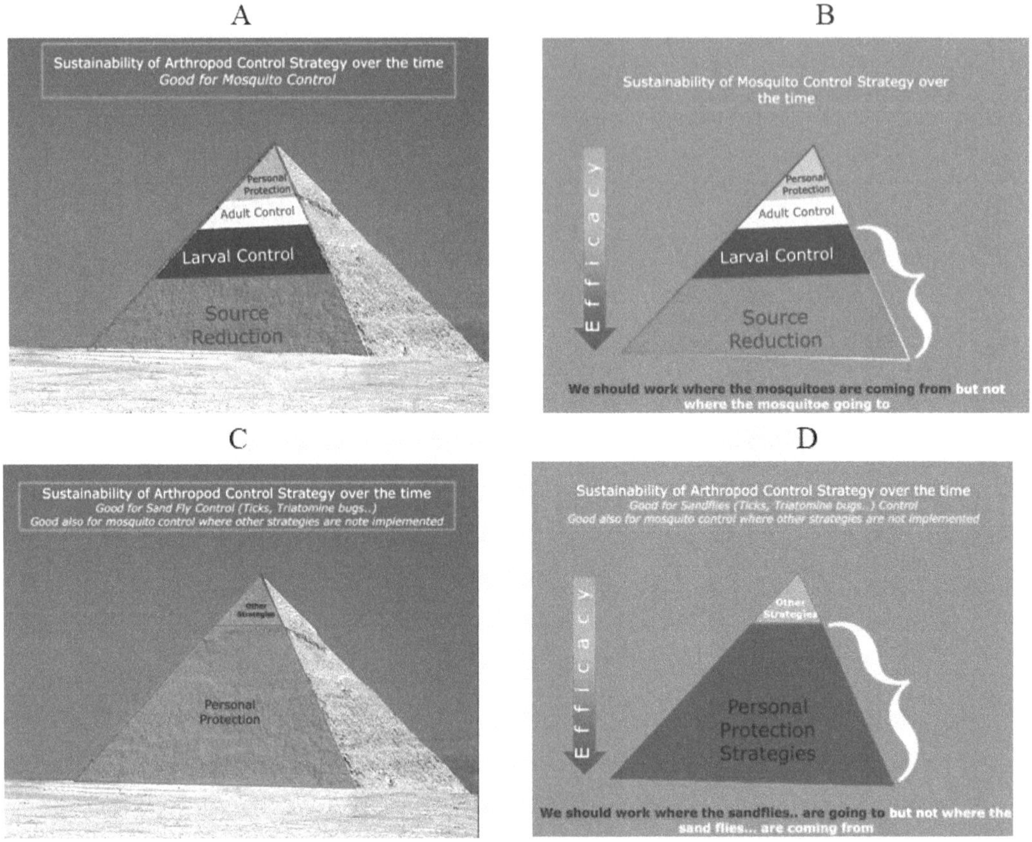

Figure 4.1: Control strategies.

The personal-protection-based control strategy, over time, is a suitable option for the control of sandflies, ticks, triatomine bugs (Figure 4.1 C), which also could be good for mosquito control as a unique available approach due to the pertinent difficulties and lack of products and tools or just inserted in an Integrated Pest Management (IPM) strategy. Despite the indication given for a rational mosquito control strategy for sandfly control,

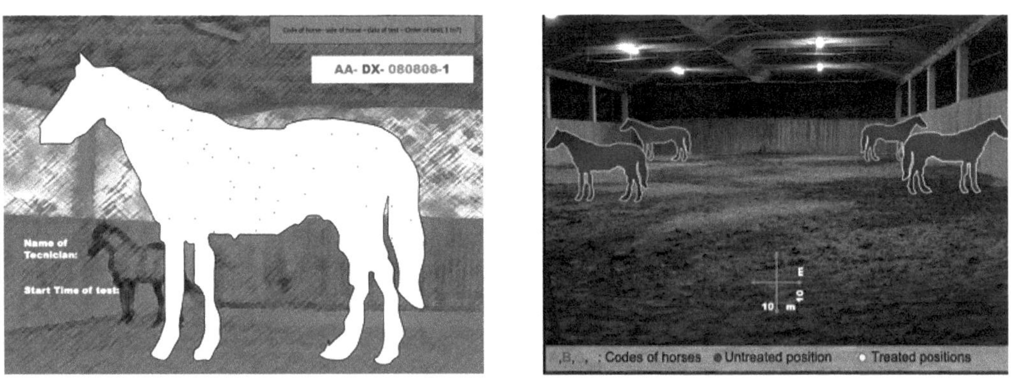

Figure 4.2: Repellent evaluation on horse.

the strategies of sources reduction or larviciding may not justify the cost effectiveness of a long-term vector control initiative, so we should work on where the sandflies are going to but not where the sand flies are coming from Figure (4.1 D).

Various measures of personal protection, both empirical and scientific, are proposed and used in any part of the world, to keep away unwanted arthropods or organisms in general. The methodologies and materials for this purpose range from the use of scents, sounds, ultrasounds, lights, physical-mechanical impediment barriers and mostly repellents, both the botanically based and those of purely chemical origin, obtained from industrial synthesis processes. Typical available repellents are the forms to be released into the area or simply the topical ones. The use of repellents against the bite of arthropods to lower, the risk of diseases transmission, are nowadays, part of the consolidated medical prevention protocols recommended by national and world health bodies that deal with public health. The literature on the effectiveness of personal protection products against arthropods is mainly limited to studies of prevention of bites, rather than prevention of disease (Debboun and Strickman 2012).

Scientists have suggested that cotton fabrics might be enhanced to more effectively repel mosquitoes by using microencapsulation (Grancaric, Laird, Botteri, Shen and Laatikainen 2019). In addition to the use of textiles, some of the advances to improve the efficacy of products and methods with an eye toward ecologically friendly outcomes include the use of nanotechnologies in combination with traditional repellents. While insecticide-based vector control strategies are important for the management of vector-borne diseases, the advent of insecticide-resistance threatens the effectiveness of this approach in the future (Peter, Bossche, Van Den and Sharp, 2005). Besides humans, numerous animals including horses with relatively large bodies suffer from mosquito bites and mosquito-related transmission of diseases (Talbalaghi, Ali and Hassandoust 2018) hence, innovative methods for animal control such as the use of repellents are strongly recommended.

In vector control, the different situations faced demand different solutions in the right ways meaning creating purpose built strategies that fit the context in which people are living. Insect repellents are therefore an alternative to the use of insecticides. They may be applied to the skin to protect an individual from the bites of mosquitoes, mites, ticks and lice or, less commonly, may be used to exclude insects from an area such as in packaging to prevent infestation of stored products (Peterson and Coats 2001).

4.3 INSECT REPELLENT MODE OF ACTION

The act of repelling insects is an age long practice. In many cases, it has been found that the behavior that has been labelled as repellency may be the result of any number of physiological or biochemical events. Hematophagous insects have been the subject of documented attempts of pest control. Among the earliest reports of repellent use are from Herodotus, a Greek historian (Paluch, Bartholomay and Coats 2010). The testing of over 6000 chemicals from 1942 to 1947 in a variety of research institutions led to the identification of multiple successful repellent chemistries (Morton, Travis and Linduska 2017).

The use of repellent is considered the main control means against the kissing bug Triatoma infestans, that transmits a protozoan, Trypanosoma cruzi, which can infect animals and people and are found only in the Americas causing Chagas disease. (Reynoso, Seccacini, Calcagno, Zerba1, and Alzogaray 2017).

Plant-based repellents have been used for generations in traditional practice as a personal protection measure against host-seeking mosquitoes. Knowledge on traditional repellent plants obtained through ethnobotanical studies is a valuable resource for the development of new natural products. A report has demonstrated the efficacy of botanical compounds as insect repellents on domestic animals (Talbalaghi, Ali and Hassandoust, 2018). Recently, commercial repellent products containing plant-based ingredients have gained increasing popularity among consumers, as these are commonly perceived as "safe" in comparison to long-established synthetic repellents although this is sometimes a misconception. To date, studies have followed standard WHO Pesticide Evaluation Scheme guidelines for repellent testing. There is a need for further standardized studies in order to better evaluate repellent compounds and develop new products that offer high repellence as well as good consumer safety (Maia and Moore 2011). Botanical repellents are numerous and target a wide variety of physiological targets and odorant receptors, suggesting that the potential for resistance to these chemistries is sufficiently low. Current and future technologies directed toward the development of long-lasting botanical or biorational repellents could lead to promising alternatives to repellent formulations that are currently in the market.

One of the major problems of natural repellents is how to establish a standard of its efficacy action, to be reported in the description of the repellents or to be shown on the label that promotes it. The molecules extracted from botanical essences, which form the basis of certain repellents even from the same origin, growing in same latitude are grown on different soil nutritional composition. The same plant species growing in different climatic conditions, with alterations in compound composition of the repellent property and efficacy may be as a result of different factors such as light, humidity, temperature and also different processes involved in the preparation, which in extension alter the components of the repellent itself.

4.4 TEXTILE AND PERSONAL PROTECTION

Many repellents can be applied to field clothing for protection against military important arthropods, especially those that crawl or hop (e.g., mites, ticks, fleas, body lice). Repellents that are or have been widely used for clothing impregnation include sul- fur, dimethyl phthalate, dibutyl phthalate, benzyl benzoate, deet, and permethrin. These materials are also effective when applied to bed nets, curtains, window screens, ground cloths, tents, and protective over garments (Gupta, Gambel, Bernard and Schiefer 2006). Many innovative initiatives have been proposed by the University of Zagreb to make various fabrics repellent against arthropods in recent years. The attempt of chemical and textile engineers to combat Arbovirus mosquitoes through textiles and paints explains the repellent efficacy of fabric cotton samples (Grancaric, Botteri, Ghaffari 2019).

4.5 IMPREGNATION OF TEXTILE

Impregnation of fabrics with repellents is a method reported to reduce bites by insects. This method works just like the impregnation of mosquito nets with Pyrethroid derivatives like Permethrin making them Long-Lasting Insecticide-Treated Nets (LLITNs) which is considered an efficacious vector control strategy especially for indoor feeding vectors. A large percentage of the human skin is covered by the treated fabric thus reducing exposure to the disease vectors. Imparting the mosquito repellents onto the textile and cloth-impregnating laundry emulsions application is one of the innovatory and practical approaches in daily routine to driving away blood-sucking arthropods from people (Brown and Hebert 1997; Maheshwari and Ramya 2014).

Permethrin, first marketed in 1973, a laboratory-manufactured pyrethroid insect repellant and contact insecticide; derived from the crushed dried flowers of Chrysanthemum cinerarifolium is a broad spectrum, non-systemic, synthetic pyrethroid insecticide that targets adults and larvae of many species of biting, chewing, scaling, soil, and flying invertebrates (Diaz 2016). Permethrin is approved by the United States Environmental Protection Agency (EPA) as an insecticide for use on crops, animals, buildings and fabric. It is not absorbed topically therefore it requires direct contact; the reason why it is referred to as a contact repellent. It's mechanism of action is through altering the nervous system by modifying the nerve membrane sodium channel. When applied to clothing, bed nets, tents, and sleeping bags, permethrin and other synthetic Pyrethroids (Allethrin, Alpha-cypermethrin, Cyfluthrin, Deltamethrin, Etofenprox, Lambda-cyhalothrin, and Metofluthrin) all provide very high-level protection against mosquitoes, flies, biting midges, chiggers, fleas, sandflies, and ticks, especially when combined with topically applied insect repellents (Diaz 2016).

There are numerous ways to assess the efficacy of treated textiles for impregnated textiles. The methods are cone test, cage test, field test and excito chamber (Sritabutra et al. 2011; Standards 2006; Tawatsin et al. 2001; WHO 1996). Textiles impregnated with repellents like LLINs drive the vector away from the treated surface, or depending on the concentration may cause knock down or mortality. The interruption of host-seeking requires proper understanding of host-seeking behaviors employed by disease vectors and is very promising in the development of vector control strategies. The applications of the mosquito repellent feature must not damage the original characteristic of the textile materials itself. Approaches aimed at curtailing wild vector populations inevitably rely on the prevention of host-seeking or biting as an endpoint.

4.6 EVALUATION OF REPELLENTS

There are many disciplines involved in studying the use of a given repellent, the manufacturing process and in evaluating it's performance; Chemistry, Engineering, Biology and Entomology. Entomologists have to evaluate the necessary capacity to measure the effectiveness of a repellent against mosquitoes or arthropods, and to give indications to other figures to improve the characteristics. The extracts of plants which are basically essential oil, have delicate physical and chemical properties, therefore during the engineering, preparation and technical process of impregnation and incorporation; in order for an impregnated repelling fabric to be of good performance, the following considerations must be made during the manufacturing process:

(1) Quantity of Active ingredient or adjuvants in the textile (dose)

(2) Dimension of Textile to be used

(3) Volatility of the active ingredient

(4) The temperature during the preparation of textiles

(5) Timing of preparation of textile

(6) The property of textile (fitness and property of absorption of repellent used)

(7) Need for long lasting repellence and slow release

To better describe the importance of the metric evaluation of the effectiveness of a repellent and to better focus on insect repellents and more precisely, in our case, on the evaluation of innovative repellents as fabrics, it is useful to start from the general meaning of repellents and to detail, the rational methods and specific protocol to be used for the evaluation of innovative textiles against vectors. As a general definition from *www.dictionary.com*, a repellent in our cases, is “something that repels, as a substance that keeps away insects”. A repellent should cause disgust or aversion; initiate repulsive force or cause rejection, serve or tend to ward off or drive away:

- Logical and relevant considerations for a repellent
- Beneficial effect
- Safe and not dangerous for the user (potential effects on human health and the environment associated with the use of the product)
- The percentage level of repellency and hours of persistency

Effectiveness and usability are the primary factors that determine a repellent’s success among the numerous brands available in several markets. Disease vector or not, insects are a source of constant annoyance. The use of repellents therefore serves to keep the vectors away and ensures little or no transmission is made on contact by disease vectors because the repellent serves to keep the insects away from the surface on which it has been applied. Repellents are becoming more portable, thanks to innovations in the development and design, making it easy to use, practically anywhere and at any time.

Repellents just like pesticides are subject to authorities of the country of manufacture. Like any pesticide, the registration process is ruled by law, it is a scientific, legal and administrative procedure which must be examined and followed to the letter. Study of fiscal and chemical parameters, toxicity study (acute-chronic), the entomological performance, the ingredients of the product in question (repellent in this case) and the dermal sensitivity of the skin surface on which it is to be applied, the quantity to be used (dose), the frequency and timing of its use; and the alterability in storage and the non-dangerousness if it must be disposed of must be evaluated in the process of registration. These studies are used to decide whether a product and its intended uses meet the scientific and safety standard and whether specific use restrictions are necessary for the safe use of the product.

4.7 MEASURING THE ENTOMOLOGICAL PERFORMANCE OF TEXTILES

For preliminary outcomes, in order to better investigate the efficacy of repellent fabrics, and in the absence of precise measurement protocols of efficacy, some attempts have been made in the past two years in order to establish a valid methodology for efficacy measurement of repellent textiles. These evaluations, carried out in the open field in Italy, 2019 and in the laboratory in the United States, 2020 have given interesting indications about the performance of samples carefully tested. The methodology used are those applied for the efficacy tests of topical repellents that are applied directly to the skin. The evidence resulting from these efforts are bellow reported.

4.7.1 Open field, Italian Mosquito Control Association Alessandria Italy, 2019

Following the activities carried out in the last 2 years which include laboratory tests, semi field tests and field tests of textiles are compulsory tentative to measure the efficacy of a certain sample. There are not established protocols to measure the efficacy of textiles to repel arthropods. Thus, during an evaluation it is necessary to reduce as much as possible the variables that may affect the results. These factors include but are not limited to: target species, number of species present during a test, age of species, climate pattern factors and light intensity. A field pilot study was set up in 2019 intended for the preparation of a well-designed protocol for the evaluation of effectiveness of the samples of textiles.

With regards to the aims of the COST Action project titled; Investigation and Mathematical Analysis of Avant-garde Disease Control via Mosquito Nano-Tech-Repellents, a field test of the efficacy of nano- and micro-particles used in textile has been performed. These materials are prepared to release repellents at a known rate, in order to undergo a protocolled efficacy studies, set up by personnel of the Mosquito Control Team of Alessandria. Such Avant-Garde measures carried out within technically sound strategies can help to reduce disease burden of vector borne diseases.

Cotton fabrics treated by different repellents prepared using the Pad-dry impregnation system, underwent a field efficacy test in the Province of Alessandria Italy in August 2019. The location was the Sport Field of Alluvioni Cambio, Province of Alessandria Piedmont Region Via Camillo Benso Conte di Cavour, 25, 15040 Alluvioni Cambio AL. Every year, in this location is held the famous “Sagra del Sedano” (Cosine Festival of Celery). This location is located a few kilometers from the southern banks of the Po river and from Europe’s largest rice paddies, vast areas of wetlands. These rice fields provide ideal habitats for the breeding of several mosquito species specifically, several generations of Ochlerotatus caspius, Culex spp and Anopheles maculipennis. Ochlerotatus caspius can migrate

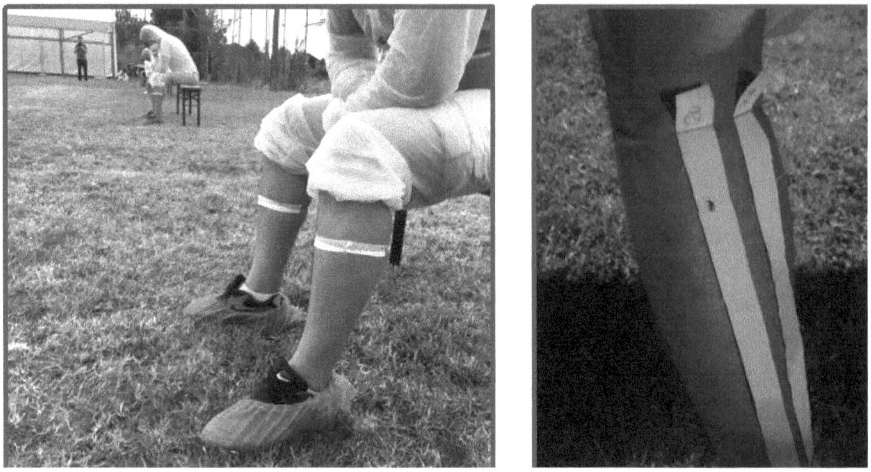

Figure 4.3: Textile evaluation on human.

up to 30 km or more from the breeding source and create a heavy infestation in Alluvioni Cambio, which was in the past, the ideal place for similar investigation for our tests.

Groups of four people in the hours of greatest infestation, after having dressed in a white suit, covered to the shoes, sit on a chair at a distance from each other, exposed to mosquitoes, from knee down for 10 minutes. For four nights, diverse horizontal and vertical fabric notes treated with repellents were fixed to one leg (right leg) on the bare part of the shin of the study participants. Untreated fabric of the same surface were attached to the left legs. The number of mosquito landings on the treated legs (right leg) with test strips were counted in order to compare the treated legs (right leg) with the untreated legs (left leg) and to observe the repellency demonstrated. At the same time as the evaluation in the same 10-minute interval, the prevalence of the nearby mosquitoes will be measured with two fixed CO_2 traps (Figures 4.3 and 4.4),register the temperature, wind velocity and lightness parameters.

4.7.2 Laboratory test at Anastasia Mosquito Control District St. Augustine, Florida, USA 2020

I. Measuring the efficacy of textile samples already treated for wrapped arm test (Figures 4.5 and 4.6)

II. Measuring the efficacy of textile samples already treated for glove test (Figures 4.7)

III. Measuring the efficacy of textile samples treated with 2 types of micro spraying treatment before the test (Figure 4.8)

IV. Evaluation of lotions of botanical-based repellents (Figure 4.9)

V. Measuring the efficacy of repellents by use of olfactometer (Figure 4.10)

VI. Measuring the efficacy of ultrasound watches (Figure 4.11)

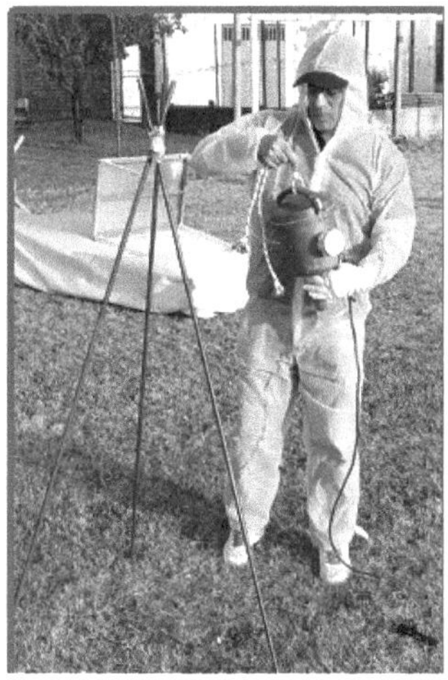

Figure 4.4: Trap installation for prevalence observation.

4.7.2.1 Measuring the efficacy of textile samples already treated for arm test

The novel evaluation of the repellency generated by innovative textiles already incorporated with nanotechnology use of some repellents against Aedes egypti Linnaeus in lab conditions carried out at Anastasia Mosquito Control District of St. Johns County 120 EOC Drive, St. Augustine, Florida, USA, with the following objectives:

a. Perform the best approaches for the evaluation of incorporated nano- and micro-particles of mosquito repellent in textile

b. Carry out lab tests, according to standard recommended procedure for the evaluation of the provided protection of 12 different impregnated fabrics

c. Determine mathematically, the measure of protection and duration of protection provided by single samples

d. Elaboration of the information results from the test results

e. Observe the consideration on efficacy performances of materials used; both textiles and products

A set of 11 cotton fabric samples of 30 x 40 cm were previously prepared in the Faculty of Textile Technology, University of Zagreb through Pad-dry laboratory with impregnation baths followed by drying at 120 °C for 2 minutes. The repellents used are basically of botanical origin: Immortelle Essential, Clove Essential oil, Repel Care® (Turmeric-Eucalyptus) and IR3535. The use of these four basic repellents and their combination to further products, Water-glass (Sodium Silicate) and Polyurethane were prepared to be impregnated in fabrics.

Experimental Details
Test organism: *Aedes aegypti* (2 - 5 days post-emergence adult)
Source of insects: AMCD Insectary, St. Augustine Florida, USA

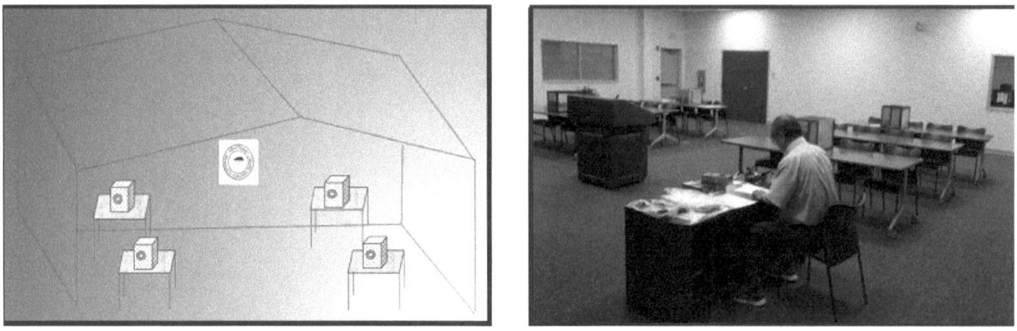

Figure 4.5: Design of cage test.

Start date: 25th March 2020
Date of the conclusion of lab test:3rd April 2020
Place of Test: Temperature 24 C° Day light illumination
Treatment of textile: According to processes proposed by the Faculty of Textile Technology, University of Zagreb for the impregnation in a unique concentration.
Number of participants: Four men over 50 years old (Figures 4.5 and 4.6)

4.7.2.2 Measuring the efficacy of textile samples treated with 2 types of micro spraying treatment before the test

Micro-spraying is done directly on textile samples in an open area and in an envelope in order to avoid the drift effect of repellents. Immediate measurement in the cage is done as with the procedure for other tests. Comparison of fresh samples and those already previously treated with the same amount of essential oil for both tests (Figures 4.7).

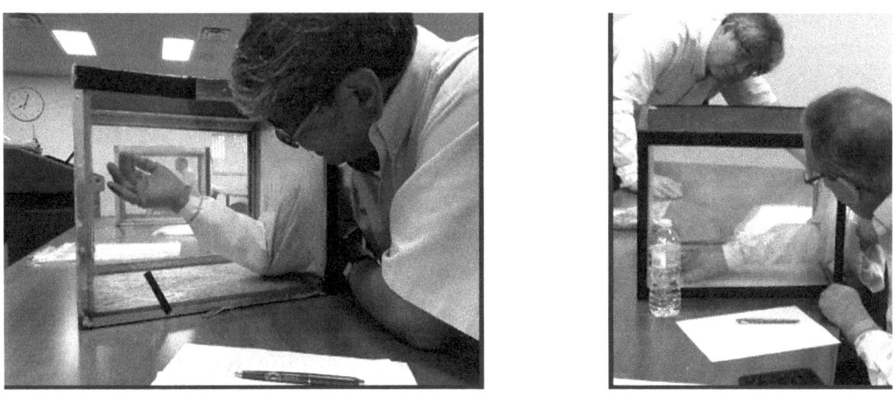

Figure 4.6: Arm textile test.

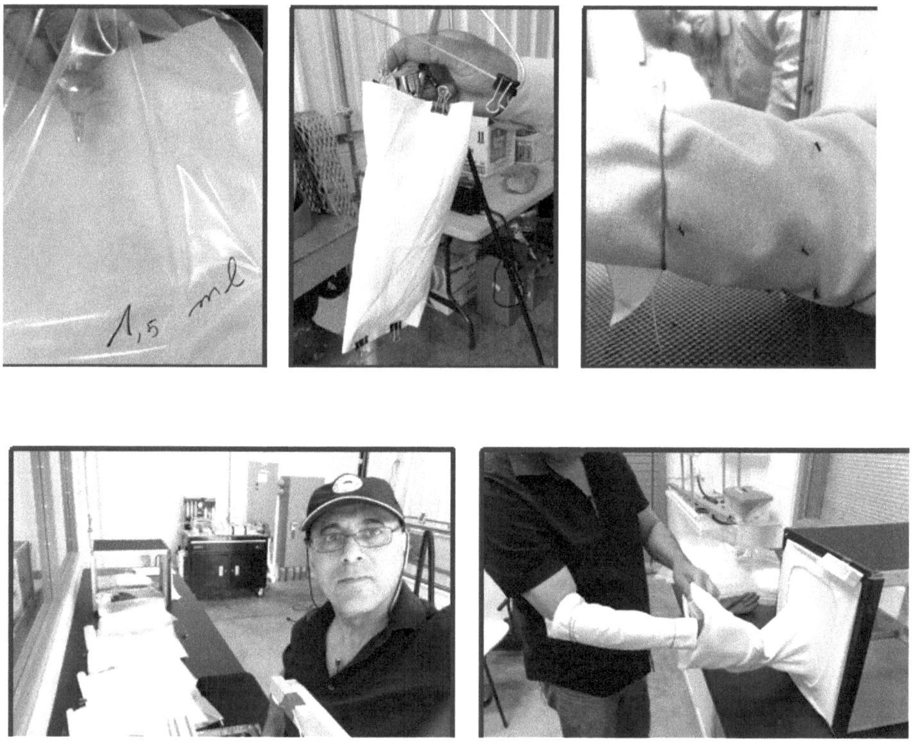

Figure 4.7: Comparison of fresh samples and those already previously treated with the same amount of essential oil for both tests.

4.7.2.3 Measuring the efficacy of textile samples already treated for glove test (Figures 4.7 and 4.8)

This method has been suggested for repellant bioassays against Asian tiger mosquito (Aedes albopictus): IR3535 applied on textile fabrics (A. Michaelakis et al. 2019). The evaluation of sample repellence is done using the glove and a cut window where samples are positioned and inserted in a cage with 200 Aedes aegypti following the abovementioned procedure (Figure 4.8).

4.7.2.4 Evaluation of lotions of botanical-based repellents

This evaluation was carried out, during a 3-month activity as "visiting scientist" at AMCD, Florida, USA, 2020, where many botanical repellent compounds were evaluated against laboratory-reared *Aedes aegypti* L (Whitney A. Qualls, Rui-De Xue, Muhammad Farooq, Steven T. Peper, Vindhya Aryaprema, Kai Blore, Richard Weaver, Dena Autry, Asghar Talbalaghi, James Kenar, Steven C. Cermak, Junwei J. Zhu 2020) (Figure 4.9).

4.7.3 Measuring the efficacy of repellent by use of olfactometer

Verifying the presence of odors with repellent nature and measuring the efficacy or persistency of a product separately is mandatory before the impregnation and incorporation into a fabric . Olfactometer test serves to fulfill this task (Figure 4.10).

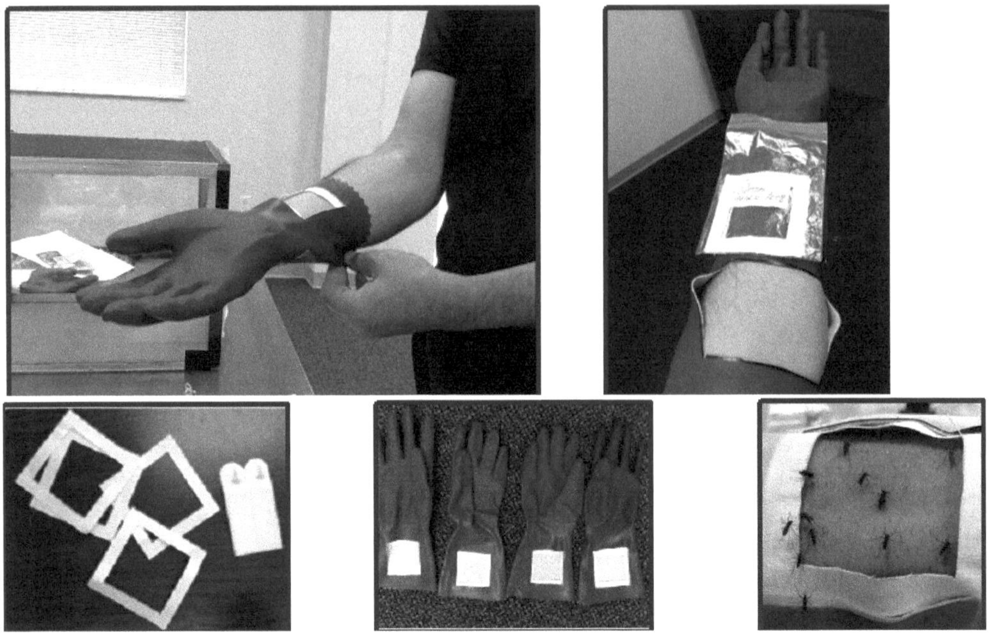

Figure 4.8: The evaluation of sample repellence is done using gloves and cut windows.

4.7.3.1 Measuring the efficacy of Ultrasound devices

Entomologists scientifically verify the functionality of some devices designed to be functional in repelling mosquitoes. A similar watch device is worn in a cage and the protocol used to investigate the effectiveness of the repellence that may have been generated is followed (Figure 4.11).

4.8 DISCUSSION ON LAB TEST

The processes involved in the design and production of textile can be exploited to promote the impregnation and incorporation of repellents on textile to achieve desired results

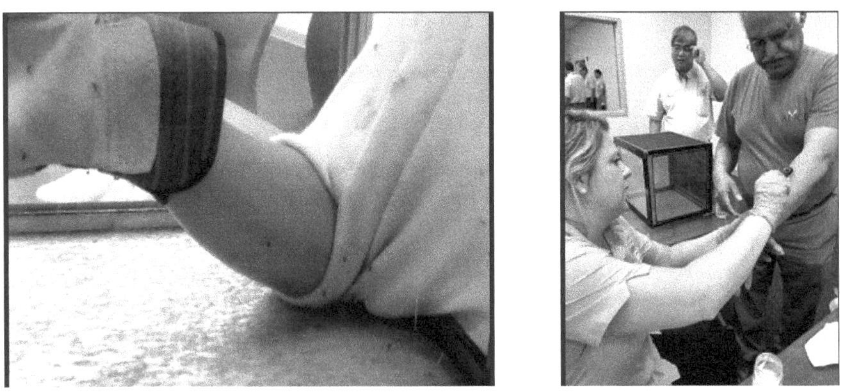

Figure 4.9: The evaluation of samples in AMCD, Florida, USA, 2020.

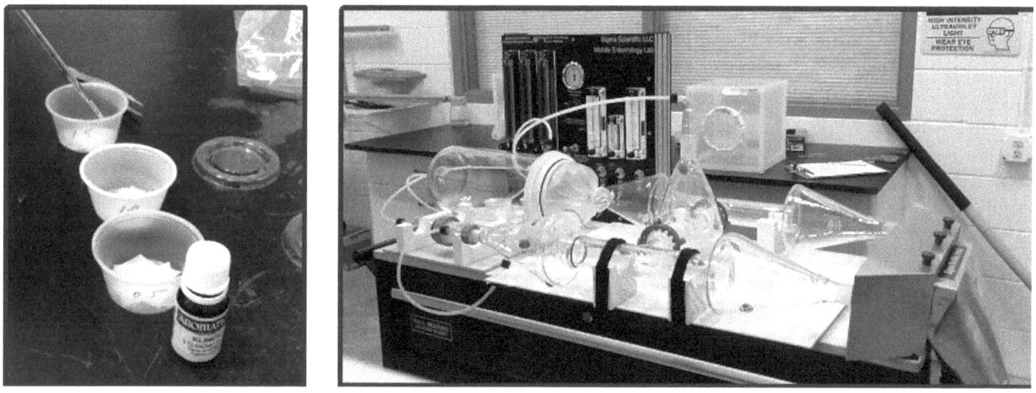

Figure 4.10: Verifying the presence of odors with repellent nature and measuring the efficacy.

for the control of vectors. This however involves prior entomological evaluation of the efficacy of the repellents and the repellency generated by innovative textiles already incorporated with repellents against vectors. Guidelines involving the testing of the efficacy of repellents has been laid down by the WHO (2009) but requirements for registration are still subject to national regulatory authorities of the particular country or territory in question.

In this study, the cage test method was used to determine the efficacy of four selected repellents impregnated on textiles. Results from this study has shown the validity of protocol The conventional impregnation and coating method in addition to an innovative technology based on prior modification of fabric using Limonene as insecticide has been reported (Hebeish, Moustafa, Fouda, Hamdy, EL-Sawy, Abdel-Mohdy 2008). The procedure for running repellents efficacy tests has been reported by a few other studies but based mostly on topically applied repellents (Barnard Donald Roy, Ulrich Bernier, Rui-De Xue and Mustapha Debboun 2007).

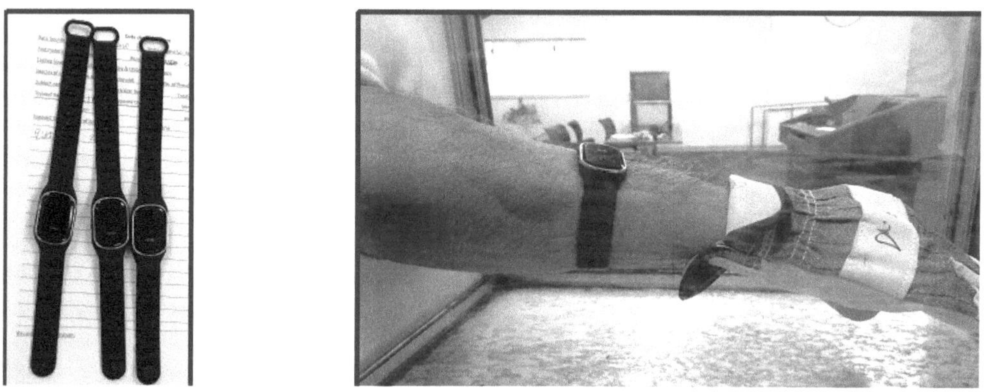

Figure 4.11: A similar watch device is worn in a cage and the protocol used to investigate the effectiveness the repellence.

This new innovative textile repellent strategy is a relatively new approach to vector control that has not been utilized extensively as it encourages the use of nano- and micro-particles in textile production for various purposes, and can be used to release chemicals like repellents and insecticides in a well-controlled rate; such that does not leave harmful residual effect in the environment. Previous studies in this capacity have been made. This includes the evaluation of the mathematical models of effectiveness of repellents where the probit plane model and exponential decay models were validated with original data from tests of DEET (N,N-diethyl-3-methylbenzamide) and ethyl hexanediol (2-ethyl-1,3-hexanediol) in the forearm against the yellow fever mosquito, Aedes aegypti (Rutledge LC, 1985). The spectrum of combinations of nano- or micro-particles, repellents, insecticides and types of textiles has not been extensively studied. Applications though not quite extensive, of repellent-impregnated textiles have been made.

Repellent-impregnated textiles will serve to protect human beings from the bite of insects. This has promises of some level of protection against vector borne diseases such as malaria, human African trypanosomiasis, leishmaniasis, lymphatic filariasis, Loa loa filariasis, onchocerciasis, dengue, yellow fever which pose serious public health problems in tropical regions, especially in Africa and Asia. In Asia, the impregnation of army uniform by repellents against *Aedes aegypti* has been reported (Banks et al. 2014 and Faulde, Michael & Uedelhoven, Waltraud 2006).

Outlook for the adoption of repellent-impregnated textiles or fabric for use in Africa is a promising one putting into consideration its tropical climate which favors the high diversity of developing vector-species complexes that have the potential to redistribute themselves across different regions leading to new disease patterns. Climate change and global warming increases average global temperatures thereby increasing the likelihood of many vector-borne diseases in new areas. This calls for the adoption of local botanical repellent productions across several regions and the collaboration of industries and private sector to develop and promote the use of repellent-impregnated textiles, this time not just for military uniform but also for extensive use especially across regions affected by vector borne diseases.

4.9 RESULTS

According to the protocol used for the evaluation, the number of landing on both treated and untreated textile examined within 3 minutes, were counted and recorded. All the operation was repeated after one hour unless the first bite is occurred within 3 minutes. From the beginning of each test, the test will be stopped as a first bite occurs. Two data were calculated. First, the "Protection Time", PT (the time from treated time to the first bite), and the "Percentage Protection", PP which is calculated using Mulla Formula (Reison, 2004; Talbalaghi, Ali, and Hassandoust, 2018). Thus, the raw data is transferred in the formula:

$$R = 100\frac{C-T}{C}.$$

where
C = number of landing counts in untreated group
T = number of landing counts in treated group

4.10 FUTURE PERSPECTIVE AND OUTLOOK

Analogous to the consolidated use of repellents to ward off mosquitoes, in sand fly control and as an extension, control of sandfly-transmitted infections in humans and animals alike, one of the effective control measures is through the use of repellents. This method is important because man is a dead-end host of a number of Leishmania species therefore treatment of existing cases may prove an abortive control measure as it generally does not affect the transmission cycle. In zoonotic visceral leishmaniasis, control of the infection and reduction in transmission is achieved through protecting animals from sandfly bites. This can be achieved through the use of insecticide impregnated collars and textiles used to create a physical barrier between the animal and the feeding sandfly. This form of interruption of transmission cycle by personal protection and creating physical barriers as with Leishmania is effective in vector control of different vector species eg ticks, mosquitoes, bed bugs. This is particularly important in humans and animals as multi-pathogen hosts because contact between the vector and the host is interrupted consequently leading to a disruption in pathogen transmission and hence, a reduction in VBD transmission, reducing overall disease burden.

Thanks to the technology of incorporating repellent materials in fabrics, ensuring that the repellent material is slow in release and long lasting; the fabric as well attains repellent quality. Textile technology may be promising with better repellence effect on the sand fly more than on mosquitoes (usually a topical repellent has more repellence effect on sand flies than with mosquitoes). It is necessary to run the test against sand fly in the fight against leishmaniasis (cutaneous CL and visceral VL) which affects thousands of persons and a properly evaluated and effective product may create a revolutionary approach to fight against this debilitating disease in many countries of the Middle East.

Middle Eastern countries are at greater risk from leishmaniasis because this region is endemic for cutaneous leishmaniasis and sees a great deal of human migration from other parts of the world. Countries with ample resources, like Saudi Arabia, have taken good measures to control the disease, evident by a gradual decline of cases reported in the past few years. Other countries, like Syria, Iran, and Iraq, should put an emphasis on health care facilities for the control of leishmaniasis. Also, a massive effort on reservoir and vector control along with actively pursuing diagnosis in endemic foci will be helpful.

Current and future technologies aimed at the development of botanical repellents are promising alternatives to the repellent formulations currently in the market. Odorizing receptors on the antennae of arthropods differ and are more sensitive in sand flies than in mosquitoes. The use of textiles impregnated with repellents as socks could be utilized to avoid attack by ticks. Similarly, with materials such as repellent infused textile bracelets,

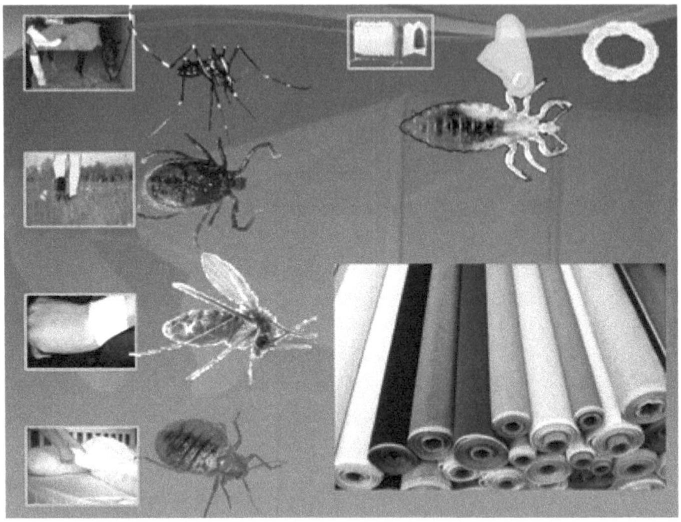

Figure 4.12: Textile treated with repellents.

sand flies and a host of other arthropods are prevented from biting a great percentage of the exposed part of the body. The usage of repellent bedsheets and pillow-cases reduces the colonization of bed bugs which are difficult to get rid of once the presence is established. Running of efficacy tests to measure entomological repellency and persistency is highly recommended. Measurement of textile repellent efficacy requires a standard cage test with a solid protocol to ensure that proper test results are obtained. From repellent treated textile, the approaches to ward off arthropods, vectors of disease is promising. (Figure 4.12).

4.11 CONCLUSION NOTE

The proven standard cage test method is the necessary step, for repellent textile efficacy approval and the determination of level of persistence (Figures:4.13 and 4.14).

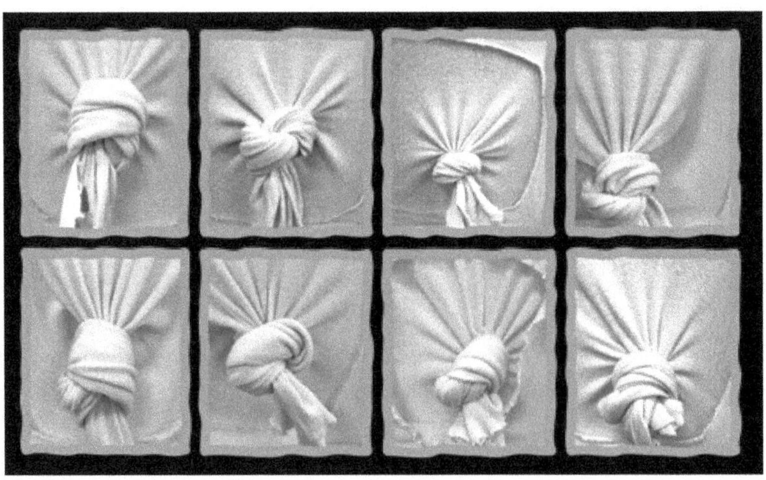

Figure 4.13: Standard cage tests.

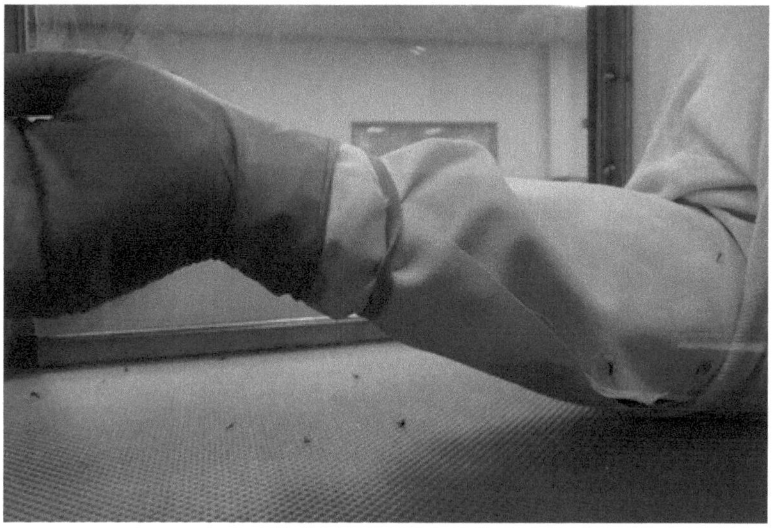

Figure 4.14: Repellent textile efficacy approval.

ACKNOWLEDGMENTS

This chapter is partly based on work performed within the framework of IMAAC (`https://imaac.eu/`) related to COST Action CA16227 (*Investigation & Mathematical Analysis of Avant-garde Disease Control via Mosquito Nano-Tech-Repellents*, `https://cost.eu/actions/CA16227/`), supported by COST Association (European Cooperation in Science and Technology). We would also like to thank Dr Mirjana Milijevic from University of Banja Luka, Bosnia and Herzegovina and Dr James R. Bozeman from American University of Malta (AUM), Malta for proofreading and translating parts of the documents into Latex.

CHAPTER 5

Biology, Surveillance and Control of Mosquito Vectors

Elton Rogozi*

Vectors' and Rodent's Control Unit (VRCU),
Control of Infectious Diseases Department (CIDD),
Institute of Public Health (IPH), Tirana, Albania
** corresponding author, e-mail: eltonrogozi@yahoo.com*

CONTENTS

5.1 Introduction on the mosquito biology 48
5.2 Biology of mosquitoes (*Culicidae*) 49
5.3 Life stages of mosquitoes 49
5.3.1 Eggs stage of mosquitoes 50
5.3.2 Larval stage of mosquitoes 51
5.3.3 Pupal stage of mosquitoes 51
5.3.4 Adults stage of mosquitoes 52
5.4 Mosquitoes concerns from the public health overview 53
5.5 Role of mosquitoes in disease transmission 54
5.6 Mosquitoes as vector of diseases 55
5.7 Vectorial capacity and competence of mosquitoes 55
5.8 Pathogens that can be transmitted by mosquitoes 55
5.8.1 Parasites 55
5.8.2 Viruses 56
5.8.3 Bacteria and other pathogens 56
5.9 Biting activity of mosquitoes 56
5.10 Mosquito as nuisance 57
5.11 Surveillance and entomological studies of mosquito vector 57
5.12 Mosquito surveillance and collection 58
5.12.1 Light traps 58
5.12.1.1 CDC light traps 59
5.12.2 Human landing catch (collection) 60
5.12.2.1 Resting catch 60
5.13 Other techniques used for mosquito collection 61
5.13.1 Adult sampling 61
5.13.2 Gravid Trap Box 62
5.13.3 The ovitraps 62
5.13.4 The Fay Prince trap 62
5.13.5 Precaution during human landing catch 63

DOI: 10.1201/9781003035992-5

5.14 Mosquito preservation, labeling and transportation 63
5.14.1 Preservation 63
5.14.2 Labeling 64
5.14.3 Mosquito identification 64
5.14.4 Dynamic and density of mosquito population 64
5.15 Data processing and field evaluation of mosquito bites via HLC method for testing repellent treated textiles 64
5.15.1 Calculation for the efficacy 64
5.16 Mosquito landing rates for the evaluation of repellent impregnated textiles efficacy! 65
5.16.1 Mosquito biting activity 65
5.16.2 Main objectives 65
5.16.3 Study site 66
5.16.4 Technique used to measure the mosquito landing bites rates 66
5.16.4.1 Results from Divjake study site 67
5.16.4.2 Results from Durres study site 68
5.16.4.3 Results from the Darzeze, Fier study site 69
5.17 Conclusion 70
5.18 Prospective for future study 71
5.18.1 The protocol used to test the repellent treated t-shirts 71

5.1 INTRODUCTION ON THE MOSQUITO BIOLOGY

Mosquitoes are important vectors for the transmission of infectious diseases in human and animals. Female mosquitoes after mating feed on human blood or warm-blooded animals for eggs development. They mate only once, and after the first batch of eggs, they seek for another warm blood animal or human to take another blood meal for the second batch of eggs development, and so on. But scientists have discovered mosquito species feeding even on reptiles' blood, even to the amphibians' blood like frogs and toads. Feeding on blood behavior is really important for the public health, as they serve as a bridge for liking the pathogen agents with humans or other animals. Knowing the attractiveness of mosquitoes from different traps augmented with dry ice or pheromones, with light and suction ventilation systems; provides data on the different mosquito species to study their host preferences, feeding behavior and their role as vector of pathogen agents like viruses, protozoan, bacteria and other parasites in human and higher animals. It is very important to know the whole life cycle of the mosquitoes, their bio-ecology, feeding behaviors, habitat preferences, ecological requirements, biting activity, reproduction, breeding seasons, number of generations, in order to draw a very good strategy for the control program.

Repellents are chemical substances which are extracted from different plants, and are used impregnated in textiles and treated bed nets or doors and windows screening to prevent mosquito bite and enter the house. Repellents are even used as sprays and creams or lotions to be applied in hand and bare body parts when resting in a place where adult mosquito are high and can bite human actively. Repellents are very good option in the strategy of mosquito control, they do not kill them, but just repel and prevent them to land in bare body parts.

The process of the impregnation of extracted repellent chemical substances by different plants like Citronella etc., is complicated and should have been taken by very professions chemists or chemical engineers. Knowing these important data of mosquitoes, their control can be more successful. Except optimal temperature and of many pond, pool or dams; humidity is one of the most important ecological factors for the survival of the mosquitoes. It is not just the humidity of the air that cause this successful life of mosquitoes, but the humidity conserved in the low grassy vegetation, tree holes, tree dense vegetation leafs, which can really be very good places where humidity can be sufficient for their growth in recreational parks near by the jungles, forests or even in the yards with dense vegetation and flower pots.

5.2 BIOLOGY OF MOSQUITOES (*CULICIDAE*)

Mosquitoes belonging to the phylum Arthropoda, class Insecta, subclass Pterygota, order Diptera and the suborder Nematocera. There are some 3500 species of mosquitoes belonging to 41 genera, all contained in the family Culicidae of which about 100 are vectors of human diseases. Control measures are generally directed against only one or a few of the most important species and can be aimed at the adults or the larvae. Culicidae family is divided into three subfamilies: Toxorhynchitinae, Anophelinae and Culicinae (Service 1993ab; Harbach & Kitching 1998).

Mosquitoes have a worldwide distribution (Knight and Stone 1977). They occur throughout the tropical and temperate regions and extend their range northwards into the Arctic Circle. The only area from which they are absent is Antarctica, and a few islands in pacific. They are found at elevations of $5500\,m$ and down mines at depths of $1250\ m$ below sea level (Harbach & Knight 1980, 1998). Mosquitoes are important vectors of several tropical diseases, including malaria, filariasis, and numerous viral diseases, such as dengue, Japanese encephalitis, Chikungunya, Zika and yellow fever. In countries with a temperate climate, they are more important as nuisance pests rather than as vectors (Service 1993, Harbach & Kitching 1998).

5.3 LIFE STAGES OF MOSQUITOES

The mosquito has four distinct stages: eggs, larvae, pupa, and adults (Figure 5.1). For more information please have a look at the given reference (Ferguson College website).

The adult is an active flying insect, while the larvae and pupae are aquatic and occur only in water. Depending on the species, eggs are laid either on the surface of water or are deposited on moist soil or other objects that will often be flooded (Service 1993). There are 4 instars of larvae, in each of them a molting event occur, where the growth of the larvae body is associated with the molting event. Depending on the species, a female lay between 30 and 300 eggs at a time. Many species lay their eggs directly on the surface of water,

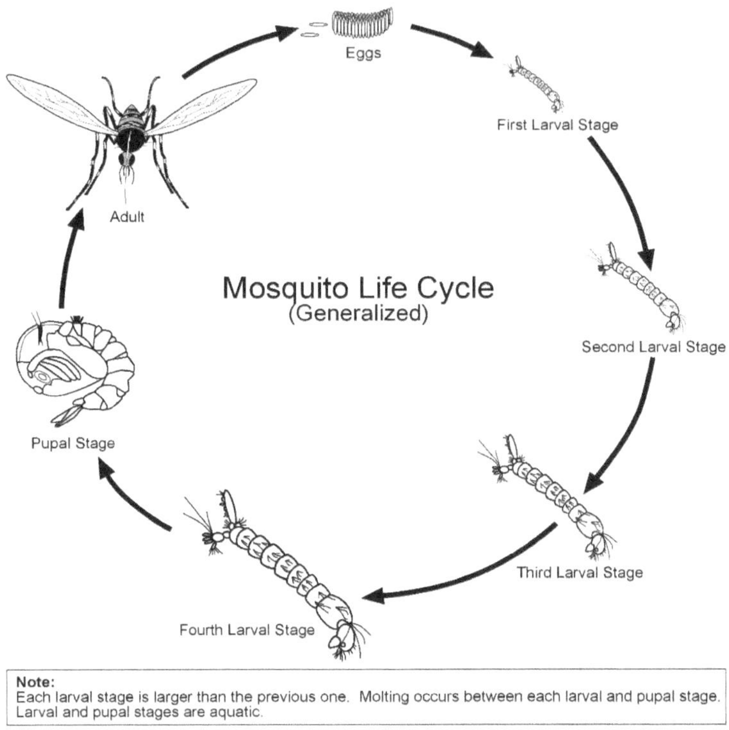

Figure 5.1: Schematic life cycle of mosquitoes (Source: *www.mosquitoes.org/LifeCycle.html*).

either singly (*Anopheles*) or stuck together in floating rafts (e.g., *Culex*). In the tropics, the eggs usually hatch within 2–3 days. Some species (e.g., *Aedes*) lay their eggs just above the water line or on wet mud; these eggs hatch only when flooded with water. If left dry they can remain viable for many weeks (Service 1993).

5.3.1 Eggs stage of mosquitoes

One factor common to all mosquito species is that eggs are laid in association with free water or on a moist surface. Eggs are white when first deposited, darkening to a black or dark brown within $12 - 24$ hours. Single eggs are about $1/50\,inch\,(0.5\,mm)$ long and those of most species appear similar when seen by the naked eye, one exception is the *Anopheles spp.* (Figure 5.2 a) whose eggs have floats attached to each side of the egg (Harbach & Kitching 2005). Eggs are laid singly by some species, such as *Aedes albopictus* (Figure 5.2 b) and others lay eggs together to form rafts such as *Culex* species (Figure 5.2 c). The incubation period (time between when eggs are laid and when they hatch) may vary considerably among species. Eggs of permanent-water mosquitoes where eggs are deposited on the water surface may hatch in $1 - 3$ days depending on temperature. Floodwater species deposit their eggs on moist soil or another wet substrate and have a wide variation in incubation periods. These eggs will not hatch until submerged by rising water caused by rainfall, melting snow in the spring, or other floodwater. Depending on the

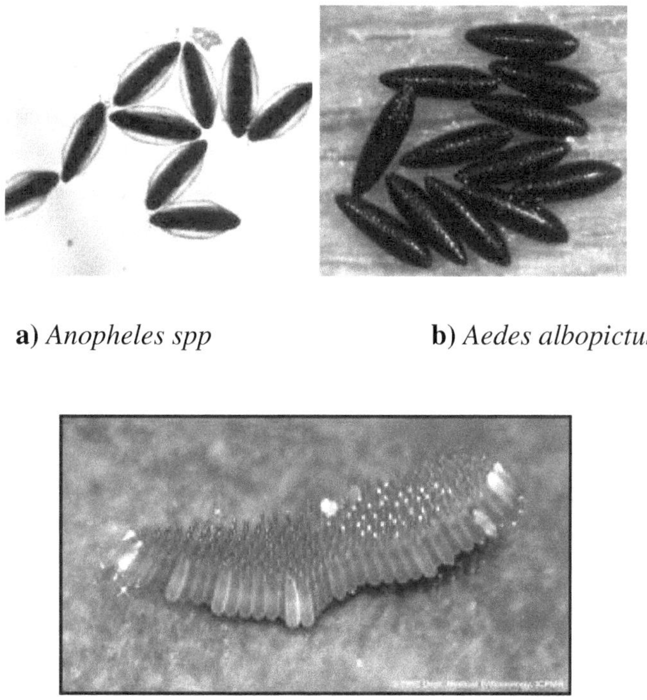

a) *Anopheles spp* **b)** *Aedes albopictus*

c) *Culex spp*

Figure 5.2: Eggs of a) *Anopheles*, b) *Aedes*, and c) *Culex* mosquitoes.

species and conditions, these eggs may hatch the next time they are flooded, as soon as ten days, or may not hatch until they are flooded one year or later (Harbach & Knight 1980, Jorge 2001).

5.3.2 Larval stage of mosquitoes

The larvae (wigglers or wrigglers) of all mosquitoes live in water and have four developmental periods or instars. These are called 1st, 2nd, 3rd, and 4th instars with each succeeding stage larger than the last. At the end of each instar, the larva sheds its skin by a process called molting. The larva is an active feeding stage. Larvae feed on particulate organic material in the water (Figure 5.3 and 5.4). The larvae of most species have breathing and must occasionally come to the surface of the water to get oxygen. The total length of time that larvae spend in the larval stage depends on the species and the water temperature. Some can develop in as little as 5 or 6 days. Upon maturity the 4th instar larvae molts into the pupal stage (`fmel.ifas.ufl.edu/key/anatomy/larval.shtml`, Harbach & Knight 1980, Jorge 2001).

5.3.3 Pupal stage of mosquitoes

Unlike most other insects, the mosquito pupa is very active, and, like the larva, lives in water. It differs greatly from the larva in shape and appearance. The pupa has a

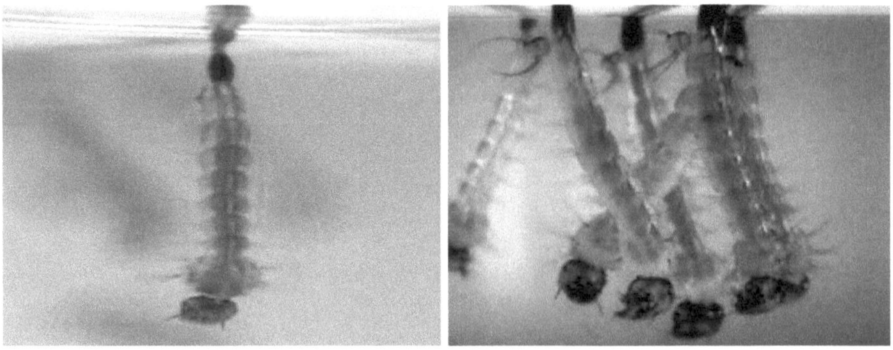

a) *Aedes albopictus* **b)** *Culex spp*

Figure 5.3: a. larvae of *Aedes albopictus* and b. of *Culex spp.*

comma-shaped body divisible into two distinct regions. The front region consists of the head and thorax (cephalothorax) and is greatly enlarged. It bears a pair of respiratory trumpets on the upper surface (Figure 5.4 a, 5.4 b). It must periodically come to the surface to get oxygen. The second region is the abdomen which has freely-movable segments with a pair of paddle-like appendages at the tip. Feeding does not take place during the pupal stage. The pupal stage only lasts for a few days and is the stage when all the larval tissues change into the adult tissues. The adult emerges directly from the pupal case on the surface of the water (`fmel.ifas.ufl.edu/key/anatomy/pupae.shtml`, Harbach & Knight 1980, Jorge 2001).

5.3.4 Adults stage of mosquitoes

The adult mosquito (Figure 5.5) is entirely terrestrial and is capable of flying long distances. Both females and males feed on nectars which they use for energy. Males and females mate during the first 3 to 5 days after they have emerged. Females mate only once. Males generally live for only a week. Only the females feed on blood, which is what is oc-

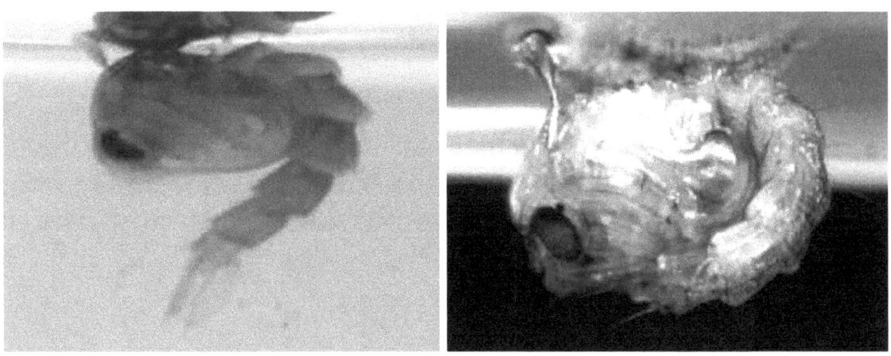

a) *Aedes albopictus* **b)** *Anopheles spp.*

Figure 5.4: Pupae of a. *Aedes albopictus* and b. *Anopheles spp.*

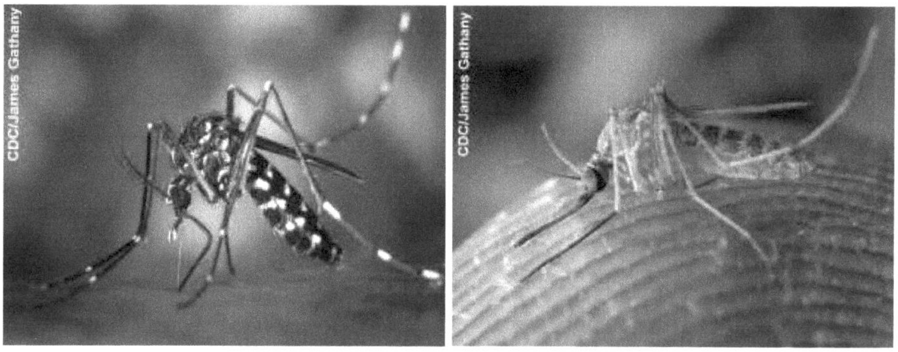

Figure 5.5: Adult of *Aedes albopictus* and *Culex pipiens*.

curring when they are biting. Females evidently gain little nourishment from blood meals but need them in order to develop eggs. Many mosquitoes feed on any warm-blooded bird or mammal. However, some prefer cold-blooded animals. Some species also prefer birds and seldom feed on mammals, which is the case with *Culex spp.*

Unfortunately, many species feed on a wide range of warm-blooded mammals and humans are often attacked. Once a female has completely engorged, it flies to a shaded environment until her eggs are completely developed, usually 3 to 5 days. Once the eggs are developed the female is called a gravid female and she begins to search for a desirable place to lay her eggs. If a female survives her egg laying activities, she will very soon start searching for another blood meal after which she will lay another batch of eggs. She does not need to mate a second time (Harbach & Knight 1980, Jorge 2001).

Generally, a female will only live long enough to lay 1 to 3 batches of eggs. Most of mosquito species are actively searching for a blood meal in the evening hours from just before dark until 2 to 3 hours after dark. During the daytime the females normally rest in cooler vegetated areas where the humidity is higher and they are protected from drying out. Females will often bite in the daytime if humans or animals invade the wooded areas where they are resting. However, *Aedes albopictus* is an aggressive biter which prefers to feed during the daylight hours and is often a nuisance in urban areas (`fmel.ifas.ufl.edu/key/anatomy/adult.shtml`, Harbach & Knight 1980, Jorge 2001).

5.4 MOSQUITOES CONCERNS FROM THE PUBLIC HEALTH OVERVIEW

Mosquito-borne diseases are not usually considered important problem for public health worldwide, but there should be awareness of their potential on vectorial capacity and competency to carry and transmit pathogen agents, which are the main cause if these infectious diseases in human. These diseases are dynamic and their potential, either in the resort, camping areas or their vicinity, can generate adverse publicity that often has a severe economic impact on recreational facilities (Newson 1977, Rohani 2008).

One of the most complaints from people tries to enjoy the outdoors activity, concern the annoyance caused by mosquito bite. In addition, recreational parks, forests close to the beach are located close to the major natural breeding sites of mosquitoes. Many people try to avoid rustic vacation areas with known mosquito problems and not realizing that these diseases are also transmitted in urban and suburban areas (Rohani 2008). In response to community concerns about the health and wellbeing of visitors to the recreational park, studies should be undertaken to consolidate and amplify information on distribution and abundance of mosquitoes in these areas (Newson 1977, Rohani 2008).

Mosquito-borne diseases are a real public health problem worldwide. There are many parasites, viruses, bacteria that can be transmitted by insects, and mosquitoes are the most predominant insects in the way of the transmission to the human beings. These pathogens can cause very severe diseases to humans with a high mortality rate.

The science that studies the mosquitoes and other insects of public health is called Medical Entomology. It provides basic concepts of entomology like the knowledge on morphology, taxonomy or systematic, bio-ecology, distribution, habitat preferences, that are good and important information for medical entomology to know the whole life cycle of mosquitoes in order to control their uncontrolled population growth. Identification, distribution, habitat preferences, bio-ecological data and the systematic or taxonomy of mosquitoes play an important role in order to control and prevent infectious diseases caused by them.

Seasonality and circadian rhythm of mosquito populations, as well as other ecological and behavioral features, are strongly influenced by climatic factors such as temperature, rainfall, humidity, wind, and duration of daylight (Reiter 2001). Both seasonal and daily activity patterns of mosquito vectors are required as baseline knowledge to understand the transmission dynamics of vector-borne pathogens (Reiter 2001), and have been widely studied for many mosquito species throughout the world (Guimarães et al. 2000 a,b).

5.5 ROLE OF MOSQUITOES IN DISEASE TRANSMISSION

Mosquitoes are included in the insects that live in human inhabited areas or near them. Living near humans is very important for their life and surviving. As human belonging to the warm-blooded animals, they can serve like possible host for mosquito females to take a blood meal before they lay eggs. They need the blood for the development of their eggs. The most preferable hosts for mosquitoes are the animals; bovine, cows, pigs, ships, goats, horses and birds too, man is not a principal mosquito's host, he can be accidentally a mosquito host, but for some mosquito species man can be an important host (Reiter 2001, RKPBV 1997, CDCP 2005).

The most important problems that mosquito can cause to human are listed here: annoyance, biting, toxicity, allergic reaction, invade of the host tissue, diseases caused by mosquitoes, contamination of food, fear from them, false parasitosis, toxins and poisons, protection of the host (Reiter 2001, RKPBV 1997, CDCP 2005).

5.6 MOSQUITOES AS VECTOR OF DISEASES

The most important pest and vector species belong to the genera *Anopheles*, *Culex*, *Aedes*, *Mansonia*, *Psorophora*, *Haemagogus*, *Sabethes*, *Anopheles* etc. species, as well as transmitting malaria, are vectors of filariasis (*Wuchereria bancrofti*, *Brugia malayi* and *Brugia timori*) and a few arboviruses. Certain *Culex* species transmit *Wuchereria bancrofti* and a variety of arboviruses. *Aedes* species are important vectors of yellow fever, dengue fever, encephalitis viruses, Zika and many other arboviruses, and in a few restricted areas they are also vectors of *Wuchereria bancrofti* and *Brugia malayi*.

Species in the very closely related genus *Aedes* also transmit filariasis and encephalitis viruses. *Mansonia* species transmit *Brugia malayi* and sometimes *Wuchereria bancrofti* and a few arboviruses (Reiter 2001, RKPBV 1997, CDCP 2005). *Haemagogus* and *Sabethes* mosquitoes are vectors of yellow fever and a few other arboviruses in Central and South America, while the genus *Psorophora* contains some troublesome pest species, as well as a few transmitting arboviruses. Many species, although not carriers of any disease, can nevertheless be troublesome because of the serious biting nuisances they cause (Reiter 2001, RKPBV 1997, CDCP 2005).

5.7 VECTORIAL CAPACITY AND COMPETENCE OF MOSQUITOES

Mosquito species have a high vectorial capacity and competence in transporting and pathogens' transmission to humans and other animals. They are the most predominant group of insects and arthropods that can serve as vector of many pathogen agents. Different pathogens can live and reproduce inside the vital organs of mosquitoes, as well as they can be fed there. High vectorial capacity of a mosquito means the opportunity that they have to carry, develop and serving like mechanical and infected transporter of different pathogens like viruses, bacteria, parasites etc. The life cycle of a pathogen agent can occur in two or more host and mosquitoes are the principal reservoirs and hosts (Reiter 2001, RKPBV 1997, CDCP 2005).

5.8 PATHOGENS THAT CAN BE TRANSMITTED BY MOSQUITOES

There are a tremendous number of different infectious and non-infectious diseases that can be transmitted by mosquitoes. These diseases can be classified in viral infectious diseases, parasites infectious diseases, bacterial infectious diseases and other infectious diseases caused by other pathogens agent. These diseases, some of them, have a very high mortality rate to humans.

5.8.1 Parasites

Parasites are worldwide, they can be carried by mosquitoes, can be fed and reproduced in the mosquito host vital organs, as well as they can be transmitted to other hosts causing severe diseases. Human is involved as host in these cycles, too. From parasites groups we can mention the group of filarial parasites, where the most predominant parasites species present are *Brugia malayi*, *Wurchereria bancrofti* and *Brugia pahangi* (Reiter

2001, RKPBV 1997, CDCP 2005). These parasites can cause filariasis in human if the mosquito is infected. When the infected mosquito is sucking blood in man the filarial worms can get out from the infected mosquito proboscis and can get in the wound or the small hole that the piercing-sucking mouthparts of mosquito proboscis has done until it was sucking a blood meal. The most important vector of filarial worm is the species of *Mansonia* genus (Reiter 2001, RKPBV 1997, CDCP 2005). Another very important parasite which can be transmitted by mosquitoes is malaria parasite. It is smaller than filarial worm and a very slender parasite. The most important vector of malaria is the species of *Anopheles* genus (Rohani 1999). These are a very severe infectious disease that can result in high mortality rate in humans.

5.8.2 Viruses

Viruses many viruses can be carried and transmitted by mosquitoes to human and other mammals and other animals. *Culex* is the most predominant species that serve as the main vector of Japanese Encephalitis. *Aedes* are the most predominant species that serve as the main vector of Chikungunia fever, dengue fever and dengue hemorrhagic fever, which are the most spread viruses in Malaysia (Reiter 2001, RKPBV 1997, CDCP 2005). These viruses can cause a very severe hemorrhagic fever disease. *Aedes aegypti* and *Aedes albopictus* are the most predominant vectors in Malaysia (Reiter 2001, CDCP 2005).

5.8.3 Bacteria and other pathogens

Bacteria and other pathogens there are a lot of different bacteria and other pathogen agent's species worldwide that can be carried, transported and transmitted by mosquitoes. In humans these bacteria can cause very severe infectious disease with a high mortality rate (Reiter 2001, CDCP 2005).

5.9 BITING ACTIVITY OF MOSQUITOES

Biting activity, the time and the frequency of biting activity depend on the mosquito species, environment conditions, ecological conditions and requirements. *Aedes* mosquito bites mainly in dusk hours 6 pm to 9 pm and in dawn between 6 and 8 am. *Culex* can bites from 9 pm to 11 pm and sometimes during the early hours of morning. *Anopheles* can bite after 11 pm, as well as the in early hours of the morning like 2 - 4 am (Reid 1968, Loong 1998). Other species of mosquitoes like *Mansonia*, *Amigeres* genera etc., have different biting time and frequency (Cheong et al. 1984, 1988). Biting activity and frequency depend on the gonotrophic cycle of mosquitoes.

After the first bite eggs can develop very fast and after 2, 3 or more days depending on the species, food, temperature, humidity (Cheong et al. 1988, Onyido et al. 2009). Eggs are laid in the water or water surface and then the mosquito can go to feed again for another blood meal. They mate just one time. The shorter the gonotrophic cycle, the shorter the eggs' developing time. The need for another blood meal is higher followed by high frequency of biting activity. Female mosquitoes feed on animals and humans.

Most species show a preference for certain animals or for humans (Cheong et al. 1988, Onyido et al. 2009). They are attracted by the body odors, carbon dioxide and heat emitted from the animal or person. Some species prefer biting at certain hours, for example at dusk and dawn or in the middle of the night. Feeding usually takes place during the night but daytime biting also occurs. Some species prefer to feed in forests, some outside of houses, and others indoors (Cheong et al. 1988, Onyido et al. 2009).

5.10 MOSQUITO AS NUISANCE

Mosquitoes can cause nuisance and fear to humans. Recreational and forest parks, and other recreational areas can be very good places where mosquitoes can breed and live. High humidity, hiding places in branches, dense leaves trees and the grassy vegetation can be very good places for protecting the mosquitoes from the sun light and high temperatures (Cheong et al. 1988, Onyido et al. 2009). Many kinds of swamps, streamlets, ponds, pools full of water can be very good places for development of the eggs, larvae and pupae mosquito's life cycle stages. All these optimal conditions in recreational areas are very favorable ecological condition for the development of the whole mosquito life cycle (Cheong et al. 1988, Onyido et al. 2009). Mosquitoes can be a very high nuisance to human in tourist recreational areas and parks. The mosquito biting activities can inflict the presence and the coming of the tourists in recreational areas. Except transmission of the pathogen agents, mosquitoes can cause parasitosis, false parasitosis, inflammation and the irritation of the human skin, allergies to sensitive people, toxins etc. (Cheong et al. 1988, Onyido et al. 2009).

5.11 SURVEILLANCE AND ENTOMOLOGICAL STUDIES OF MOSQUITO VECTOR

Mosquito surveillance should be a routine part of any mosquito program. A good surveillance program provides information on a list of local mosquitoes (including distribution and population size estimation), and effectiveness of the control strategies being used. Information on the epidemiology of insect-borne diseases is essential if the disease is to be controlled. Entomological, parasitological and clinical studies provide useful information on the characteristics of disease transmission in an area as well as the habits and habitats of the specific vector species.

Entomological studies have several important roles to play in vectors of diseases control, including the following (WHO 1992): i) identification of the vectors responsible for transmission of the disease; ii) provision of basic information on the habits and habitats of vector species for purposes of planning effective control measures; iii) monitoring the impact of control measures (for example, by determining changes in vector population density, rates of infection, susceptibility of vectors to insecticides, and residual effects of insecticides on treated surfaces) and iv) contributing to the investigation of problem areas where control measures prove unsuccessful.

Entomological studies must not only be carried out to provide a practical answer to clearly defined control-oriented research questions when data is unavailable or inadequate. Entomological studies are also important in the estimation the expected impact of the various control measures. This helps to decide whether some measures are more useful than others and whether some control measures are dangerous to implement (AFPM 2002).

5.12 MOSQUITO SURVEILLANCE AND COLLECTION

Collecting and evaluating information on adult mosquitoes is important for decision-making on deployment of appropriate control activities. The association between species of mosquitoes can provide clue to an understanding their biology and their role in the transmission of pathogen. Adult collections are most frequently conducted because adult mosquitoes are generally easier to survey, collect and identify, than the immature stages. A trapping device is the most common and the simplest tool for the collection of mosquitoes, mainly for its surveillance, vector relative density, abundance and its control (Cameron & Russell 2005). Collection of mosquitoes could be performed from 18:00 to 06:00 for the landing and the resting catch and the same period time for the CDC light traps baited with dry ice. The three main collections methods and other methods of mosquito collection use in other studies by other authors are shown in the pictures and paragraphs listed below:

- CDC-light traps baited/augmented with CO_2
- Human landing catch or bare lag catch and
- Resting catch

5.12.1 Light traps

Light traps are limited to gathering data on density and species composition of nocturnal adult mosquito species that are attracted to light. Some *Anopheles* and *Aedes* mosquitoes are poorly attracted to light; therefore, light traps are ineffective in collecting these species. Although light traps are generally not recommended for use in collecting these genera, some *Aedes* are strongly attracted to light traps (e.g., *Ae. vexans*, *Oc. sollicitans* and *Ae. taeniorhynchus*) (WHO 1975).

Because of these behavioral differences, other of adult mosquito collection methods (e.g., resting stations or landing counts) are needed to obtain a valid index of the total population. A variety of light trap types exist. Wide differences in capture efficiency have been noted between species due to differences in their reactions to light. Some species are caught in great numbers while others are rarely taken even though they may be plentiful in the vicinity (e.g., *Ae. aegypti* mosquitoes).

Therefore, to increase their effectiveness, various modifications have been added such as CO_2 or dry ice and other components of host odor. The established role of CO_2 as a mosquito attractant (Service 1993, Cameron & Russell 2005) makes it feasible to use as a standard in the sampling of mosquito population. Vythilingam et al. (1992) reported that light traps supplemented with CO_2 showed synergistic effect toward various species of mosquitoes.

5.12.1.1 CDC light traps

CDC light traps baited with CO_2 (dry ice). Traps can be set and fix in metallic stick as holder. Batteries were used for the functioning of the traps' light and ventilation system. Insects are attracted to the light during the night and from the smell of the CO_2 (dry ice), which imitates the exhaled CO_2 from animals, who is a very attractive smell for the mosquitoes. It has been well established that CDC trap without CO_2 is not attractive to mosquitoes (Oli et al. 2005). CDC traps augmented with CO_2 from dry ice is an efficient trap (Figure 5.6). However, since it is difficult to obtain dry ice in many remote areas in tropical countries, yeast generated CO_2 traps could be used since it is easily available and cheap (Oli et al. 2005).

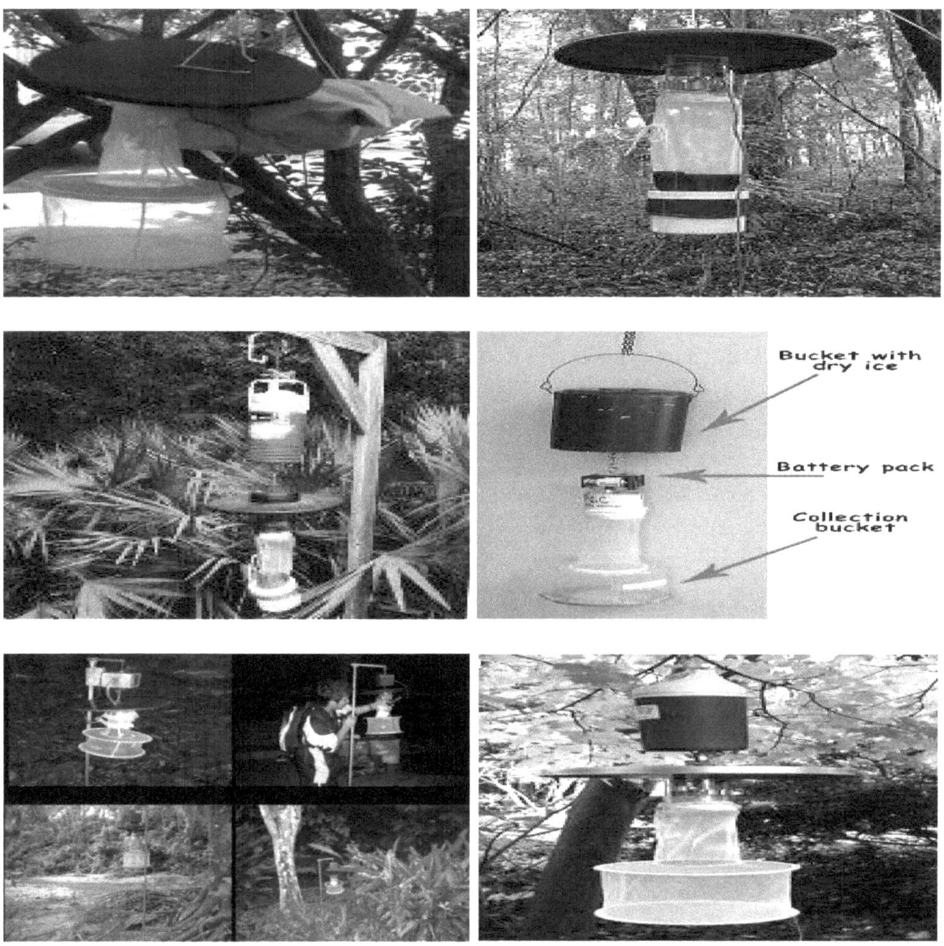

Figure 5.6: Different CDC light traps baited or not with CO_2.

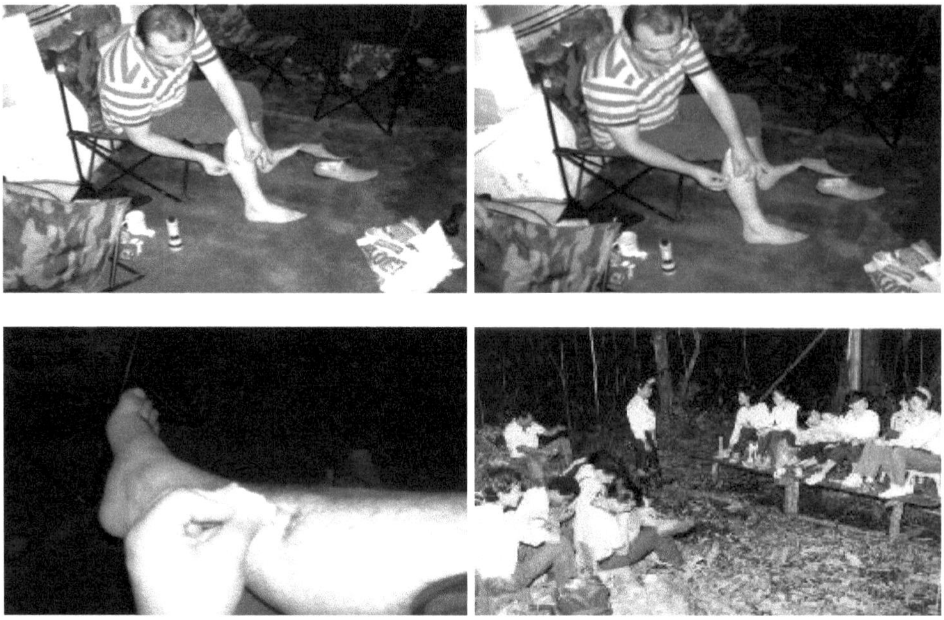

Figure 5.7: Human landing catch method, and mosquito catching into the vial.

5.12.2 Human landing catch (collection)

Landing counts on humans are useful for determining population densities of anthropophagic (human biting) mosquitoes that are not attracted to light traps and for rapid checks of mosquito populations (Figure 5.7). The use of this method is recommended when complaints or suspicions are not corroborating by light trap collections. This survey technique establishes an index or landing rate by counting the number of mosquitoes landing on the collector during a specific period of time. However, landing count surveillance is time intensive, inconvenient and difficult to standardize (WHO 1992). This technique may increase the exposure of survey personnel to disease. Therefore, during a mosquito-borne disease outbreak, survey personnel must use personal protective measures, such as wearing head nets and rolling down sleeves, but do not use repellents. All survey personnel should be on any chemoprophylaxis recommended in the area being sampled.

If a mosquito-borne disease is present for which no vaccine, chemoprophylaxis or treatment is available (e.g., many viral diseases), this sampling technique should not be used (WHO 2002). This method has to leave the legs or arms bare or undressed in order that female mosquitoes to approach to the human body alight to the leg or arm, but not allowing them to bite. Then a $50 \times 19\, mm$ glass vials could be used to catch them inside, after that a piece of cotton pad is used to plug in the vials. The HLC method could be used even by groups of people or volunteers in different habitats and recreational places for human.

5.12.2.1 Resting catch

Torch lights are used during the night to see and collect for the female and male mosquitoes (Figure 5.7). They can be hidden in the tree leafs, tree branches, tree holes,

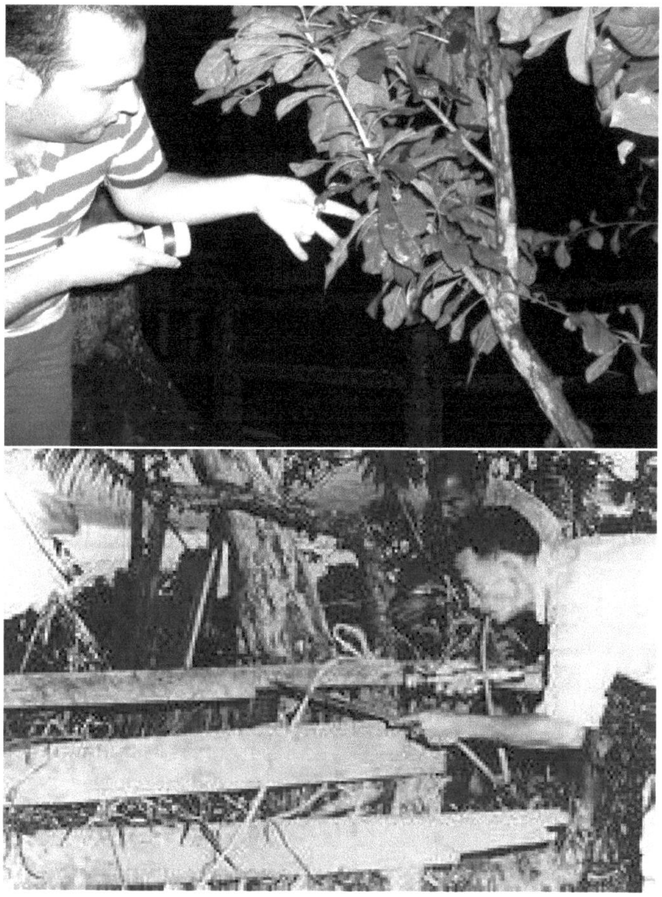

Figure 5.8: Resting catch or torch light mosquito collection method.

grassy vegetation, inside human dwellings on the wall, ceiling, rocky crevices and holes and other places where mosquitoes can be surely protected and hiding from nocturnal predators, from low temperatures etc. Then a mechanical aspirator or sucking tubes are used to suck them inside the tube, after that a $50 \times 19\, mm$ glass vials is used to catch them inside, after that a piece of cotton is used to plug in the vials. A 10 minute per hour time might be performed from 6 pm to 6 am to collect for female and male adult mosquitoes.

5.13 OTHER TECHNIQUES USED FOR MOSQUITO COLLECTION

5.13.1 Adult sampling

According to Eliningaya & Aneth 2009, the four sampling methods evaluated were operated in the same time. Human landing catch (HLC), odor-baited trap (OBET), pit shelters (PS) and indoor resting collection (IRC). IRC can be performed in the morning from 6:30 am to 8:30 am of every experimental day in cowshed and indoors using mechanical aspirator as described in entomological manual book (Eliningaya & Aneth 2009).

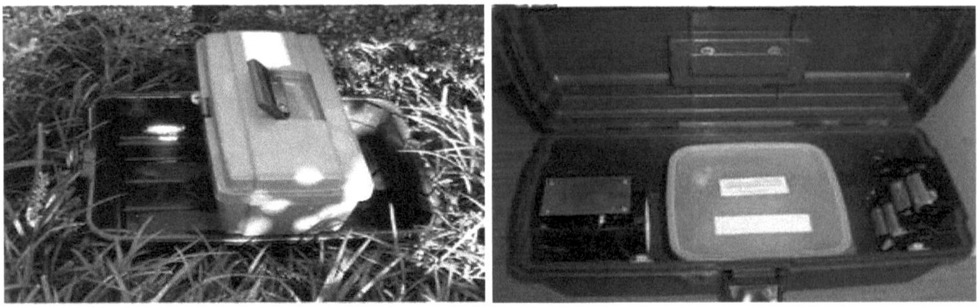

Figure 5.9: Gravid trap boxes used to collect adult mosquitoes.

Pit shelters can be sampled every morning from 7:00 am to 7:30 am, the pit dimensions were as described in entomology manual for collecting outdoor resting mosquito's density (Eliningaya & Aneth 2009). OBET, the trap is composed of a tent with either a man or cow whose odors are drawn to a cage trap by a fan via polythene tunnel. OBET dimensions were height 2 meters, length 2 meters and width 1.5 meters (Eliningaya & Aneth 2009). For HLC, the same man can expose his feet while using mechanical aspirator for collecting landing mosquitoes at each collection site, one collector worked from 6:00 p.m. to 6:00 am, mosquitoes were sorted by an hour interval. OBET used both man and cows: the mosquitoes seeking for hosts were collected in a protected chamber before reaching the host (Eliningaya & Aneth 2009).

5.13.2 Gravid Trap Box

This trap looks like a tool box sitting on top of a tray. The tray contains a mixture of fermented grass and straw which has a powerful smell (disagreeable to people) but attractive to mosquitoes. The tool box contains a collecting pod, and a small fan that is powered by four "D" cell batteries (Figure 5.9). When the mosquitoes are attracted to the water to lay eggs, they pass by the trap opening and are pulled into the collection pod. The mosquitoes are removed in the laboratory for examination and analysis. These traps are usually used when intending to collect *Culex* gravid female mosquitoes.

5.13.3 The ovitraps

The ovitraps are a small water-containing vessel that looks like a stadium cup with a surface inside it (such as a tongue depressor) for mosquitoes to lay their eggs on (Figure 5.10 a). The surface containing the eggs are collected and counted to determine the density of the reproductive mosquito population. These ovitraps will provide initial and ongoing data on mosquito populations. Ovitraps are mainly used to collect *Aedes albopictus* eggs.

5.13.4 The Fay Prince trap

The Fay Prince trap is a daytime trap that is used to collect the Asian tiger mosquito, *Aedes albopicuts*. These traps are suspended from low branches and trees and work much like a CDC miniature light trap except it uses contrasting black and white surfaces to attract

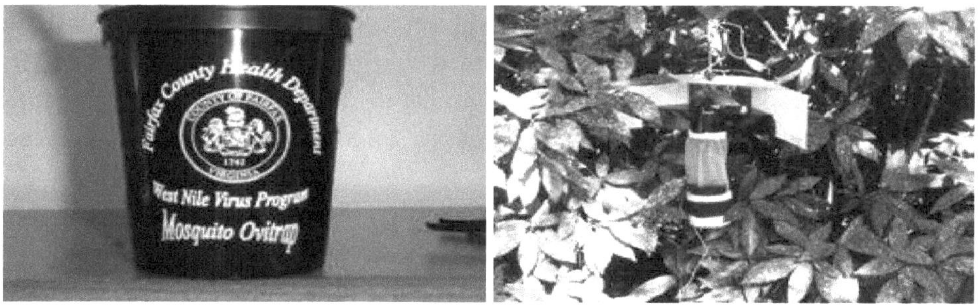

Figure 5.10: a) Ovitap used to collect mosquito eggs and b) CDC miniature light trap (Fay prince).

mosquitoes rather than a light bulb (Figure 5.10 b). The trap was designed for mosquito abatement operations and arbovirus survey purposes (Hock 2004). These traps are commonly suspended from tree limbs that hang above the ground and are powered by a battery. Traps attract mosquitoes by a light bulb and CO_2 that is emitted from the dry ice in a cooler. When the mosquitoes get close to the light they are pulled into the container by a small electric fan where they are captured for analysis (Hock 2004).

5.13.5 Precaution during human landing catch

During the human landing catch, there should be some awareness about the mosquito catching with this method and the time that the mosquito must be allowed to bite. As a possibility of the infectious from an infected mosquito, when it alight and bite to the leg, arm or body, the time that mosquito must be allowed to bite must be as shorter as possible. The mosquito must not be allowed to stay long to the biting site of our body, it must not be allowed to manage to bite or to bite and stick with its proboscis to our skin. As shorter the time the mosquito rest in our body, as lower the possibility for the mosquito to bite and the possibility of an infectious if the mosquito is infected with any kind of viruses or other pathogen agents. Persons whom apply this method should be very careful from the undetectable mosquito biting and the time that mosquito must stay in their arms, legs or body surface or skin during catching of them.

5.14 MOSQUITO PRESERVATION, LABELING AND TRANSPORTATION

5.14.1 Preservation

After the collection of the mosquito specimens with the HLC method described above, they should be put into small vials covered with a small cotton pad. At the bottom of each vial, a small piece of wet tissue should be placed, in order to keep the mosquito specimens alive during the preservation and the transportation to the lab. The wet piece of tissue can provide such humidity, as to keep the specimens alive until the lab. This is because the living specimens can be easily identified. Many of the bristles, hairs and bands can better be distinguished in the living specimen than in the dead one. This is the main reason why we have kept them alive during the time of the preservation and the transportation to the laboratory to proceed with further procedure and the identification purposes. When mosquitoes are collected with adults' traps, they should be kept in small container in thermobox with dried ice to preserve them before transporting to the lab.

5.14.2 Labeling

After the specimens have been put inside the vials (HLC collection) or inside small containers (adults' traps collection), every vial and small container should be labeled with the date, locality or station, collection method used, and time of capturing to better analyze them later.

5.14.3 Mosquito identification

The adults' or larvae mosquito specimens, should be transported to the lab, before identification procedure. The identification of every specimen of mosquito caught, should be carried out after every field trip using a stereomicroscope with light. Identification should be performed based on adults' or larva's characters using established taxonomic keys (Reid 1968, Schaffner et al. 2001).

5.14.4 Dynamic and density of mosquito population

Mosquito dynamic has to do with the 24 hours' activity and movement of the individuals of one population for food, water, shading, hiding places, breeding, laying eggs, taking of a blood meal for female mosquito etc. Mosquito density has to do with the number of mosquito individuals present and active in one area. The higher number of the individuals in one population in one area, the higher will the mosquito density be.

5.15 DATA PROCESSING AND FIELD EVALUATION OF MOSQUITO BITES VIA HLC METHOD AS A STANDARD TECHNIQUE FOR TESTING REPELLENT TREATED IMPREGNATED TEXTILES

5.15.1 Calculation for the efficacy

Bites/man/hour formula should be used to calculate the biting activity cycles of female adult mosquitoes. This formula gives in real time the exact number where a man can get bitten from adult mosquitoes in a specified time period of the day, in a specified site and mosquito habitat. This does not give the efficacy, but gives us a clear overview on the most anthropophilic mosquito species present, their biting activity cycle and their biting behavior. After getting these results, it is easier to test the treated textiles or t-shirts with a specific density and a specific or different repellent concentration on it, which will get tested wash after wash, to see even the number of wash that the treated textile can handle with still effective repellency feature.

Calculation for the efficacy tested on repellents impregnated textiles is performed by the formula of $R_{\%}$ below:

$$R_{\%} = \frac{C - T}{C} \times 100 \tag{5.1}$$

where

- C – is the average number of the total number of mosquitoes biting on the lower legs of the persons with the control treatment (untreated).
- T – is the total number of mosquitoes biting on the lower legs of the repellent-treated subject (treated).

5.16 MOSQUITO LANDING RATES FOR THE EVALUATION OF REPELLENT IMPREGNATED TEXTILES EFFICACY! A SIMPLE FIELD TRIAL DURING 2019 SEASON IN SOME REGIONS OF ALBANIA

5.16.1 Mosquito biting activity

The biting activity of mosquito depends on many factors. Biting activity, the time and the frequency of biting activity depend on the mosquito species, environmental and ecological conditions and requirements etc. It is mostly depending on the mosquito species; different mosquito species have different biting activity time. Sometimes the biting activity is depending on the weather conditions, too. Bad weather condition can directly influence in the timing of their biting activity for different mosquito species. Determination of the biting activity of one mosquito species is a very important data, because this determine the timing when mosquito species start to feed on blood. This will lead to nuisance for the human population living in certain areas or touristic and recreation ones, limiting their movement and activities. Furthermore, knowing of the biting activity of mosquito is very important for the program of mosquito control with insecticides. This program must be undertaken during the biting activity time of one certain mosquito species. In this way the control insecticides program would be more efficient.

5.16.2 Main objectives

The Objectives of this research trial was aiming the species composition and presence, biting activity of different mosquito species, evaluation on the human biting or landing rates, as well as to determine the best testing time of each mosquito species according their biting activity and gonotrophic cycles. At first, some criteria for the site collection, as well as some principal habitat composition related to human recreational and touristic areas were previously studied and described as follows: presence and density of human settlements, density of human/tourists in the respective site, distance from the urban/suburban/rural areas, history of mosquito presence in the past, mosquito collection and their data analyzing throughout the years (2006 - 2019 in Albania), and possibility of mosquito bite related to their habitat preferences and distribution in the country.

5.16.3 Study site

The data on the collected mosquitoes were set at the most appropriate sites from our long year's study on the adult and larvae mosquito collection from the Institute of Public Health Albania. Those data were collected from:

- **Lushnje:** Divjaka Beach and Resort, coastal area some of the characteristics of the habitat were the high and dense coniferous forest of pines, sandy ground composition, presence of recreational areas and settlements, high presence of larval breeding sites inside the forest (where human penetration is impossible), presence of nocturnal and diurnal mosquitoes.
- **Durres urban coastal area:** some of the characteristics of the habitat were high, dense and isolated deciduous forest, sandy ground composition, urban area with dense human settlements, presence of larval breeding sites inside the forest and human houses (manmade hole, basement), presence of nocturnal and diurnal mosquitoes.
- **Fier:** Darzeze Beach and Resort, coastal area some of the characteristics of the habitat were the high and dense coniferous forest of pines, sandy ground composition, presence of recreational areas and settlements, high presence of larval breeding sites inside the forest (where human penetration is impossible), presence of nocturnal and diurnal mosquitoes.

5.16.4 Technique used to measure the mosquito landing bites rates

The human landing catch counts the number of bites from female adult mosquitoes in human bared limbs in a specified period of time; generally, it is measured with the number of bites/men/hour. The picture 5.11 show the mosquito suction with mechanical aspirator. At the same site, other traps for adults' collection and eggs collection were used.

As mosquito collection is varied and different for species; this was done to compare the attractiveness, trappability and capturability of adults' mosquito related to methods used for their collection (Rogozi 2012ab). The other techniques of the adult, larvae, pupae and mosquito eggs collection were performed parallel in the same sites where the human landing catch collection method was tested. This was, to see a broad collection way in order to capture a broad range of mosquito species in the most appropriate sites. As well, the different collection techniques were used to see attractiveness of adult mosquitoes and to reveal the species most present with the most antropophilic behavior features (Rogozi 2012ab).

Several types of mosquito species do not feed on human blood, as they are better attracted by birds, the so-called the mosquito with ornitophilic behavior. Several other species take blood from animals, cattle, domestic animals etc. (Rogozi 2012ab). The ones that are of our study interests are only the antropophilic behavior. Mainly the widest spread mosquitoes in Albania are *Aedes caspius*, *Aedes albopictus* and *Culex pipiens*. But,as well, several other species, which are less abundant than the three above mentioned species, are the ones of the genera like *Uranotaenia*, *Culiseta*, *Anopheles*,*Coquillettidia* etc.

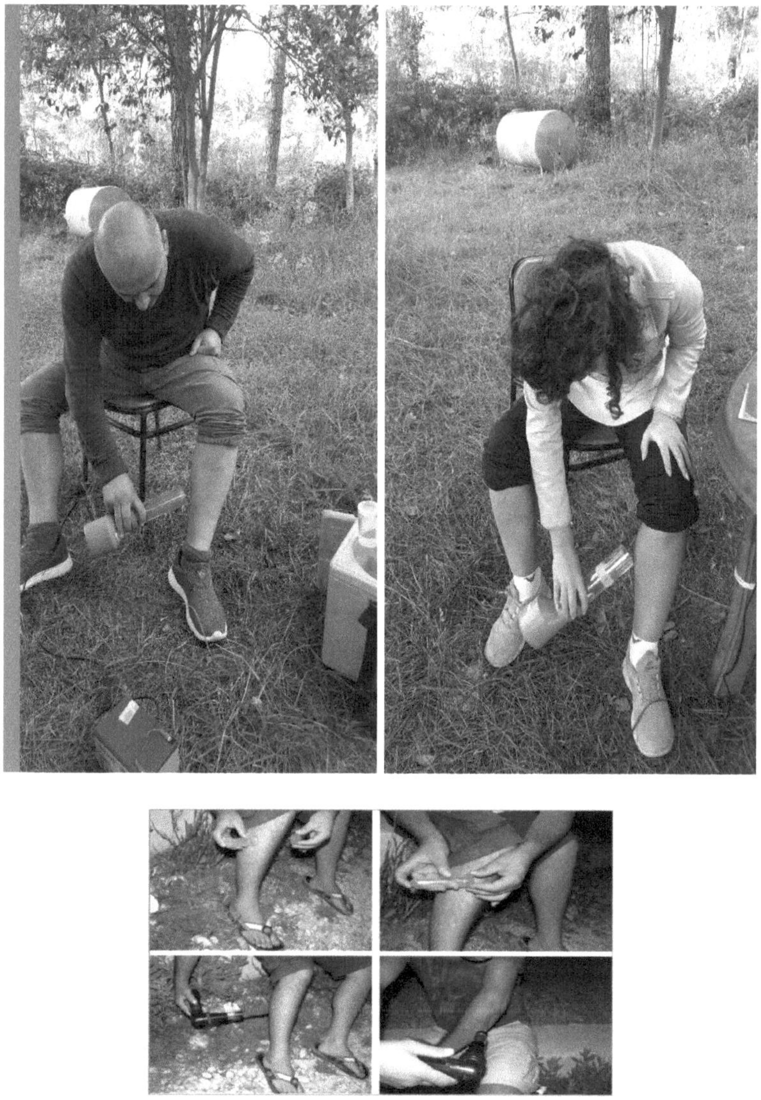

Figure 5.11: Mosquito suction with different battery aspirator, while putting them in small tubes/vials.

5.16.4.1 Results from Divjake study site

In total 488 adult mosquitoes were captured with HLC technique performed by the person-1. All these mosquitoes after identification belonged to *Aedes caspius* species. Out of them 113 adult mosquitoes were captured for a period of 30 minutes with the HLC technique, where only one person was used as bait during dawn in 10 minutes' intervals between 07:30 - 08:20 time. A number of 375 adult mosquitoes were captured during 50 minutes HLC by one bait person during dusk in 10 minutes' intervals between 17:30 - 19:15 time. In total 1565 adult mosquito were captured with CO_2 light traps during 14 hours from 17:00 - 07:00 in 17 - 18 October 2019, where 1558 belonged to *Aedes caspius*

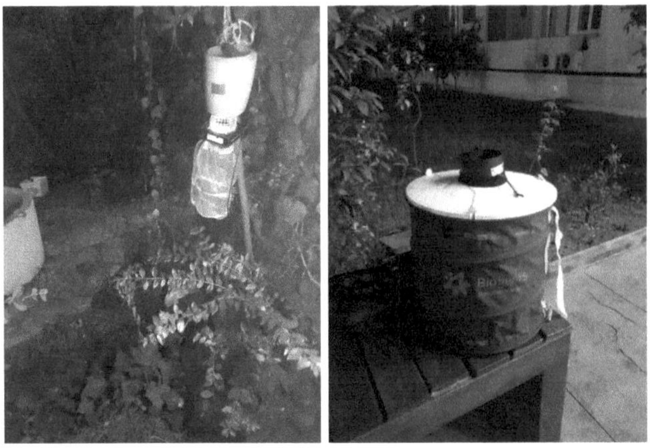

a) IMT light CO_2 traps b) BG-Sentinel CO_2 traps

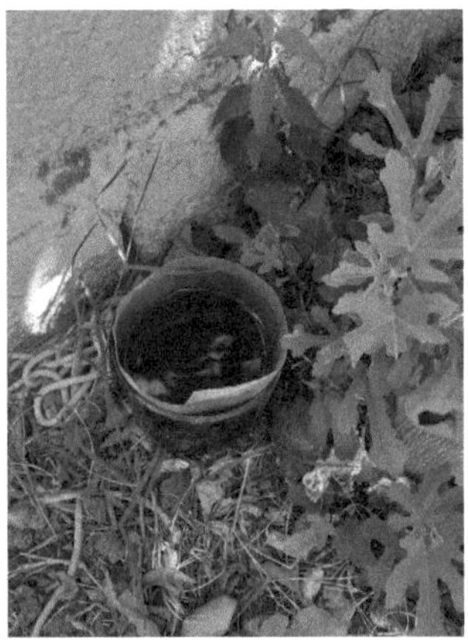

c) Ovitraps

Figure 5.12: IMT-CO_2, BG-Lure-CO_2 adult traps and ovitraps. Different traps for the monitoring of mosquitoes to compare with the adult mosquito captured with the HLC collection ones.

species and 7 individuals *Culex pipiens*. Most of adult mosquitoes captured with light trap technique belonged to *Aedes caspius*, all females and only one male specimen, where only 7 females belonged to the *Culex pipiens* species.

5.16.4.2 Results from Durres study site

In total 94 adult mosquitoes were captured with HLC technique performed by two persons (Person-1 and Person-2), where, 74 individuals belonging to *Aedes albopictus* species, 7 individuals *Aedes caspius*, and 13 individuals *Culex pipiens*. Adult mosquitoes were captured during a total timing of 110 minutes with HLC technique by two bait persons during dusk in a 10 minutes' intervals between 16:10 - 19:05 time. In total 13 adult mosquitoes were captured with CO_2 light traps duirng 3 hours from 16:00 - 19:00 in 24 October 2019,

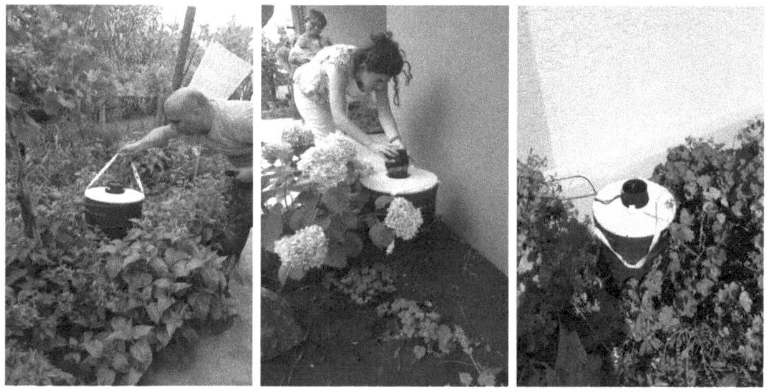

Figure 5.13: BG Sentinel traps set for adults of *Aedes albopictus* monitoring and presence to compare with the adult mosquito captured with the HLC collection technique.

respectively, 10 individuals *Culex pipiens*, 1 individual belonging to *Aedes albopictus*, and 2 individuals *Aedes caspius*.

5.16.4.3 Results from the Darzeze, Fier study site

In total 10 adult mosquitoes were captured with HLC technique performed by 1 person (Person-1). Adult mosquitoes were captured during a total timing of 20 minutes HLC by one bait person during dusk in two intervals of 10 minutes each between 16:30 - 16:50 in 20 October 2019 (heavy rain started): 8 individuals *Aedes caspius*, 1 individual belonged to *Aedes albopictus*, and 1 individual of *Aedes sp.* (specimen not identified, due to its damaged body parts). In total 7 adult mosquitoes were captured during 2 hours from 16:00 - 18:00 in 30 October 2019 with 2 IMT light CO_2 traps and 1 EVS CO_2 light trap. 5 individuals *Aedes caspius* and 2 individuals of *Aedes sp.* (specimen not identified, due to its damaged body parts).

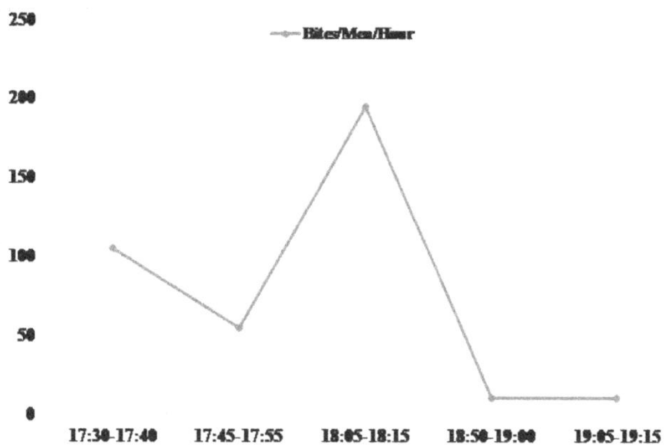

Figure 5.14: Biting activity of adult mosquitoes in Divjake on 17th October 2019 *Aedes caspius* – Bait: Person-1.

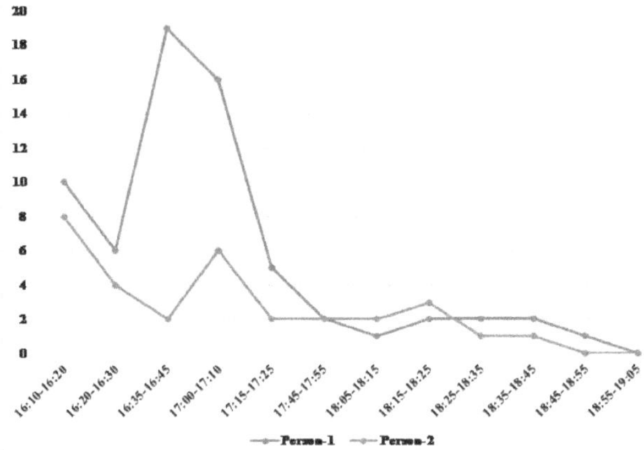

Figure 5.15: Biting activity of adult mosquitoes in Durres on 24th October 2019 *Aedes albopictus* and *Culex pipiens*- Bait Person-1 and Person-2

5.17 CONCLUSION

We concluded that the most present species in Divjaka and Darzeze (Fier) was *Aedes caspius*. The biting activity for *Aedes caspius* peaked 30 minutes before sunset and 30 minutes after sunset. Exactly 17:30 - 18:15 interval in 17 October 2019. Biting activity of this species was depended on the sunset time, not the exact timing. For example, in 17 October the peak was reached within 17:30 - 18:15, meanwhile earlier this date or during September the peak shifts in accordance with the sunset time.

We also concluded that *Aedes albopictus* was the most present species in Durres in 24 October 2019 from 16:10 to 18:30. The biting activity for *Aedes albopictus* peaked at dusk and right after the sunset while getting fully dark, they stopped biting. *Culex pipiens* was another species, biting activity peaked after the biting time of *Aedes albopictus*. The biting time was overlapped for both species after sunset.

In Divjake and Darzeze (Fier), the testing time could be performed within 1 hour; 30 minutes before sunset and 30 minutes after sunset. *Aedes caspius*, is the mosquito species, where the test would be performed. *Aedes caspius* is a very aggressive biter in the areas of Divjaka and Darzeze (Fier).

The testing of textiles efficacy should be performed within the timing of a certain mosquito species biting activity. In Durres region, the testing time could be performed within 1-2 hours before the sunset if the test would be performed against *Aedes albopictus* species. Testing time could be performed within early dark and 1 hour after sunset, if the test would be performed against *Culex pipiens* species. Repellent impregnated textile test efficacy in Albania in the areas of Divjake and Darzeze (Fier) would have to consider *Aedes caspius* species. The efficacy test in Durres would have to consider it against on both *Aedes albopictus* and *Culex pipiens* species.

The HLC would be better performed in more urban areas related to altitudes, vicinity from sea, marsh lands and lagoons. To have a better efficacy test of repellent treated textiles, the HLC would be better performed throughout the night and the day, to see the diurnal and nocturnal biting activity of mosquito species in a specified are. This could provide better data for the test efficacy, knowing the most nuisance species and the time they bite more aggressively.

5.18 PROSPECTIVE FOR FUTURE STUDY

During the future summer seasons, aiming would be to perform the test of treated t-shirt or other treated textiles. We agreed to test the treated t-shirts with two concentrations of repellent, but, more different repellent concentrations would be tried. The treated t-shirts efficacy tests in Albania, would be performed in the same sites where the evaluation of the mosquito landing bites and their biting activity was done before. A group of 3 - 4 people (depending on the availability going to the field) will participate to this study.

We think to try and test the t-shirts in three different regions starting from the Southern part of the country in the coastal areas, close to the border with Greece, following with the central part of along the coast, as follows (subject to change more or less in accordance with the possibility for field trips:

- The first study site could be Butrinti National Park, an isolated forest of different oaky dense forest, where species like *Aedes caspius*, less the Asian tiger mosquito *Aedes albopictus*, and rarely several other mosquito species of the *Culiseta*, other *Aedes*, *Culex* and other mosquito genera.
- The second study site could be set at the pine forest of Divjaka (Lushnje) beach, a site with a sandy ground composition and a dense forest of pine with dense herbaceous and shrubby vegetation, which is an optimal habitat for the mosquito *Aedes caspius* in Albania.
- The third study site could be set at the poplar forest of the Villas areas in the urban city of Durres along the coast and the beach zone with a sandy ground composition and a dense forest of poplar with dense herbaceous and shrubby vegetation, which is an optimal habitat for the mosquito *Culex pipiens* and *Aedes albopictus* in Albania.

5.18.1 The protocol used to test the repellent treated t-shirts

The protocol for testing the repellent treated t-shirts, is still developing and we aim to finalize it before starting the test in the field. Anyway, we aim to use three or four people, where one of them will wear an untreated t-shirt without repellent to use it as the control to compare it with the bites with the two or three other people. The people will stay $10-15m$ far from each other wearing the specific t-shirts for each, and start count their bites in the same interval of 10 minutes. Each of the persons involved in the study will wear a long-sleeved t-shirt and will cover all the other bared parts of the body like hands, legs, face and head, to prevent the mosquito to bite them and to avoid a possible mosquito landing interference with the treated parts.

Each of the people will have a mechanical aspirator equipped with a big tube and a fully charged battery to work properly during the collection of the mosquitoes that land in the t-shirt. This procedure will be realized exactly in the same 10 minutes' time for all the persons involved in the study. If there would be two different concentration of repellent in the t-shirts, we will test them in 10 minutes' interval for each of them, independently. After all the collection period of 10 minutes, all the tubes would be coded with the name of the location, date, time, name of the person, t-shirt code, repellent concentration 1 and 2, without wash, after wash nr. 1, wash nr. 2, wash nr. 3, wash nr. 4; and if the repellency efficacy will still be effective after the 4th wash, we will still continue to wash them and test them till no repellent effect will be observed. We will mark the t-shirts with the code or name of each person, in order that the same shirt to be used from the same person during all the period of the study.

Mosquitoes collected and labels tubes would be later identified in the Laboratory of Medical Entomology up to species level, and noted at the total data recorded. The data about the repellent and the impregnation procedure will be provided from the person in charge for this procedure. The detailed data of this will be later noted and provided during the field study and at the end of the research for a complete data set of it. The textile of the t-shirts would be sent to the Textiles Department in the Polytechnic University of Tirana for all probable and needed performance and measurements features before starting the test in the field. As well, washing procedure will be realized in the Textiles Department in the Polytechnic University of Tirana. The data will be collected and noted in excel sheet to be later analyzed and find the efficacy of the repellent treated textiles or t-shirts.

ACKNOWLEDGMENTS

This short field trial was kindly supported by the Institute of Public Health Albania in the frame of the National Program of the Mosquito Control in the Urban and Coastal Areas of the Country. This chapter is partly based on work performed within the framework of IMAAC (`https://imaac.eu/`) related to COST Action CA16227 (*Investigation & Mathematical Analysis of Avant-garde Disease Control via Mosquito Nano-Tech-Repellents*, `https://cost.eu/actions/CA16227/`), supported by COST Association (European Cooperation in Science and Technology).

II

Mathematical Modelling of Immunity: An Overview based on Malaria

CHAPTER 6

Models of Acquired Immunity to Malaria: A Review

Miracle Amadi*
LUT School of Engineering Science,
Lappeenranta University of Technology,
Lappeenranta, Finland
** corresponding author, e-mail: miracle.amadi@lut.fi*

Gerry Killeen
AXA Research Chair in Applied Pathogen Ecology
at the Environmental Research Institute and School of Biological,
Earth & Environmental Sciences,
University College Cork, Cork, Ireland

Heikki Haario
LUT School of Engineering Science,
Lappeenranta University of Technology,
Lappeenranta, Finland

CONTENTS

6.1 Introduction 76
6.2 Complex factors of acquired immunity and their modeling approaches 79
6.2.1 Misleading binary view on malaria immunity 80
6.2.2 Functional immunity/clinical immunity 84
6.2.3 Unfounded assumptions about what protective efficacy of immunity constitutes 85
6.2.3.1 Transmission-blocking immunity (TBI) 85
6.2.3.2 Increase in recovery rate/Decrease in infection duration 86
6.2.4 Age and acquired immunity 87
6.2.5 Duration of acquired immunity to malaria 90
6.2.6 Malaria parasite variants 92
6.2.7 Acquired variant-specific and variant-transcending immunity 94
6.2.8 Superinfection/ Reinfection and acquired immunity 96
6.2.9 Other factors influencing the acquisition of immunity 97
6.2.9.1 Effect of intervention measures on immunity acquisition and malaria prevalence 97

DOI: 10.1201/9781003035992-6

6.2.9.2 Climatic driving effect on immunity acquisition 98
6.2.9.3 Effect of population dynamics on immunity acquisition 99
6.2.10 Summary of modelling approaches 100
6.3 Discussion 102
6.A Methods for literature search 107
6.A.1 Literature search strategy and selection criteria 107
6.A.2 Outcome of literature search 107
6.B Detailed model descriptions 109

6.1 INTRODUCTION

Malaria is a considerable health threat to almost half of the world's population, especially in sub-Saharan Africa [29]. According to WHO, the number of reported malaria cases has not significantly changed from approximately 216 million cases in the periods 2015 to 2017. However, the global burden has significantly reduced over the last decade as malaria mortality rates have globally declined by 60% since 2000 [2]. In 2017, malaria-related deaths were estimated to be about 435 000 of which over 90% of the estimated deaths occurred in Africa [1]. The burden posed by malaria is greater in Africa because the majority of infections in Africa are caused by *Plasmodium falciparum*, the most dangerous of the known human malaria parasites. Again, the most effective malaria vector *Anopheles gambiae* is the most widely spread in Africa [29]. The groups most vulnerable to this pandemic are usually children below the age of five and pregnant women [132], [129], which is far less true today because the effect of NAI has waned in older age groups. The socio-economic impact of malaria is so high that it measurably contributes to poverty and underdevelopment on national scales [207], [208].

A protozoan parasite, called Plasmodium, is the pathogen responsible for causing malaria. However, *P. falciparum*, *Plasmodium vivax*, *Plasmodium malariae*, *Plasmodium ovale* and *Plasmodium knowlesi* are the five species of Plasmodium known to cause malaria in humans. Each of these species are subject to genetic polymorphism resulting to multitude of variants which differ widely in virulence, response to treatment and tendency to relapse, which is equally dependent on the interactions with individual hosts [88], [89]. The predominant cause of human infection in Africa is *P. falciparum*. It accounts for both 80 percent of all recorded malaria cases and 90% of malaria related deaths in Africa [8]. *P. vivax*, is the second most significant species and is prevalent in Southeast Asia and Latin America [9], [137]. Infectious female mosquitoes of the genus Anopheles are responsible for malaria transmission between humans.

The complete life cycle of malaria parasites involves two hosts: humans and the vector (female Anopheles mosquitoes). The sexual cycle takes place in mosquito after it ingests the parasites (gametocytes) from a malaria-infected person during blood feeding which it needs to nurture its eggs. The parasites reproduce sexually, and then develop inside the mosquito gut, where they undergo meiosis and afterwards, migrate via the midgut wall

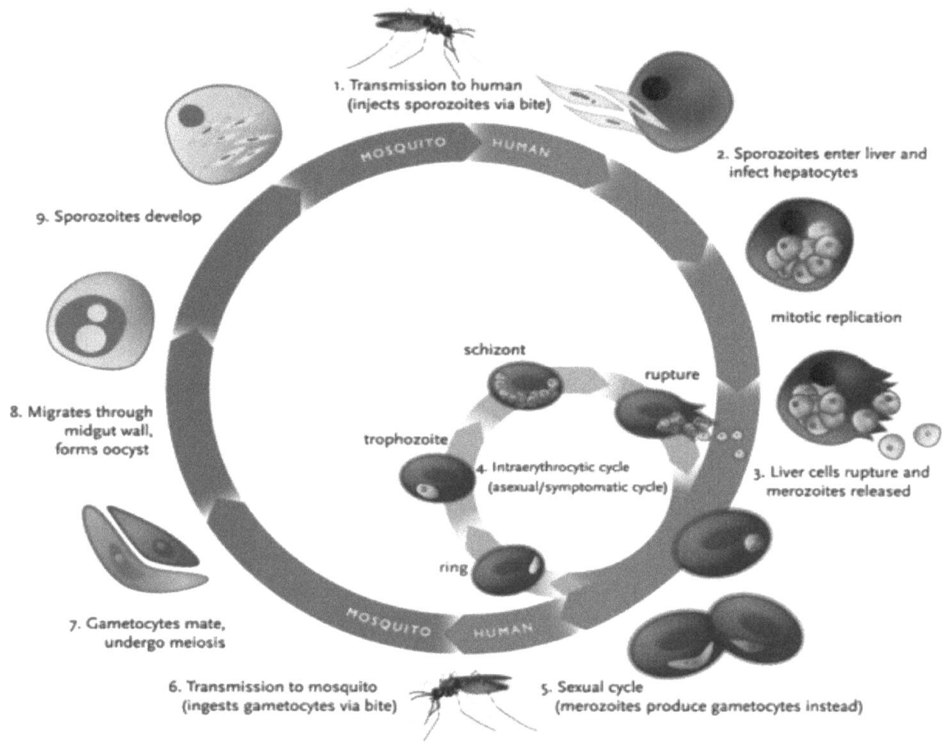

Figure 6.1: Malaria life cycle [107].

of the mosquito to form an oocyst, within which thousands of sporozoites develop. The sporozoites are moved to the salivary glands of the mosquito. Upon biting the human, the sporozoite-stage parasites contained in their salivary gland are injected into the human bloodstream from where they are transferred to the liver cells. At this stage, each sporozoite multiplies inside a hepatocyte and develops into thousands of schizonts, which rupture and give birth to merozoites that are thereafter released into the blood stream. The release of merozoites into the blood initiates the erythrocyte stages, (often referred to as asexual blood stages) where they invade and replicate within red blood cells (RBCs) causing the infected person to experience malaria symptoms. On the other hand, some of the asexual blood parasites (merozoites) can develop into gametocytes which mosquito ingests upon biting, resulting into parasite transmission to the mosquito; and the cycle continues. Thus, asexual parasites are responsible for illness, whereas gametocytes are responsible for transmission from human to vector [25] (see Figure 6.1 for more visual details).

Naturally acquired immunity usually occur when an individual is exposed to a live pathogen which as a result, brings about the creation of antibodies by the immune system [216]. According to [36], upon recovery from reinfection, there is usually rapid boosting of antibody responses to various antigens, as an indicator of the presence of memory B cells. It can take some days or weeks for the adaptive immune response generated against the pathogen to develop but may be long-lasting, or even lifelong. For example, infection with chickenpox or measles infection and subsequent recovery, gives rise to a natural active immune response usually leading to lifelong protection. However, this is not same for some diseases such as Malaria, which requires continuous exposures to sustain it's protective efficacy that is not lifelong [34]. The duration for which an individual is protected can vary markedly depending on the pathogen and antigens involved. Thus, individuals get reinfected to certain diseases either because the pathogen mutated and our immune system no longer recognizes it, which is believed to be the case with malaria.

Plasmodium parasites have developed mechanisms to down-regulate protective immune responses against ongoing and subsequent infections [20], [195]. The parasites undergo an essential expansion phase in the liver prior to the erythrocytic infections. Again, Plasmodium parasites have high level of antigenic diversity which is believed to be maintained by both gene conversion and recombination events that give rise to multitudes of variants in humans. This mechanism helps them to overcome recognition of existing antigens and makes it difficult to achieve lifelong immunity to malaria [34]. Moreso, NAI to malaria in humans comprises two stages: liver-stage and blood-stage immunity. Thus, antigenic functions are split between liver- and blood-stage parasites [197].

These mechanisms and more, discussed in the later part of this review, form the major reasons why efforts made to provide a foolproof commercial malaria vaccine have proven to be elusive [20],[21], [23], [22],[33]. Moreover, many anti-malaria drugs are becoming inefficient as a result of evolving drug resistance mechanisms by some malaria parasites [5], [25]. Universal coverage with insecticide-treated nets (ITNs) and indoor residual insecticidal sprays are currently the front-line preventive measures undertaken in malaria endemic areas [3], [4], [13]. This is because the principal malaria vectors primarily feed indoors at night when people are asleep. However, NAI (Table 6.1) to the parasite can help to limit the health burden posed by malaria in older previously-exposed individuals [34], [37]. Although the mechanisms behind this have not been fully explored, there exist some general consensus view.

This work aims at reviewing the state of research on NAI so as to have a comprehensive understanding of its underlying mechanisms and how modelling has contributed to the consensus view of NAI. By so doing, more efficient ways of studying the consequences of immunity in a given population can be suggested. Also, it will inform the research on malaria vaccine, since one of the difficulties of producing a malaria vaccine lie on the insufficient knowledge of the mechanisms behind NAI to malaria [23], [24], [101]. This is detailed in the following research questions/objectives:

- RQ1: What are the current perceptions about NAI to malaria; what is true, misleading, or yet unclear?
- RQ2: How can the modeling approaches currently used to study the impact of NAI in a population and their possible deficiencies be constructively assessed?
- RQ3: What are the opportunities for further improvement of models of immunity to malaria infection?

In the rest of the chapter, we will explain how understanding and modelling approaches have evolved together. Moreso, we will discuss how separate, parallel developments with agent-based models (ABMs) of human and mosquito populations, and populations of parasites within individual human hosts, addressed previously unresolved inconsistencies between models and empirical knowledge. We close by explaining how these modeling approaches were merged to provide the kinds of advanced, quite realistic models we rely on today, especially those included in the OpenMalaria ensemble. The materials for the discussion of the review were found by a systematic literature search and through expert knowledge (see Appendix 6.A for more details).

6.2 COMPLEX FACTORS OF ACQUIRED IMMUNITY AND THEIR MODELING APPROACHES

Various kinds of NAI against plasmodium parasites in humans have been defined: anti-disease immunity, anti-parasite immunity, and premunition (see Table 6.1). Thus, protection is defined as objective evidence of a lower risk of clinical diseases resulting from lower densities of parasitemia. Moreso, NAI to malaria in humans comprises two stages: liver-stage and blood-stage immunity (see Figure 6.1). The pre-erythrocytic (liver-stage) immunity can be responsible for lowering the probability of developing a blood-stage infection upon receiving a bite from an infected mosquito, implying that it can lower the proportion of infected bites that lead to blood-stage infection. This it does by reducing the number of infected liver cells that successfully mature to release merozoites and initiate the blood-stage infection. The liver-stage immunity can provide a window of opportunity to ultimately abort infection [136], [135]. This is because parasites are relatively few in number and confined within a single organ during liver stage development, while blood stage parasites develop in billions and spread allover the body. Upon initiating the blood stage infection, parasites grow at a rate dependent on how many merozoites successfully invade new RBCs, and this increase in parasitemia is considered as the *parasite multiplication rate* (PMR) [6]. Thus, the blood-stage immunity is responsible for reducing the probability of a mosquito contacting infection upon biting an infectious human, by lowering the number of merozoites that develop into gametocytes [34], [136], [160]. With constant exposure, the blood-stage immunity which is expressed by reduction in PMR, can suppress infection by either limiting the parasites from attaining a density sufficient to produce more than a slight clinical attack or constituting a greater delay until infection is detected [6], [159]. Thus, the most efficient role of the immune response is the ability to impede the growth of parasites in erythrocytes [78]. Hence, it is evident that antigenic functions are split between liver- and blood-stage parasites [197].

Acquired immunity to malaria is thought to be influenced by many complex factors such as climate, use of intervention measures, population (both host and vector) variation, parasite diversity, age and intensity of exposure. It is also believed to constitute some aspects of protections in humans which can wane after sometime, if not duly sustained . All of these concepts have been perceived in different ways by different researchers, some of which are either correct, questionable, or yet unclear. These complex factors associated to NAI to malaria have been included "in parts" in malaria models in somewhat different ways. Some modellers have made some artificial assumptions for simplicity. Thus, this review seeks to reevaluate these perceptions about NAI to malaria.

Table 6.1: **Glossary of definitions for commonly-used special terms**

Innate immunity	Inborn protective mechanisms which are the first line of defense against infection. It is not dependent on any previous infection [11], [199].
Adaptive or naturally acquired immunity (NAI)	Immunity that is gained through exposure [11], [199]. It constitutes anti-disease immunity, anti-parasite immunity and premunition, all of which develop in parallel, reducing the probability of experiencing symptomatic malaria upon each subsequent infection.
Clinical or anti-disease immunity	Immune responses that reduce the frequency and severity of clinical disease [200], [11], [211].
Anti-parasite or parasitological immunity	Immunity, that is responsible for parasite clearance from the body [200], [211].
Premunition	A functional immunity that reduces the frequency and severity of clinical disease but does not necessarily eliminate infections but rather allows them to remain at low density [212]. This is usually seen in endemic areas and comprises age dependent and haplotype-independent effects on parasite densities, which reflect the strength of maturity of the immune system [35], [170] and gradual acquisition with exposure [168], [169].
Pre-erythrocytic (erythrocytic) immunity	Immunity against liver-stage (blood-stage) malaria parasites; also known as liver-stage (blood-stage) immunity [34].
Asymptomatic	A case of no obvious symptoms in an individual who is a carrier of a disease[202]. Regarded as a misnomer due to the significant health and societal consequences of chronic infections which in reality are associated with considerable non-acute burden with mild symptoms [117].
Sterile immunity	Immunity that completely suppresses an innoculum of a pathogen [201]. This can be thought of as the highest attainable peak of acquired immunity which is probably never achieved. Non-sterile immunity results in persistence of the pathogen, but no symptoms of disease.
Parasitemia	Characterizes the density of parasites within a host [38]. Lower parasite density tends to confer milder symptoms but could be dangerous if not detected and treated, since it adds the number of new cases occurring within a period of time (incidence), and can become very symptomatic later [15]
Superinfection	The imposition of a second infection on a first before it has died out [88], [165]

6.2.1 Misleading binary view on malaria immunity

The early compartmental models are simplistic and oriented towards understanding how to eradicate the disease, using the transmission threshold criterion, R_0 (see Table 6.2) with little or no detail on the immune mechanism. The use of mathematical modeling in the study of malaria originated from the seminal works of Ross [95] well over a century ago. His work suggests that reducing the mosquito population to below a certain threshold can engender successful malaria eradication. The Ross Macdonald model [96] simply

Table 6.2: **Glossary of some epidemiological terms**

Basic reproduction number (R_0)	The number of secondary cases of disease that could arise from a single infected individual in a totally susceptible population, over the full duration of that infection [203].
Vectorial capacity	The number of potentially infectious inoculation of another human from a single infected human, through the vector population, per unit time [204].
Prevalence	The proportion of people affected by a disease at a point in time [217].
Force of infection	Per capita rate of acquiring new blood-stage infection per unit time[205].
Entomological innoculation rate (EIR)	The number of infectious bites sustained by an individual over a defined time period [66], [210]. It is the preeminent measure for assessing malaria endemicity and transmission intensity.
Heterologous (homologous)	Having different(same) evolutionary origin [88], [30].
Backward bifurcation	A condition where a stable endemic equilibrium coincides with a stable disease-free equilibrium when the associated reproduction number is less than one. Its epidemiological consequence is that the conventional prerequisite of the reproduction number being less than one becomes only necessary, but not sufficient, for disease elimination [206].
Holoendemic	Perennial intense transmission with protective clinical immunity among adults. It is the highest level of endemicity in which the strongest level of acquired immunity is attained. Classically, holoendemic malaria is associated with the following thresholds for epidemiological indications in the human population: spleen-rate of over 75% in children 2–9 years of age, and low spleen-rate of less than 25% in adults [209].
Mesoendemic	Variable transmission that fluctuates with changes in one or many local conditions, such as weather. It features spleen-rate of 11–50% in children 2–9 years of age [209].

captures the basic features of the interaction between the fractions of infected human and mosquito population. Macdonald attempted the subject of immunity to malaria, but he did not succeed in modelling it. Again, his model is of course highly simplified since it does not distinguish between the various infected classes of human and mosquito hosts in order to account for the different stages of the parasite development [97].

A new deterministic malaria transmission model was developed by Dietz [40] some years after Macdonald's death, in which humans can gain temporary immunity. The model has only one class "immune negatives" for the immune individuals, and at the same time it assumed that they have no parasites in their body. It also failed to account for the loss of immunity and stochastic phenomena that are particularly necessary when transmission is significantly reduced. As a result, it obviously can not apply well in low endemic areas, as demonstrated simplistically in [44]. Many other mathematical models [49], [48], [46], [62] have also made it appear that immunity is simulated as a simple binary variable, where a single class exist for the immunes. However, in reality, protective immunity to malaria is achieved in a progressive manner. At the initial stages of exposure, anti-disease immunity (Table 6.1) is acquired for protection against death or severe clinical diseases, then with more exposure to the disease at adolescent and early adulthood, immunity fights against even milder clinical attacks. Then at mid adulthood especially in endemic areas, immunity gives a stronger and wider range of protection against all circulating parasite variants [39], [68], [36], [69], although sterile immunity (Table 6.1) is probably never achieved [133], [165]. Furthermore, the mere distinction between immune and non immune is not consistent with the knowledge that immunity acquisition is a dynamic process driven by transmission intensity and the genetic complexity of circulating parasites (see Section 6.2.6). Thus, some models have considered immunity as a sequence with different levels of protection, so as to evaluate the role of repeated exposure on malaria transmission dynamics in a population [68],[40],[50], [94], [52].

The human population was classified in [103] into five different classes: susceptible to infection S_1, exposed E, infected symptomatic and infectious I_1, infected asymptomatic and infectious I_2, recovered but could be potentially infectious to mosquitoes S_2. The model by Yang [50] comprises seven human compartments where the immune class is split into three categories: immune, partially immune and non-immune but with immunologic memory. Niger and Gumel [94] also developed a deterministic malaria model which incorporates three stages of immunity. The human population comprises seven mutually exclusive sub-populations: susceptible humans $S_H(t)$, first-time infected humans $I_1(t)$, first-time recovered humans $R_1(t)$, second-time infected humans $I_2(t)$, second-time recovered humans $R_2(t)$, third-time infected humans $I_3(t)$ and third-time recovered humans $R_3(t)$. It is assumed that individuals in the R_3 class have the highest possible acquired immunity from exposure, which would be long-lived. Numerical simulations illustrate that infectious individuals with their first infection transmit the disease at a higher rate as compared to those with their second or third infections. These models demonstrated the impact of immunity boosting on delaying the entrance of a previously infected human to the susceptible class. They also extend some earlier malaria modelling studies by including multiple infected and recovered human classes in an attempt to account for the effect of repeated exposure to infection. However, it is should be taken as just an illustrative model since for instance in [94], more repeated exposure is needed to gain immunity that can last as long as was assumed for those in the R_3 class in reality. Furthermore, dividing into immune and partially immune [50] is not enough to explain the progressive pattern of immunity, but allowing some relevant change in immune function with the age of the host would be a better alternative [52], [118].

In order to validate immunological markers of protection, Filipe et al. [52] developed an age-structured malaria transmission compartmental model which combines epidemiological and immunological processes. In their SEI model for the humans, there are three classes for infected humans : infection with severe disease, asymptomatic patent infection, and infection with undetectable parasite density. Based on the model, NAI can function in three complementary ways: reducing the likelihood of clinical disease, accelerating the clearance of parasite, i.e, recovery from asymptomatic to undetectable infection, and improving tolerance to sub-patent infections i.e. controlling malaria parasitaemia at low density and slower clearance of such infection. The results of their model show that the first two mechanisms together account for the patterns of malaria by age group which match with observed data in the African settings, whereas the latter was not needed to explain the observed data. This model also suggests that immunity to symptomatic disease grows faster with higher levels of infection in the population, can last for at least five years, and increases with age-associated cumulative exposure. On the other hand, anti-parasite immunity (which results in more rapid recovery from symptomatic or asymptomatic infections to undetectable infections) develops later in life and can last for 20 years or more. Based on the model, this aspect of immunity appears to better portray the pattern of parasite prevalence and clinical disease by age than being exposure-dependent. By implicitly incorporating immunity functions, this model provides a framework to study time frames over which clinical and parasitological immunity are likely to develop and dwindle, and also the role of exposure and age on these functions. The concept of treating immunity as a function of many parameters is different from the approach used by most deterministic models which consider immune individuals as a separate class without considering the role of immunity in disease progression.

An advanced way employed by some modelers is to model immunity as a function of individual exposure history, where immunity memory can either grow by adding an exposure value or decay by a factor with each iteration, based on whether or not an individual got an infection [76], [109], [72], [102], [37]. These models represent immunity by a single effector variable which regulates the course of the disease; such that infection scenarios are different with respect to immune status accumulated over time. However there is no such thing as completely immune and completely suceptible individual as some models would assume [109], [110], [37]. In [109] for instance, Immunity ranged from 0 defined as "no immunity" to 1 defined as "full immunity". The ABM simulations of acquired immunity in [37] show a strange spiraling behavior as time increases, which might have resulted from the oversimplified assumption about NAI wherein an individual is classified as either completely immune or completely susceptible to infection, which is not biologically reasonable [68], [36].

The classification of humans into discrete categories or just adding a value to immune memory does not reveal the fact that malaria parasite populations can exist at varied densities within the human hosts [30], [43], [126], [127], [128], [146], [160]. Thus, these models give simplistic or no descriptions of the interaction between the population biology of malaria and immune responses. However, immunity to malaria in an endemic area is evident via both lower prevalence of detectable parasitemia with age and lower rates of disease [36], [92]. Moreover, the density of asexual parasites is clearly associated with disease risk, so diminished parasite counts as a result of immunity, obviously contribute to reduced disease burden [34], [76], [78]. Aron [181] demonstrated how the underestimation of the prevalence among older age groups, can also confound the statistics of prevalence, rates of infection and apparent recovery. This suggests that an more realistic model will have to follow a more detailed description in which the clinical symptoms and the immune response are dependent on the density of parasite in an individual host rather than grouping people into discrete classes of infected and uninfected hosts. Thus, immunity indicators should depend on the quantitative facets of infection, rather than on binary factors (i.e either present or absent).

Elderkin et al. [146] and Aron [43] have attempted to model malaria parasite densities in response to immunity acquisition in their so called density model. The interaction between immunity and infection is modeled by assuming that immunity increases at a rate proportional to the density of asexual parasitemia, and in the absence of parasitemia, immunity decreases. The density model did not capture the potential of reduced transmission to increase malaria prevalence in older age groups [43]] as was earlier demonstrated in [44] (see Appendix 6.B). Also, these models present a collective behavior of a group, thus, specific individual characteristics such as disease history, can not be tracked unlike in more recent models [159], [76] [56], [205], [114], [115], [160], [161], [113]. A more recent and detailed approach is seen in the OpenMalaria models where clinical symptoms and immune response are functions of parasite density in an individual host [159],[76], [214],[115], [134], [160], [114]. In those studies, empirical descriptions of within-host asexual parasite densities are embedded in the model for infection process, enabling the stochastic predictions of parasite densities as a function of age of infection. Moreso, the effect of immunity to asexual blood stages was modelled by considering how the distribution of parasite densities is modified in the semi-immune host [76]. They also analyzed the relationship between asexual parasite densities and infectivity to the vector to derive a model for the transmission to the vector [160], [114], which most models neglect.

6.2.2 Functional immunity/clinical immunity

The compartmental deterministic models mostly focus on illustrating how prevalence and parasite densities dwindle with age at a given level of force of infection [43], [44]. Thus, they can only show that immunity develops after several years but are not efficient to explain categorically how individuals mount a certain level of protective immunity after each infection episode. The reason is mainly because most compartmental models address only a single undifferentiated form of immunity [44], [62], [50], [48], [46]. However, various types of NAI against plasmodia such as clinical immunity, anti-parasite immunity (see Table 6.1) has been defined [31], [30], [32], [43]. For instance the model in [52] suggests that anti-disease immunity grows faster with higher levels of infection and anti-parasite immunity (which induces more rapid recovery from symptomatic or asymptomatic infections to undetectable infections) develops later in life. Moreso, some studies have shown that immunity to severe malaria can be acquired after one or two episodes [98]. It has again been observed that a single prior infection can induce detectable clinical immunity (Table 6.1) [31],[30]. This is based on the malaria therapy reinnoculation data examined by Molineaux et al. [30]. The study reveals that a second homologous (Table 6.2) inoculation brings about a lower first local maximum density, which is now accepted to be probably the most important effect of NAI to malaria. As a consequence, out of the 38 patients who experienced fever after the first inoculation, only 31 had it after the second inoculation (see also [126], [127], [128]). This is a particular instance of how individuals can be protected from homologous variants. It does not nullify the fact that a complete protective immunity can take several more episodes to achieve a sufficiently diverse repertoire of antigenic memory which can take considerable number of years to effect depending on the transmission intensity [159], [205], [100], [63], [52], [34].

Considering that protective immunity against blood-stage infection is achieved in a progressive manner and is never complete, a person might be free from clinical diseases without complete loss of infection, thus posing a barrier to total disease eradication [206], [95], [117], [150], [114], [160], [163], [130], [53]. Such chronic, sub-acute infections are characteristics of the widely used misnomer, "asymptomatic" malaria infections which have been recognized to result from partial immunity [117], [193] (see Table 6.1). In the theoretical sense, from the point of view of deterministic modelling approach, the humans in the so-called "recovered compartment" are still partially immune and can be infectious (see [40], [57], [160]). Thus, such compartmental models of malaria transmission with partial immunity to reinfection have noticed a phenomena called backward bifurcation(see Table 6.2), such that two steady states exists for a given value of R_0, [93], [94], [151]. This is what Smith et al. [154] referred to as the sticky situation (see the diagrammatic illustration in [154]). The numerical simulations reveal that increasing the rate of partial protection of recovered individuals engenders increase in the region of backward bifurcation. Thus, the prevalence of malaria in African countries and the evasiveness of complete control was linked to people with partially acquired immunity [16]. Such people do not visit the hospital either due to being asymptomatic or having uncomplicated clinical manifestations. This situation needs to be considered in planning for intervention measures.

From the view point of premunition (see Table 6.1), sterile immunity is never achieved. Thus, a more realistic modelling would entail a proper measure of infectivity in relation to the host disease and state, and also linking the infectivity of human to that of mosquito infection [102], [114]. Given that most deterministic models, especially those that considered immunity and infectiousness as being binary, could not include this concept in their models, some other deterministic compartmental models have done a related study in this regard [103], [52]. For instance, the human population in [103] was classified into five different classes: susceptible to infection S_1, exposed E, infected symptomatic and infectious I_1, infected asymptomatic and infectious I_2, recovered but could be potentially infectious to mosquitoes S_2. Although these models are advanced as compared to the binary models, in practice infectivity is not a collective characteristics of a group but varies with individuals, based on their parasite densities. As such, it requires an individual-based model which can study the relationship between asexual parasite densities and infectivity to mosquito [160], [114].

6.2.3 Unfounded assumptions about what protective efficacy of immunity constitutes

6.2.3.1 Transmission-blocking immunity (TBI)

Most models of malaria transmission assume that complete TBI can be acquired after repeated exposure or with age [63], [40].This does not seem to be right because of the following reasons. First, the concept that gametocyte mortality increases with host-age or with exposure is poorly understood. The epidemiological data in the Garki project [63] showed that the prevalence of gametocytes in areas of high transmission decreases more rapidly with age as compared to asexual parasites. This was viewed to directly result from increasing immunity against the pool of asexual parasites, leaving fewer to survive to produce gametocytes [185], [182], [183]. The question on whether NAI lowers survival of circulating gametocytes was considered by Diebner et al. [32] in a model comparison paper. The fits to the data on individual courses of parasitemia improved upon changing a constant mortality rate of gametocyte to one which grows with time. However, better fits were obtained when gametocyte mortality was allowed to grow with its age. This is in accordance with the concept of allowing gametocyte density to decline by natural mortality [146], [43]. This amounts to the fact that immunity is geared mainly against the asexual blood stages. In this line, some models implicitly predict infectiousness as a function of blood-stage parasite densities without invoking any acquisition of TBI [192], [114], [160].

On the other hand, children have usually been thought to mostly contribute to transmission of parasites to vectors due to their higher parasite densities [157]. Nevertheless, studies that have examined the contributions of different ages of human hosts to the infectious reservoir have found that adults also make a significant contribution (see [175], [114], [184]). The reason could probably be because: first, the body size of adults exposes them more frequently to mosquito bites [205]. Second, parasite densities decrease with age and exposure as a result of immunity in a somewhat exponential manner (i.e it never gets sterile) which can still allow infections to persist without symptoms. These reasons suggest why onward transmission to mosquitoes is plausible in adults. Boundi et. al. [174] studied TBI in relation to age, gametocyte density and transmission intensity. It was found that there was no relationship between TBI indicators and age, but a trend of increasing values as gametocytaemia increases was noticed, and regarded as a confusing factor. This seem to confirm the assumption that TBI does not apparently increase with age, and that adaptive immune responses to gametocytes are not of epidemiologic significance. These conclusions however, are based on insufficient evidence.

6.2.3.2 Increase in recovery rate/Decrease in infection duration

Most models considered increase in recovery rate as an indicator of immunity (see [122], [41], [189], [40], [72], [63]), [43], [44]. Based on Macdonald's report in [143] immunity is generally assumed to be proportional to the duration of infection, which results to a formula in which the basic reproductive number is proportional to infection duration. The model by Dietz [40] for instance, comprises two classes of humans with low and high recovery rates, which is associated with low and high immunity levels. The concept that NAI increases the rates of termination of infections in humans has been the subject of extensive debate. Acquired immunity is markedly known to increase with age, thus, infection duration may be expected to decrease as immunity rises. Again, it was expected that the decrease in parasite densities resulting from the acquisition of immunity, would lead to a decrease in detectability with age, which would also bring about an increase in recovery rate. Bekessy et. al. [41] in their catalytic model applied to microscopy data, observed that for the first 4 months of life, the durations of infection were very short, and much longer in older infants 1 - 4 years, after-which the recovery rate increased by a factor of more than 10 in older individuals. The study suggested that the fall in recovery rate in those aged 1 - 4 years could be either because of loss of maternal immunity or because of superinfection and that the subsequent rise in recovery rate in older people is due to increasing immunity (see also [189]).

On the other hand, Smith et al. [188] found in their study that the average multiplicity of infections increases at the same time as children acquire immunity. This was interpreted to be mainly because the average duration of infection increases even though children are becoming more immune (see also [191], [193]). The suggested reason is that lower parasite densities reduce the effective variant introduction rate, thereby slowing parasite and immune dynamics. Slower switching rate exhausts variants at a slower pace, prolonging infection duration until further slowing fails to subdue adaptive immunity (see [192]). They also argued that the short durations of infection in adults estimated by microscopy data [41], [189] could be due to diminished sensitivity of microscopy at low parasite densities. However, recent studies of infection duration with age (since cumulative exposure and acquired immunity increase with age) [124], [125] found no general age trend [213], [192]. An involvement of NAI would entail that short infection durations should become repeatedly common in older age groups, which has not yet been reported by any study.

6.2.4 Age and acquired immunity

The burden of malaria in humans residing in endemic areas is strongly age-determined [68]. A simplistic demonstration can be seen in the simulated solution plot of the age-specific SIRS model in [44] (given in Figure 6.2). It reveals how prevalence changes with respect to age for different values of force of infection. With a higher rate of infection (h = 5/yr), typical for endemic areas, malaria prevalence rises speedily at young age up to a peak, from where it gradually declines to a low level in adulthood, as a result of the increase in immunity. Contrarily, prevalence is shown to have an insignificant dependence on age for low force of infection (h = 0.05/yr). This model predicts that in highly endemic areas, the prevalence rapidly rises in early childhood and gradually wanes into adulthood as a result of slow acquisition of immunity with age and time. Also, it can be seen that the prevalence in adults is highest at intermediate infection rates. This is consistent with the infection pattern summarized by Boyd for tropical Africa [60] and also with the speculations of some epidemiologist that partial control, which leads to a moderate reduction of transmission from initially high levels, could increase adult prevalence [148], [63]. While immunity to malaria generally rises with age, especially in places with the highest forces of infection and stabilizes at adulthood, this increase with respect to age is not noticeable at low force of infection. In areas where the disease is not endemic and exposure is only occasional (i.e. once every few years), the burden posed by malaria extends into adulthood and similar infection levels is seen among various age groups since protective immunity is not consistently maintained [71]. See Appendix 6.B for more explanation of this model.

In high transmission areas, children below the age of five are most vulnerable to severe malaria attacks [29]. This is related to the fact that these children with the least prior

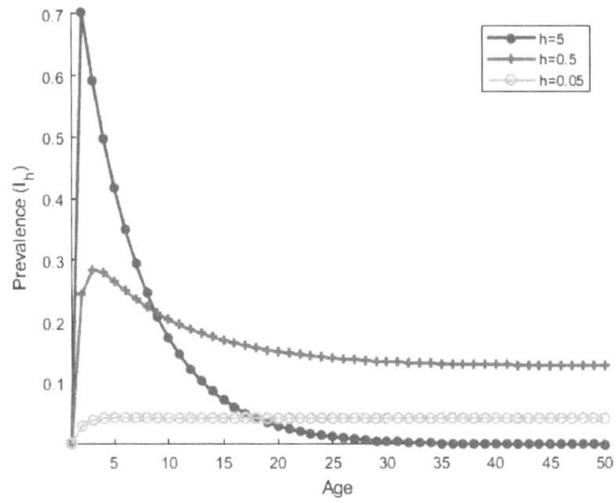

(a)

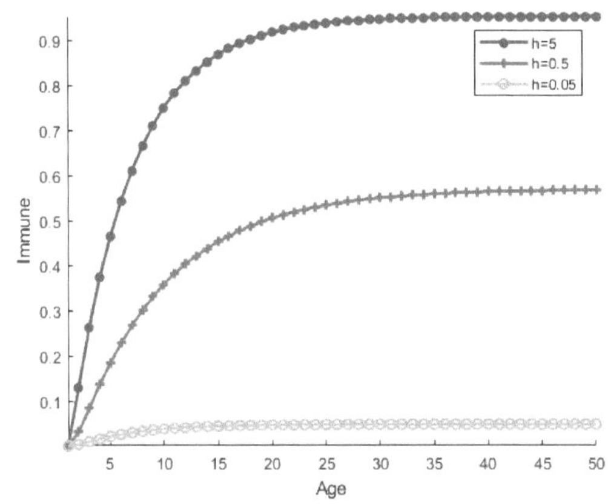

(b)

Figure 6.2: (a) Age prevalence and (b) immune curve simulated using the Aron model [44] for different forces of infection with $r = 0.9$/yr, $q = 0.25$/yr and $\tau = 5$ yrs.

exposure, have the least acquired immunity to infections and are also at highest risk of nutritional problems [115]. However, with frequent re-exposure, the vulnerability to severe clinical attacks is reduced by NAI as they age. Parasite infection prevalence begins to rise only at about 20 weeks of age, since infants are peculiarly resistant to high parasitemia and severe disease [205], [57]. This kind of protection is known to be either linked with the presence of maternal immunoglobulin antibodies such as secretory IgA and/or parasite growth-inhibitory factors such as lactoferrin found in breast milk and in the sera of mother-infant pair [74], [162]. Some models however, for simplicity, ignore this protective maternal immunoglobulin antibodies and assume that all individual lack immunity at initial stage [6], [109], [62]. Nevertheless, maternal protection has been incoporated in a stochastic model by [76] in a biologically reasonable way. The host's age was modelled to be inversely related to the amount of maternally gained protection. The extent of maternal protection is treated as independent of maternal exposure. This was based on the argument that if transmission is low, only few infants will be exposed in their first few months of life, so maternal protection is unimportant. However, in a case where transmission is frequent, then all mothers will probably have similar immune level. An exception to the age-dependence of NAI in endemic areas is seen in pregnant women. The risk of disease is much higher, even with prior immunity, because pregnant women are immuno-suppressed, so that they can carry the baby without reacting to it [142]. An additional reason is due to preferential sequestration of infected erythrocytes in the placenta [129], often referred to as "placental malaria".

Although NAI results from uninterrupted heavy exposure to infection, it appears that no amount of heavy exposure in children can induce an adult-like protective immunity for individuals in a given area [205]. Baird [170] demonstrated an approach to assess the effects of cumulative exposure and age by studying NAI among people of all ages who are shortly exposed to intense infection pressure. After a year of residing in a hyperendemic area of Irian Jaya, the frequency and density of parasitemia among newcomers from Java, decreases with increasing age. Adult newcomers manifested evidence of naturally acquired protection relatively rapidly, whereas their children remained susceptible. It is wondered why adults are resistant to infection, while children remain susceptible after a brief period of apparently uniform intense exposure among all age groups (see also [179]). This is presumed to be as a result of the difference in the structure of the immune system of a child and that of an adult [35] and age-dependent pathophysiological mechanism [99], which accounts for an immune system in children that is less capable of mounting protective response against parasites. In [102], this concept of immune maturation as humans age was accounted for by allowing a slow change of the immune stimulation parameter from a relatively low value at infant ages to relatively higher values as age increases. It allowed for more efficient "adult response" to an identical exposure, compared to that of a child. As such, the rate and duration of severe episodes decline with age due to immune maturation. Smith et al. [118], evaluated immunity to *P. falciparum* infection in African children by comparing SIS to SIRS models, allowing for heterogeneous infection rates and superinfections. In this study, the model that fitted best to the malaria data of African children was the SIS model with no immunity to reinfection. This was suggested to be because children do not acquire protection to new infections after recovering from a single infection, but protective immunity requires repeated exposure or perhaps some change in immune function with with respect to age (see [52]). However, in some models such as in [72], immunity was modelled as a function of individual exposure history only, without taking age into account; moreso in most compartmental models, time is represented through age with the assumption that the population has reached its equilibrium pattern of infection, which is erroneous. Recent stochastic models have incoporated both age and exposure history in a more practical way [114], [205].

On the other hand, the growth in body surface area with the age of a host, entails more exposure of adults to mosquito bite [7] and perhaps explain why they seem to acquire immunity faster than children when exposed to heavy malaria transmission for the first time [205]. Smith et al. [205] proposed a model for the relationship between the EIR and the force of infection in endemic areas. The model considered the effects of increased exposure to mosquito bites resulting from the growth in body surface area with the age of the host, and the reduced survival of the inoculations as the hosts acquire pre-erythrocytic immunity. This model accounted for the non-monotonic relationships between the age of the host and risk factors such as parasite prevalence and clinical malaria. This non-monotonic relation appears to be because the risk factors increases with age (accompanied with increasing body size), and at the same time, immunity decreases the risks. However, while some recent age-structured models have considered the concept of increasing human attractiveness as they age, grow and increase in biomass [114], [160], others have ignored this concept and assumed equal biting rates among individuals [6], [16], which is unrealistic.

In general, age and acquired immunity are inseparable factors that hugely determine the disease burden in a given population, especially in endemic areas [215]. This implies that increasing age does not itself result in immunity acquisition. Anderson and May [59] incorporated age structure in the classical Ross model by studying the population fraction of humans in the infected class as a function of not only time, but age as well; with the sole aim of enabling infection in a given population to depend on the age of an individual over time . However, upon matching the predicted dependence based on the their model with the observed prevalence trend in [60], it was revealed that the model is not a good fit to the data since they had not considered NAI in their model. The need to explicitly interplay NAI with age was apparent (see [16], [38]). Furthermore, the simulation studies that do not consider maternal antibodies or varied biting rates as a function of age, generate curves that reach adult equilibrium levels more quickly than are observed in real data [192].

6.2.5 Duration of acquired immunity to malaria

Immunity is generally modeled based on the fact that individuals are born susceptible and can become infected with respect to a certain rate of infection per year, h (otherwise known as the force of infection (Table 6.2)); after which they can recover within a certain period of time and can acquire a certain level of immunity with repeated exposure. People routinely exposed to malaria accumulate memory B cells specific for malaria antigens with exposure. In most mathematical models, the duration of immunity, τ is suggested without taking re-exposure to infection into account [59], [67], [65], [152]. This again stems from the binary view of malaria adopted by most modellers which wrongly suggests that there is an automatic switch between presence or absence of immunity and malaria parasites. However, epidemiological studies have proven that this approach of describing the duration of immunity could be unrealistic since it is observed that both blood-stage immunity and pre-erythrocytic protection against malarial infection are boosted with exposure to infection [61], [63], [76] (see next subsection for more details). Some models considered that re-exposure could boost immunity [79], [70], [106]. Dutertre, in his model, [64] included a discrete class of immune humans whose entrance to susceptible class is delayed by re-exposure, and calculated on a monthly basis. Aron in [45], again developed a continuous-time process of immunity acquisition based on the underlying assumption that NAI abates gradually in the absence of reinfection and suggested that immunity can last until τ years without exposure, but if there is an exposure before the time τ elapses, the immunity is strengthened and lasts longer. On the other hand, if immunity lasts for τ years in the absence of new infections, then the individual becomes highly susceptible to severe episodes (see [115]). This suggests that the rate at which the immune population become susceptible again, γ, is dependent on the rate at which they acquire new infections, h [38].

However, the average number of years without exposure that can lead to loss of protective immunity is yet unclear and it's known to vary with individuals. A related study reveals that emigrants from Africa to Europe loose much of their immunity after over 2 to 3 years of their stay while remaining protected from severe disease attacks [91]. The outbreak of malaria infection in the central highlands of Madagascar aided the opportunity to compare malaria incidence in first-time exposed children and young adults, with that in older adults who spent their childhood in the study area before the introduction of malaria control measures [215]. It was found that, individuals older than 40 years were more protected than younger adults. This increased protection was suggested to be probably due to immunological memory. These works are consistent with the evidence that fatality rates are significantly higher among non-immune individuals exposed to malaria for the first time than among previously immune humans revisiting endemic areas (see [76]), because prior exposure has a considerable protective effect [131], [130], [192]. This also suggests that clinical immunity may hardly be completely lost as most deterministic modellers assume [215]. With the assumption that mortality acts approximately equally on all individuals, the average per capita rate of losing immunity is given in [45] as

$$\gamma = \frac{he^{-h\tau}}{1-e^{-h\tau}}. \tag{6.1}$$

The changes in γ with respect to h and τ, in the absence of re-exposure, are presented in Figure 6.3. The model demonstrated that with a high force of infection as a result of continuous exposure, the rate of losing immunity could almost get to zero but appreciable rates of immunity loss are noticeable with lower force of infection and short durations

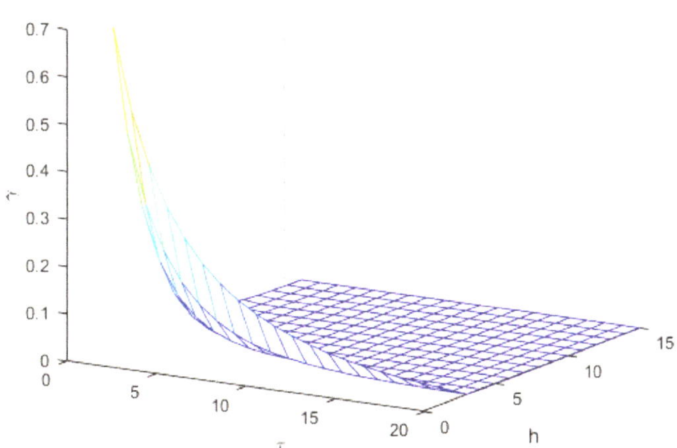

Figure 6.3: Changes in the rate of immunity loss γ with different values of h and τ.

of immunity. The study in [45] is just illustrative without any field data and it handles a single undifferenciated form of immunity. There is limited quantitative data from which to estimate rates of decay of immune protection against malaria.

6.2.6 Malaria parasite variants

Malaria parasite diversity and transmission intensity affect the acquisition of parasitological immunity (Table 6.1) [104]. The time needed to develop this immunity is thought to be directly proportional to parasite diversity (i.e., genetic diversity of *Plasmodium* infection) and inversely proportional to transmission intensity [90], [164]. As earlier mentioned, there are five species known to cause malaria in humans, each of which comprises multitudes of variants. The strain theory by Gupta and Day [123] assumed that malaria comprised of discrete, independently transmitted, immutable strains [121], [122]. This definition entails that a strain retains its identity in a locality where other strains occur such that the gametocytes of one strain should be resistant to fertilization by another. The theory has been considered inappropriate since *Plasmodium*, just like other protozoan and bacterial pathogens, has the ability to modify surface protein expression, and thereby alter the profile of antigens that are exposed to the immune system of a host [138], [180]. This results in the amplification of extensive repertoires of multi-copy, hyper-variable gene families that encode infected erythrocyte or merozoite surface proteins. Thus, a single parasite genotype can express numerous and diverse antigenic and functional phenotypes upon re-infection [180].

Additionally, when mosquitoes acquire gametocytes of two different clones in a blood meal, crossing generates recombinant clones differing from their parental genotypes [176], [177], [178]. The high level of antigenic diversity is believed to be sustained by both gene conversion and recombination events [105], [139], [138]. This mechanism of antigenic variation enables malaria parasites to succeed in bypassing the immune response of a host, to establish long-term, persistent infections, thereby increasing the efficiency by which they are transmitted to mosquito vector [173]. This genetic diversity of the parasites is one of the major causes of the slow acquisition of immunity to malaria [167]. Thus, the more individuals are exposed to diverse circulating parasites, the more they develop effective anti- malarial immunity [77], [34], [86], [95]. On the other hand, increasing the number of locally circulating variants can prolong the time needed to develop broad immunity [192].

Thus, the term strain can be used for a freely mixing unstructured population of parasites, recovered from a source in a given geographical area, that possesses confirmed or suspected distinctive characteristics that may be the results of the pressure of natural selection [164]. This idea of freely mixing strains implies that the control of malaria may be far more difficult than previously assumed. Strains of a given species of Plasmodium can be viewed in this context as different races of the same Plasmodium species which apparently share common antigens [141], [88]. This suggests that if a definite immunity is built against a strain of *P. falciparum* for instance, it extends to the strain of same species in several hundred miles away. In the experiment conducted in [141], the different response to infection appeared to be much more dependent on the quantitative degree of immunity of the patient, than on the origin of the strains used (origin in this context is defined based on the common assumption that in each region, malaria has a character of its own conferred upon it by the peculiarities of the local parasites [141]). This, to a large extent, renders the concept of discrete and independent strain inconsequential. Thus, the concept of malaria parasite strains should instead be understood as variants of a given *plasmodium* species, since they are dynamic entities resulting from the interaction between parasite genomes and the human immune system [42], [76], [164], [138].

Milligan and Downham [70] demonstrated how increase in the number of circulating strains in a population results to slower rate of reduction in susceptibility. Individuals are considered to be immune to infection with strain k, if they have experienced at least N_k infections with that strain after say, W bites from infected vectors. In a simple case where vectors can host at most one parasite strain, and infection with different strains in a single contact are mutually exclusive, the multinomial distribution can be employed while summing over different strains. Hence, the probability of getting infected with any strain at the $(W+1)$th infectious bite is given as

$$P(W) = \sum_{k=1}^{s} q_k \sum_{r=0}^{\min(W,N_k-1)} \binom{W}{r} q_k^r (1-q_k)^{W-r}, \tag{6.2}$$

where q_k is the probability that an individual acquires an innoculum of strain k upon receiving an infection bite. For simplicity, with a constant $N_k = 2$ for all strains k (although it is host dependent), and equally abundant strains ($q_k = 1/S$ for all k), the plot of $P(W)$ against W with 3 different numbers of circulating strains, S is given in Figure 6.4.

The above demonstration can only be appropriate if malaria variants are discrete and immutable as applicable in some viruses. Based on the current understanding of malaria parasite variants, it follows that exposure to more diverse variants would progressively reduce the repertoire of parasites clones that may be capable of establishing patent and virulent infections [140], [88].

However, it is possible for a primary infection with a given parasite species to confer protection against a secondary infection with heterologous species if the species share

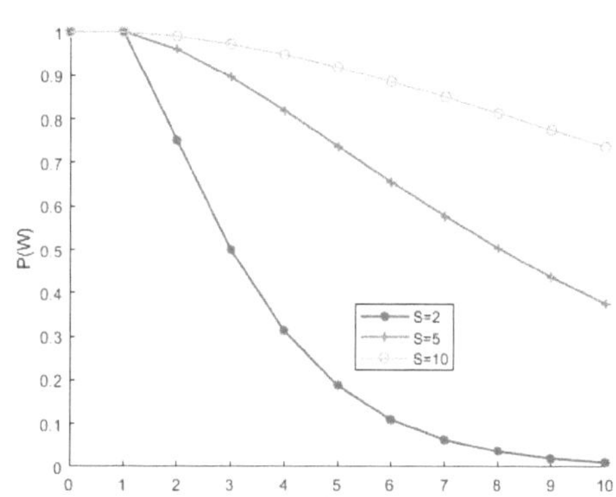

Figure 6.4: Probability of getting infected at the $(W+1)$th bite from an infectious vector when assuming mutually exclusive strains.

common antigens. This situation was suggested to be true for *P. falciparum* and *P. malariae* in a retrospective examination made to determine parasitemia and fever episodes, since parasitologic and clinical immunity was evident when infection with *P. falciparum* follows that with *P. malariae* [127], [165].

6.2.7 Acquired variant-specific and variant-transcending immunity

Acquired immunity to malaria has mostly been modeled as a general phenomenon without considering any defined variants ([43], [44], [50], [109], [72], [37], [108]). However, malaria parasite diversity is known to affect the development of parasitological immunity since an individual may have to be exposed to the entire (or almost) diversity of the antigenic make-ups in parasite populations in order to develop effective protection, [165], [77], [34], [167], [86], [95]. Smith et al. [165] demonstrated this schematically using overlapping/non-overlapping blobs on two frames representing a hypothetical immune space comprising the total repertoire of immune responses within a host. The two frames were used to illustrate the concept of immunity acquisition by showing the dramatic difference between very young children and older people. In infants or susceptible individuals, the mechanism which allows the persistence of chronic infections has not come into play and the immunologic space is still sparse because the strong anti-parasitic effect of fever itself or the cytokines released during fever [172], prevents the establishment of chronicity (This cytokine-mediated effect is a sign of their inability to control parasite densities, thus persistent infections do not exist). However, in older individuals residing in high transmission areas, the immunological space is already broadly occupied and new infections can hardly be established. A similar schematic diagram as in [165] is reproduced in Figure 6.5.

The mistaken assumption by some investigators that NAI is strictly strain-specific and lifelong (see [120], [121], [122]) was conclusively addressed in an insightful critical appraisal over 20 years ago [119]. It became clear that the basic model of lifelong strain-specific immunity leads to impossibly dynamic predictions, which conflict with the notorious observed stability of malaria transmission (see [63], [173]). Considering that the stability of a process relies on negative feedback loops, it follows that if strain-specific immunity which can be rapidly acquired, limits the transmission of malaria, then it must be down-regulated equally rapidly for malaria prevalence and transmission to be as resilient as has been proven by thousands of epidemiological studies.

A mathematical model of *P. falciparum* asexual parasitaemia was developed and fitted to 35 malaria therapy cases [31]. The model included three internal mechanisms that aided its simulation of the courses of asexual parasitaemia in human host in a more realistic way: innate, acquired variant-specific and acquired variant-transcending immune responses, all of which are believed to control the peaks of parasitaemia at certain levels and stages. According to this model, the innate immune response is responsible for early control, and thereafter becomes progressively less relevant, while the acquired variant-transcending immune response is relatively inconsequential for early control but dominates in the later stages of the infection. On the other hand, variant-specific immunity regulates the density of a specific variant and eventually eliminates it. A general conclusion from a review of

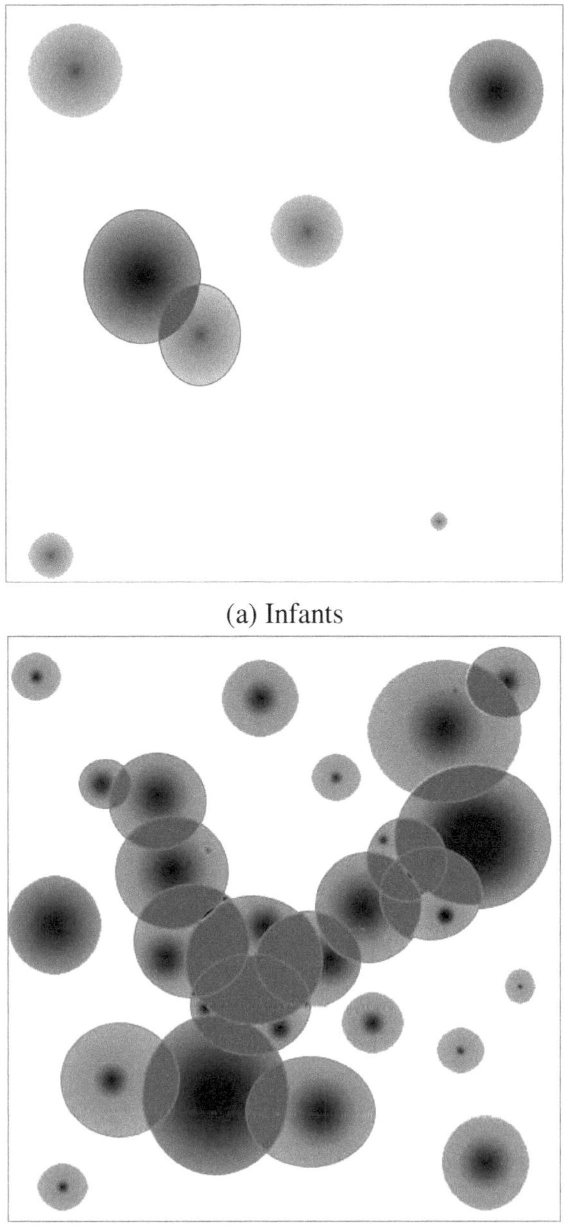

(a) Infants

(b) older people

Figure 6.5: Schematic illustration of malaria premunition reproduced from [165].

intra-host models of malaria [112] is that with time, NAI moves from variant-specific to variant-transcending, as accumulated diversity of exposure increases.

In the same vein, a stochastic model of within-host immunity was employed to explore which form of immunity could account for the observed rates of reinfection in adults and children in field data [6]. The model focused on the immunity impacting the growth of blood-stage parasite, where such immunity might either be variant-specific (resulting from the infection with a certain variant and neutralizes the parasites of that variant), or general (i.e., variant-transcending as in [31]; resulting from the infection with any strain and neutralization affects all strains equally) (see also [156]). The existing level of immunity was assumed to decay at some constant rate in the absence of re-infection. The impact of variant-specific immunity was apparent in that, one can repeatedly see the clearance of one parasite peak, while another grows immediately. However, incorporating only rapidly accumulated variant-specific immunity was helpful to demonstrate the clearance of individual parasite peaks but cannot explain age-associated variations in reinfection and parasitaemia. This is because variant-specific immunity has to be short-lived [186] in order to allow for effective clearance and also for reinfection. This suggests the need for a general slowly accumulated immunity that decreases the growth of all variants; which must be long-lived. Thus, incorporating both the rapidly-induced strain-specific immunity which wipes out individual infections, and general immunity that accumulates slowly and reduces the mean parasite growth rate with age, gives model outputs that are consistent with the observed data. In general, the role of antigenic diversity whereby existing infections contribute significantly to protection, contrasts with the theory that NAI to malaria is-strictly strain-specific and long-lasting [165].

6.2.8 Superinfection/ Reinfection and acquired immunity

In malaria-endemic areas, an individual can receive hundreds of infectious bites each year, thereby increasing the risk of superinfection (Table 6.1) which results from consecutive infectious bites [88], [80], [85]. In practice, an individual can host more than one plasmodium species or variants of the same plasmodium species, at a time [182], [173], [165], [81], [57], [187], [88] in endemic areas. In areas of low or moderate level of endemicity, it is likely that re-inoculations would be infrequent within a short interval so that the first infection would have become latent, or even have been cleared, before re-inoculation.

Several opinions of the mechanism associated with superinfection in malaria exist. One idea from Macdonald's model [143] was that successive infections are effectively "stacked", waiting to express themselves at the end of the previous infection. This idea was also adopted in [72] by resetting the infection date of the individual, so that courses of different infections proceed without interference, such that recovery from superinfection happens when the course of the last infection is completed. Another related suggestion by Dietz [144] is that infections arrive and run their course completely independent on each other. Neither of these two models appears to be correct (see [40]). For the former model, there is no evidence for an infection waiting for another to be completed. The latter model by Dietz, on the other hand, ignored the concept of immunity and possible competition among parasites. Richie [84] in his suppression hypothesis postulated the tendency of malarial species to exclude each other and thereby appear chronologically in the blood. This he presumed to be caused by competition for host cells or nutrients, or by heterologous immunity. However, the repressed species bounce back after the previous species has dwindled, and can result in prolonged infection. His hypothesis is supported by experimental data obtained from the simultaneous inoculation of two Plasmodium species into laboratory animals; which show that one of either species is suppressed. This mechanism seem to benefit both the host and the incumbent parasite by keeping parasite density at levels that are not severe before the role of NAI activates. A similar study by Portugal [81], [82] who explored the possibility of the liver-stage of infection to be modulated by the presence of an ongoing blood-stage infection and contribute to acquisition of immunity, explains that this mechanism arises as Plasmodium in the blood strives to protects its niche, perhaps ensuring transmission on the basis of first-come, first-served. This appears to enable the host immune system to fight one circulating parasite at a time, consequently raising thc host's chances of survival. In addition, the number of scenarios of liver-stage infections would be more than that of blood-stage infections, boosting the immune response to the liver stage without exposing the host to blood-stage infection. This action seems to contribute to the more rapid acquisition of immunity to severe disease (see also [111]).

On the other hand, some deterministic models which consider malaria infection as binary, assume that an individual can be completely protected from superinfection after attaining a certain threshold of parasite density [108], [106]. In [108], individuals whose parasite density are below a defined threshold are described as primary infectious and are prone to superinfection, whereas secondary infectious individuals are assumed to be completely protected from superinfection [81], [82]. These theories and studies try to explain the how the impact of superinfection and can be suppressed; and how NAI to severe diseases can be boosted in non-naive individuals even during the occurrence of superinfection, but the underlying mechanisms seems either unclear or unrealistic.

In general, the idea that already present chronic infections can protect against superinfection dates from the work in [168] where the concept of premunition was brought up, and was used by Cohen and Deans [169] to refer NAI which frequently controls parasite densities, but does not eliminate infection. However, in [165], the concept of premunition is used as the limitation of superinfection. Thus, the outcome of superinfection is controlled by limiting the rate of newly infecting homologous and even heterologous (Table 6.2) haplotypes that could get established in the host. This implies that parasites which have similar antigenic properties with those already existing would be suppressed or controlled based on the extent of overlap of their antigenic haplotypes i.e the degree of relatedness of the antigenic repertoire of the incoming infection, with prior experienced antigens [192], [173], [165], [166], [190], [70]. However, it should be noted that the maximum number of superinfection decreases with age due to the acquisition of immunity (See also [80], [165]). This is because chronic malaria infection is known to occur in older individuals who have mounted immune response which controls parasite densities sufficient enough to avert clinical attacks but allows the infection to remain at low density [171], [169], [168], [173]. On the other hand, in non-immune individuals, superinfection poses a high risk of hyperparasitemia and mortality [82].

6.2.9 Other factors influencing the acquisition of immunity

6.2.9.1 Effect of intervention measures on immunity acquisition and malaria prevalence

Populations utilizing intervention strategies which reduce malaria transmission and subsequently immunity, such as insecticidal-nets and drug treatment, may also be prone to have rebound effects, especially in endemic areas [113], [102], [55], [57]. An illustration was captured in individual-based model simulations in [102] which indicated that protection against new infections reduces the acquisition of asexual blood-stage immunity. This causes accumulated immune memory to wane, such that a compensatory rise in clinical incidence may result when protection measures are not available (see also [113], [194]). The same case is postulated for the use of bednets, as it may only shift the age of the incidence of severe disease without considerably reducing the overall disease burden.

In the individual-based model of malaria transmission developed in [72], a short-lived effect of the intervention program was noticed which could be due to a rebound after immunity has waned in the population [113], [116], [102]. On the contrary, no rebound effect was noticed with administering a hypothesized vaccine which was assumed to not only provide an immediate boost in immune response, but also brings about the early maturation of the immune response, normally associated with aging. This suggests that the use of intervention should be effective and long-lived [154], [153] (see the diagrammatic illustration in [154]). On the other hand, reduction in the use of short-lived intervention measures will reduce drug pressure and the emergence of parasite variants resistant to the widely used anti-malaria drug treatment [17], [18], [108], [106], [149]. This is because immunity acts especially by reducing the frequency and severity of clinical attacks, and thus the drug pressure. The same case is applicable to chemicals used in treating insecticidal-net. The negative effect of having small number of immune individuals in low transmission areas, can be counterbalanced by the sustained implementation of very effective transmission-reducing interventions for an indefinite period [154], [54]. This can also be augmented by a transmission blocking vaccine which enhances and artificially induces immunity.

6.2.9.2 Climatic driving effect on immunity acquisition

Although climate is the dominant driver of seasonal outbreaks of malaria, it has been demonstrated that NAI can buffer its effects [103], [26]. To clarify the differences in the impact of NAI among high and low-transmission settings, Laneri et al. [103] developed a stochastic human–mosquito model to fit the data from two unique adjacent cohorts in settings with mesoendemic (Table 6.2) seasonal and holoendemic (Table 6.2) perennial malaria transmission in Senegal, which were followed up for two decades, recording their daily malaria cases. Thus, for the cohort in which epidemic transmission is limited by mosquito density and rainfall, the highly dynamic pattern of cases is climate-driven whereas the impact of climate on incidence was largely buffered by clinical immunity in the endemic village where mosquitoes are present year-round. This is consistent with the field observations in [147], suggesting that places with dry season transmission are associated with stable hotspots of largely asymptomatic parasitaemia and robust immunity acquired early in life.

Yamana et al. [26], [27], [28] developed a coupled hydrology and agent-based entomological model that uses environmental data (such as temperature, rainfall and topography) which typically regulates mosquito population dynamics, to simulate the mosquito biting rates and subsequently the malaria prevalence alongside the level of NAI in the human population. The model demonstrates the impact of NAI on malaria prevalence in two Niger villages that are entomologically and hydrologically disparate. The model suggests that the NAI depends on hydrologically driven mosquito abundance over previous years. Thus, greater acquired immunity is obtainable in the wet village due to more mosquito bites as compared with the dry village. However, the model also shows how NAI dampens the effect of increased biting, since without the effects of immunity, the wet village would have much higher prevalence than the dry village.

6.2.9.3 Effect of population dynamics on immunity acquisition

The assumption of maintaining a constant population size, made in most models for simplicity, needs to be addressed since it's unclear if it matters or not, even though it seems to be artificial. It is known that human population is characterized by birth, mortality and immigration. Some modelers believe that the consideration of these factors in the models entails a more realistic modeling of the acquisition of immunity with time since for instance, malaria is an endemic disease which has a high mortality rate [72], [46], [48], [109]. Moreover, the interaction between the vector and human populations instigates a considerable level of variability on especially the mosquito populations for which the assumption of constant population may not be realistic [46].

Ngwa and Shu [46] developed a SEIR model which assumes density dependent death rates in both the human and mosquito populations, with the total populations varying with time. Chitnis [49], [48] on the other hand, developed a model with constant immigration for the Susceptible class such that people enter the latter class either by birth or through immigration. To account for population dynamics, age-specific fertility and mortality rates are calculated for each individual and an additional mortality component, specific for each individual (such as malarial related death), is incorporated in an individual-based malaria risk assessment model [109]. The model demonstrated the creation of individual disease history (immunity, infectedness and illness) depending on their circulation behavior (e.g going to work, traveling) and residence over a given period of time. The model in[103] includes the variability of both the human and mosquito population; the former, through yearly census and the later, either measured directly through landing catches or estimated based on the variability in meteorological conditions (rainfall and temperature).

Some of these models produced results which show the impact of including demographic effects in predicting the rate of fatalities that could arise from the disease. Incorporating population variability of humans might seem pointless in cases where the quantitative influence of human population growth is small enough to neglect and deserves far less attention. However, most models considered mostly the human population dynamics with little emphasis on the dynamics of the vector population [109], [110] which is the major driver of malaria transmission. The emphasis on the mosquito population dynamics dates back from the work of Ross [95]. His work suggests that if the vector population can be reduced to below a certain threshold, then malaria can be successfully eradicated. This threshold is typically dependent on biological factors such as the biting rate and vectorial capacity Table (6.2) which solely depends on the vector population dynamics. In [40], the immune status of the population was viewed as a function of the vectorial capacity (Table 6.2), which drives incidence of infection in humans. However, MacDonald [143] on the other hand demonstrated that reducing the number of mosquitoes would have little effect on the epidemiology of malaria in endemic areas. This, in fact, depends on the extent of reduction.

6.2.10 Summary of modelling approaches

In this review, the epidemiological models of NAI to malaria have been grouped in terms of the realism of immunity acquisition scenarios accounted for. This idea is engendered by the assumption that more realistic models would boost the understanding of how immunity effects transmission dynamics at both the individual and population level. These models range from deterministic to ABMs and they have played substantial roles in developing epidemiological understanding of the disease. Considering that the mechanisms of natural acquisition of immunity to malaria are so complex, the discussion of both the deterministic and ABMs depends apparently on the scope of the questions asked. For instance in [42], the earlier model of the full course of parasitemia in non-immune individual [31] was restricted to the first wave of parasitemia in same persons. By so doing, the description of acquired immunity was simplified, reducing it to a single dimension, with no distinction between variant-specific and variant-transcending immune response and also ignoring decay of immunity.

Compartmental SEIR models, in general, are not sufficient for reproducing the real dynamics of malaria as they allow only a limited account of the complex process of malaria transmission, and NAI in particular. They make clearly artificial assumptions that seem to make them conceptually compelling, but are actually inefficient. One considerable reason is that malaria modelling requires an indepth study of in-host parasite dynamics rather than a mere presence or absence of infection and prevalence in a group of population. Again, the important sources of heterogeneity, spatial and temporal scales of transmission remain inadequately addressed using deterministic models. A general interest for the deterministic models is geared at knowing if one infection in one person in an entire parasite population across an entire endemic setting will varnish or persist in a population. This is usually assessed by computing the R_0, which is somewhat governed by immunity status, since most of these models assume that an individual's probability of infecting a mosquito reduces as immunity increases. In the deterministic models, immunity is either included by considering a separate human immune class (R_h) [51], [50],[75], [19], [39], [48], [49],[47], [46], [43], [44] , [40] or by integrating an immunity function in existing models [59], [53], [52], [55], [57], [58].

Agent-based models of malaria transmission, however, have become an attractive alternative in the evolution of malaria models in recent times. This is because they allow simulation of heterogeneous communities subjected to more realistic transmission scenarios and can incorporate complex and stochastic issues affecting malaria spread. Thus, any kind of heterogeneity (such as heterogeneous intervention measures, host movement, multiple parasite variants) and stochasticity (such as inter-patient variability in duration of infection and virulence) relating to malaria transmission and interactive variability in parasite-host dynamics can easily be modelled. Another strength of this modeling approach is that it enables the simulation of the interaction of individuals and vectors in the domain of interest, which can in itself be heterogeneous, and stores information about each agent (mosquito and/or human). Protective efficacy of immunity varies between individual humans [42], so it may be misleading to ignore individual variations in biologically important parameters while this can be efficiently addressed by ABM simulations. Decay rates of Immunity, for instancc, varies in humans and should be sampled from a suitable distribution with an assumed mean. The flexibility of agent-based approaches in modifying model attributes to reflect local individual features and geographical factors, allows the construction of models that can handle realistic questions relating to malaria control in specific local contexts. A considerable disadvantage is the higher computational burden, especially with increasing population size.

Most individual-based models focus more on increasing the immune status of an individual as they age and get more exposed, without considering how parasite densities changes. However, the models which meet the kind of realistic expectation of the dynamics and complex structure of NAI to malaria are those suggesting that immunity indicators should be functions of parasite density and diagnostic detection sensitivity rather than binary factors. Most of these models are those included in the OpenMalaria ensemble [159], [194] which are the advanced, quite realistic individual-based models we rely on today. The programming of the models was done in C++ as part of the open source software platform (`http://code.google.com/p/openmalaria/`), hence the name, OpenMalaria. A compelling strength of this model is that it couples an ensemble of 14 associated submodels that have been validated with real field data from various African settings. The integrated mathematical models are used for predicting the epidemiologic and economic effects of malaria vaccines both at the individual and population level. The model simulations use a function that reduces asexual parasite densities to model important concepts such as: the transmission to mosquito [160], [114], the degree of severity of episodes based on the parasite load [115], [134] and how the distribution of parasite densities is modified in the semi immune host [76]. Additionally, the model considers the effects of factors such as heterogeneity in transmission [198], body surface area [205], [114], [160], maternal antibodies [76], stage-specificity of immunity and superinfection [115], [76], [205]. However the aspect of the decay of NAI in the absence of exposure is yet to be properly addressed. This is because there is limited quantitative data from which to directly estimate this rate of decay of immune control of parasite densities. Overall, there still remain other unclear mechanisms of malaria immunity which have not yet been properly explained (by the aforementioned model), mainly due to limited field data, but they remain a reliable basis for further research on this topic. Closing these gaps so as to facilitate the development of malaria vaccines remains the main target of tropical diseases research.

Most of the models discussed in this review were approximately fitted to available epidemiological data, where the infection incidence determines the status of either stable endemicity and widespread immunity or an unpredictable pattern of sporadic epidemics in a population lacking sufficient regular exposure to maintain immunity. Moreso, while some models were fitted to data from many sites, others were fitted to single-site data. In as much as fitting to single-site data does not necessarily limit relevance of the models themselves, it is difficult to exclude the possibility that they are only applicable to the specific context of the studied data-set, and predictions may not be extrapolated to different areas/scenarios. Another interesting thing to do considering the pitfalls of both deterministic and agent-based modeling approaches is to tactically combine the two, so as to capture the desired population size, heterogeneity and study period [196].

6.3 DISCUSSION

Naturally acquired immunity against malaria plays an important role in the reduction of the health burden posed by malaria, as it protects numerous people who are routinely exposed to the infection against severe disease and death. In this review, the principal features of NAI to malaria have been reevaluated in terms of how different modellers perceive them and how the ideas have evolved. However, some of the underlying mechanisms behind this protection are not yet clear. Owing to the need to understand NAI on an individual level, modelling strategies have gradually evolved from deterministic compartmental models to stochastic ABM which build on more advanced knowledge base than the purely deterministic models that preceded them for decades. The ABMs came in nicely but quite late in the evolution of malaria models, as needed to cope with issues like interactive variability in parasite and host dynamics that were first identified with deterministic model fits to data sets for single individuals. Thus, more recent idea of modelling suggests that immunity indicators should be functions of parasite density and diagnostic detection sensitivity rather than binary factors.

Contrary to the suggestion that protective immunity is acquired after one or two infections, more recent studies demonstrated that immunity to severe malaria is more gradually acquired with exposure. While it is believed that sterile immunity against infection is never completely achieved, chronic, subacute carriage is the rule among adults. Such chronic carriers are less vulnerable to the parasite infection and have partially reduced infectivity to mosquitoes. Given these dynamics, it is easy to understand how malaria transmission is so robust and difficult to eliminate. This review considers the opinion that adults in endemic areas are completely immune and do not contribute considerably to the infection reservoir as unreliable. Thus, recent models such as those of the OpenMalaria models, are adopting the concept of modeling infectivity in relation to the asexual parasite densities of hosts, and also linking the infectivity of human to that of mosquito infection. There is still a need for improved models explicitly describing the impacts of age and exposure in the infectivity of humans to mosquitoes in endemic areas.

Furthermore, the mechanism of control of malaria parasites upon reinfection or superinfection in semi-immune individuals, has been addressed. The convincing account is that superinfections or infections that share antigens recognized by the already existing immune responses can be controlled such that it would not be severe. There is very little evidence that NAI has much impact on the duration of infections since models that have evaluated this concept found no general trend with age. It is accepted that naturally immunity is acquired at a rate which is dependent upon the degree of exposure and is highly effective in adults after uninterrupted lifelong heavy exposure but can also be lost to a considerable extent upon cessation of exposure. Although the rate of loss is yet unclear, it is expected that realistic modelling should not define immunity duration beforehand as was done by some early compartmental models. Additionally, in high transmission areas, the prevalence of malaria infection and the risk of malaria-associated morbidity and mortality is known to markedly decrease with age. Although immunity is age determined in such areas, it is clear that increasing age does not in itself result in immunity acquisition since another and major underlying determinant is not age per se but rather the accumulated infection exposure risk that come with it. Hence, the need to explicitly interplay naturally acquired immunity with age in a biologically realistic way has been emphasized. The best evidence to date clearly indicates that NAI may be considered as the product of cumulative exposure to multiple parasite variants over time, which gives rise to a diverse collection of variant-specific and a general variant-transcending immune responses. This opposes the mistaken perception of a life-long strictly variant-specific immunity. It is currently believed that variant-specific immune response is rapidly induced, but also appears to be short-lived, whereas the variant-transcending immune response takes time to develop and is long-lived. In principle, the duration of variant-specific immunity can vary depending on the frequency of antigenic variation, the polymorphic nature of the antigen, and the inoculation rate experienced by humans.

Furthermore, natural acquisition of immunity to malaria is believed to be somewhat stage specific. However, it appears that even though the liver-stage immunity is necessary as it protects against infection, the blood-stage immunity is the major force shaping the observed infection dynamics. The development of clinical and parasitological immunity to malaria is evident in the ability to control the asexual blood-stage parasite density which in turn limits disease symptoms and pathology. Thus, the most effective part of the immune response in clinical terms is its ability to limit parasite densities in erythrocytes, which is the target of ant-malaria drugs. It has also been explained how the use of intervention measures in a highly immune population which features reduction of exposure, can initially engender rapid reductions in disease prevalence, after which the previous burden of disease resurges as the immunity is gradually lost. The negative effect of then having small number of immune individuals in the population can only be counterbalanced by the sustained implementation of highly-effective transmission-reducing interventions for an indefinite period. This can also be augmented by a transmission blocking vaccine which enhances and artificially induces immunity. The crucial role of climatic factors in the acquisition and persistence of immunity to malaria has been emphasized. Additionally, the effect of population dynamics, of especially the vectors, which is the major driver of malaria transmission, should always be taken into account so as to engender a more ideal modeling of transmission scenarios.

In addressing these complex factors associated with NAI to malaria, the benefits of individual-based modelling approach are evident. The short-comings of deterministic models are not reasons for them to be rejected because they provide some quantitative understanding of malaria transmission. Instead, the focus is to debug some of the assumptions that are unrealistic for a particular population at a particular time, and also to build models with the appropriate level of complexity. Moreso, the prevailing global capacity for state-of-the-art analysis of malaria-related data is in advanced countries where there is no local malaria transmission [158]. In order to achieve improved control, elimination and maybe eventually eradication, the geographic disparities of data analysis capacity need to be addressed urgently. Otherwise malaria data analysts will continue to reside far away from the location of data collection and the field staff who understand them. This will limit their ability to adequately analyze and interpret the malaria data [158].

ACKNOWLEDGMENTS

This chapter is partly based on work performed within the framework of IMAAC (`https://imaac.eu/`) related to COST Action CA16227 (*Investigation & Mathematical Analysis of Avant-garde Disease Control via Mosquito Nano-Tech-Repellents*, `https://cost.eu/actions/CA16227/`), supported by COST Association (European Cooperation in Science and Technology).

GLOSSARY

Epidemiological Terms: The definitions of some commonly-used special terms related to immunity, and that of some general epidemiological terms are given here.

FURTHER READING

Killeen, Gerry F.; Ross, Amanda; Smith, Thomas, (2006)
Infectiousness of malaria-endemic human populations to vectors, The American journal of tropical medicine and hygiene, (2006); 75(2 Suppl):38-45.

Smith T, Felger I, Tanner M, Beck HP, (1999)
11. Premunition in Plasmodium falciparum infection: insights from the epidemiology of multiple infections, Transactions of the Royal Society of Tropical Medicine and Hygiene, (1999); 93(Supplement_1):59-64.

Smith T, Ross A, Maire N, Chitnis N, Studer A, Hardy D, Brooks A, Penny M, Tanner M, (2012)
Ensemble modeling of the likely public health impact of a pre-erythrocytic malaria vaccine, PLoS Med. (2012); 9:e1001157.

Dietz K, Raddatz G, Molineaux L, (2006)
Mathematical model of the first wave of Plasmodium falciparum asexual parasitemia in non-immune and vaccinated individuals. The American journal of tropical medicine and hygiene, (2006); 75(2_suppl):46-55.

Smith DL, Cohen JM, Chiyaka C, Johnston G, Gething PW, et al., (2013)
A sticky situation: the unexpected stability of malaria elimination, Philosophical Transactions of the Royal Society B: Biological Sciences, (2013); 368:20120145.

Appendices

6.A METHODS FOR LITERATURE SEARCH

6.A.1 Literature search strategy and selection criteria

Here, we present the main tools used in the literature search and analysis. These include:

- Web of Science
- Google Scholar
- Vos-viewer
- Snowballing
- Expert knowledge

A systematic literature review was performed through the Web of Science, using the option "all databases". No constraints were placed on publication type, dates of publication (see Appendix 6.A), publication status and study location. The search strategy fetched publications mentioning each of the following concepts in their subject heading, keywords list, title or abstract: acquired immunity to malaria, malaria model and malaria parasite density. Additional articles were found through snowballing [83] (backward and forward) literature search, utilizing the Google Scholar database and also through expert knowledge. The abstracts of all returned candidate studies were assessed for suitability. Papers that mentioned "(acquired) immunity" to malaria, malaria model or malaria parasite density, (anti-malaria) drug resistance or intervention in their abstracts were selected for full-text review. Full-text articles describing the model of acquired immunity to infectious diseases other than malaria and other than human-malaria, were excluded. Also, papers majorly describing vaccine induced immunity and the co-infection of malaria with some other infections such as HIV are excluded.

6.A.2 Outcome of literature search

Altogether, 120 literatures were included for answering the research questions. Forty models of naturally acquired immunity to malaria were explicitly studied with the key characteristics of each model in relation to quantifying the effect of immunity on malaria prevalence identified. The remaining 80 papers were included based on the insights they provided into the properties and underlying mechanisms of acquired immunity, and are essential to the interpretation and evaluation of the modelling papers. A network visualization of the most common terms addressed and/or used in the titles and abstracts of the included papers was created (Figure 7) with Vosviewer [14]. It appears that there are three main clusters of topics/terms addressed by the included papers:

- Immunity to malaria, its stages of acquisition and its level of protection with age and exposure to parasite infection (left-bottom).
- Malaria transmission and prevalence, based on transmission intensity in different settings/areas (right).

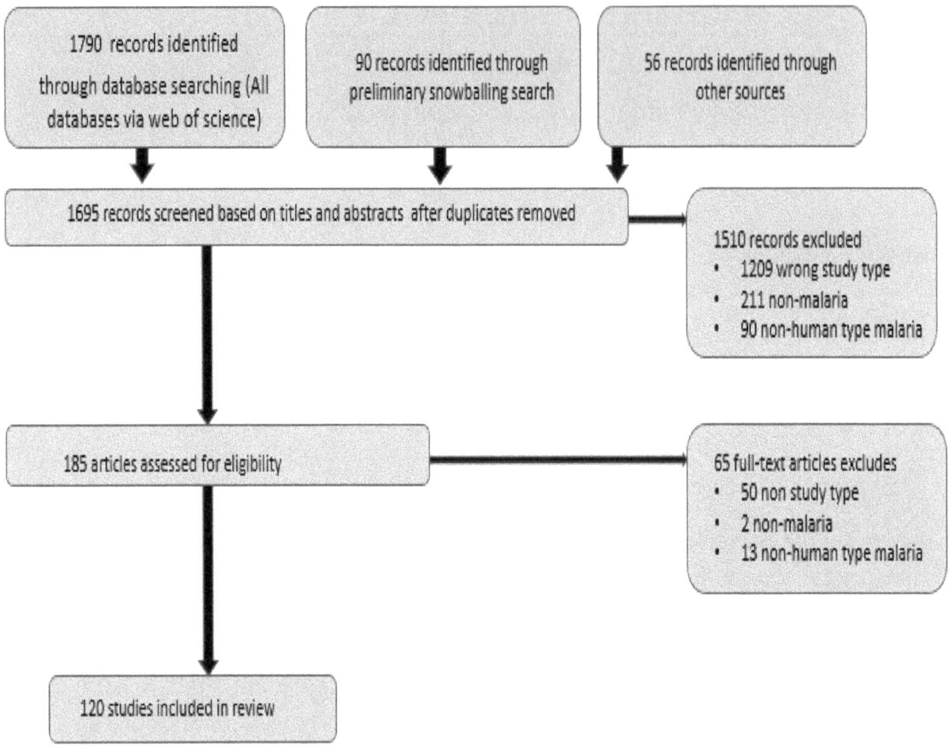

Figure 6: Search flow diagram for study selection.

- Models of immunity to malaria (deterministic and agent/individual-based), which address some dynamic topics relating to the disease infection, such as superinfection parasite strains and duration of infection (top).

The density visualization (Figure 8) also gives an overview of the important areas in the map, with immunity being the center of concentration from where all the other terms are linked directly or indirectly and thus, the thickest.

The visualization of the relatedness of included studies in terms of citations is given in Figure 9. The label may not be displayed for some of the documents in order to avoid overlapping labels. The papers are arranged in three clusters:

- The ABMs of acquired immunity to malaria (extreme right corner)
- The mathematical models of acquired immunity to malaria (left-hand side)
- Other studies that are not necessarily model-based but support and explain the underlying mechanisms of acquired immunity to malaria (middle).

The density visualization in Figure 10 reveals that not much studies have considered modeling with the agent-based approach.

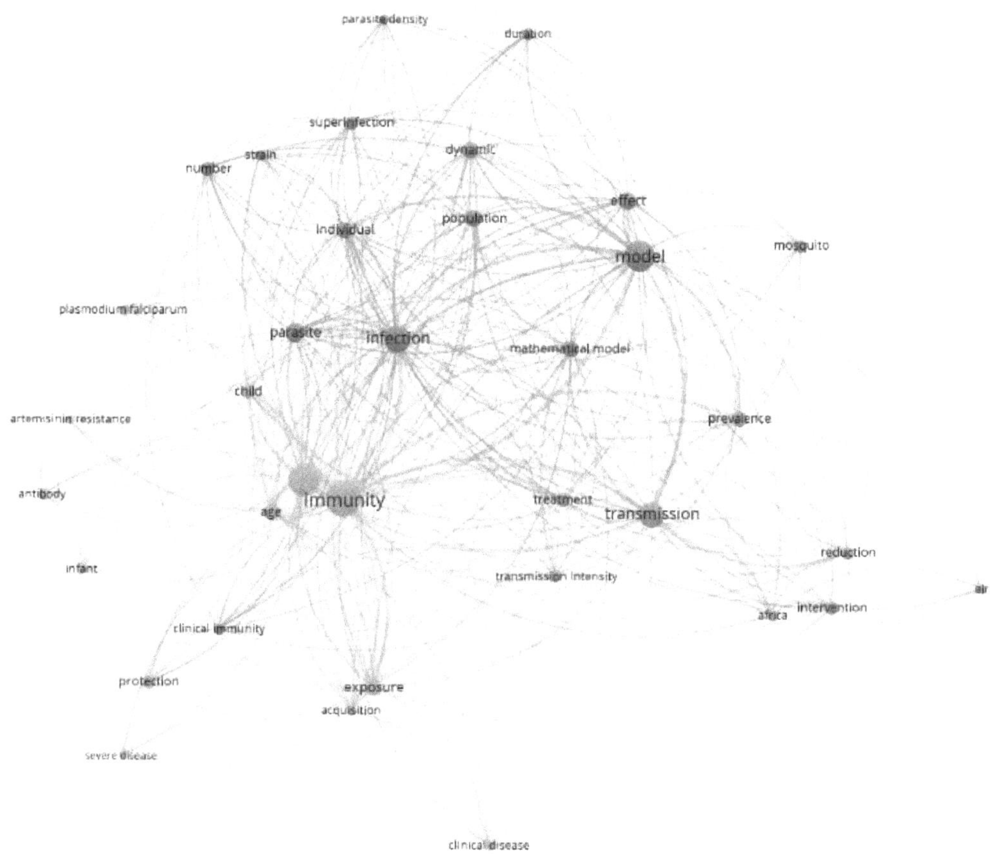

Figure 7: **Network visualization of the most common terms** (represented by circles) in the titles and abstracts of the included papers. The terms are located based on their co-occurrences in the titles and abstracts. The size of the label and circle of a term is determined by the weight of that term.

6.B DETAILED MODEL DESCRIPTIONS

Aron and May in [44] demonstrated how the burden of malaria is age-determined in endemic areas and what happens when transmission is reduced. In their age-specific SIRS model, the rate of loss of immunity γ, depends on the transmission rate h, in the manner described by Equation 6.1. In the model, time is represented via age of the cohort; typical for a population that has attained its equilibrium stage of infection. The model comprises three compartments in humans: *Susceptible* (S_h), *Infected* (I_h) and *Recovered and Immune* (R_h), where the effect of mosquito is introduced through the force of infection h. In

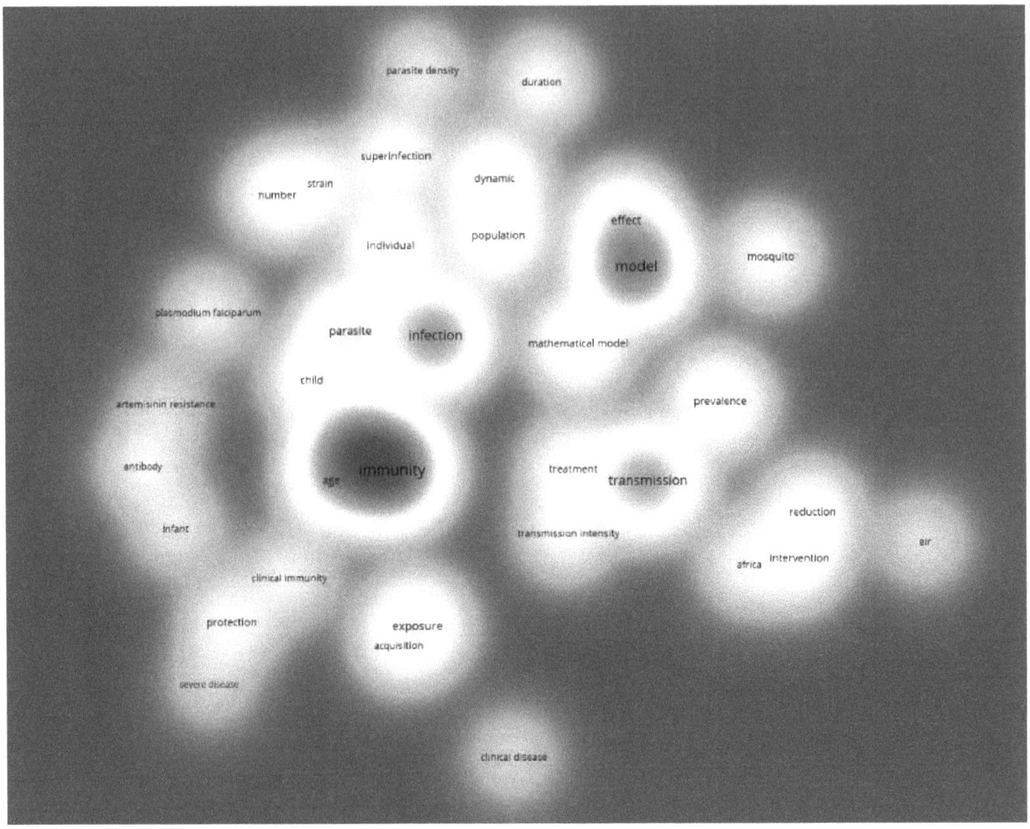

Figure 8: **Density visualization of important areas** in the map created with the most common terms in the titles and abstracts of the included papers. The density ranges from red highly dense points to low dense points [14].

this model,

$$\begin{aligned}\frac{dS_h}{da} &= -hS_h + rI_h + \gamma R_h \\ \frac{dI_h}{da} &= hS_h - rI_h - qI_h \\ \frac{dR_h}{da} &= qI_h - \gamma R_h,\end{aligned} \tag{6.B.1}$$

an infected person can recover at rate r and move directly to the susceptible class, or may slowly acquire immunity at rate q. They introduced immunity factor in their model by subtracting the people who lost immunity, γR_h from the immune class R_h and adding them to the susceptible class S_h. The plot of the simulated solution of the model Equation 6.B.1, given in Figure 6.2, reveals how prevalence changes with respect to age for different values of force of infection. With a higher rate of infection (h = 5/yr), typical for endemic areas, malaria prevalence rises speedily at young age up to a peak, from where it gradually declines to a low level in adulthood, as a result of the increase in immunity. Contrarily, prevalence is shown to have an insignificant dependence on age for low force of infection (h = 0.05/yr). This model predicts that in highly endemic areas, the prevalence rapidly rises

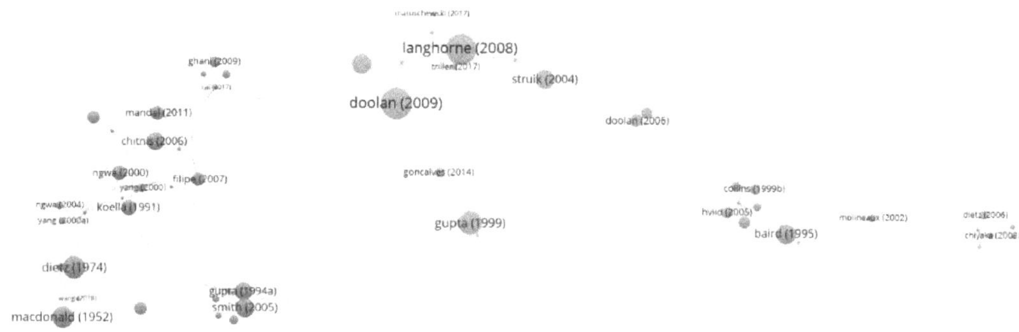

Figure 9: **Visualization of document citations and relatedness.** The distance between two documents in the visualization approximately indicates their relatedness of the journals in terms of methodology. The size of the label and circle of a document is determined by the citation weight/impact of that documents, whereas the position of a term, determines the cluster of publication year to which the document belongs. Lines between documents represent links.

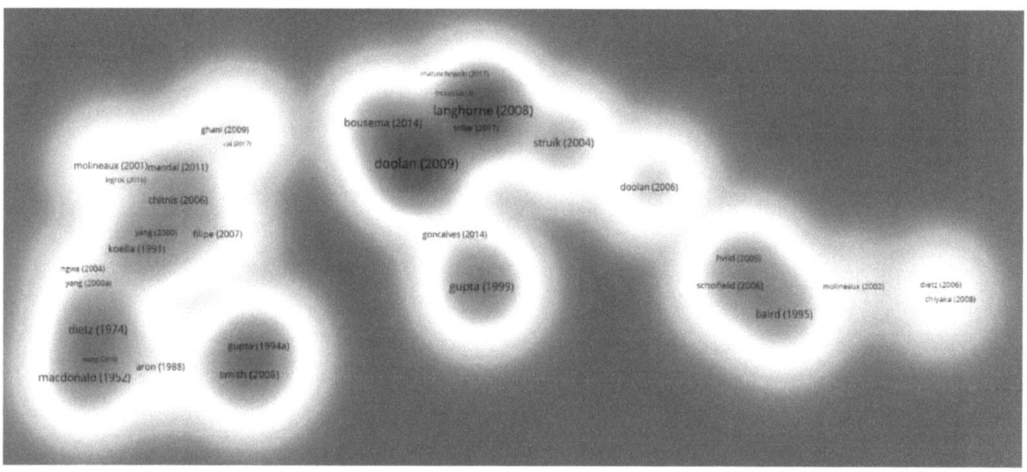

Figure 10: **Density visualization of document citations.** The positioning of the terms in this figure is the same with that of Figure 9. The density ranges from highly dense points to low dense points.

in early childhood and gradually wanes into adulthood as a result of slow acquisition of immunity with age and time. Also, it can be seen that the prevalence in adults is highest at intermediate infection rates. This is consistent with the infection pattern summarized by Boyd for tropical Africa [60] and also with the speculations of some epidemiologist that partial control, which leads to a moderate reduction of transmission from initially high levels, could increase adult prevalence [148], [63]. While immunity to malaria generally rises with age, especially in places with the highest forces of infection and stabilizes at adulthood, this increase with respect to age is not noticeable at low force of infection.

The model described in Equation 6.B.1 is an advance compared to some early models [40], [95], [203] since it illustrates how the reduction in transmission can make things worst for adults by diminishing naturally acquired immunity. Nevertheless, it gives a simplistic description of the interaction between immune responses and the population biology of malaria. This is because, the classification of humans into discrete categories does not reveal the fact that malaria parasite populations can exist at various densities within the human hosts. Aron [181] has shown how such false negatives, which result in underestimation of the prevalence among older age groups, can also confound the statistics of prevalence, rates of infection and apparent recovery. This suggests that an accurate model will need to abandon the approach of dividing people into discrete classes of infected and uninfected, and move toward a more detailed description in which the clinical symptoms and the immune response depend upon the magnitude of the parasite burden in the individual host.

In view of the above, Aron [43] developed age-specific density-dependent model as a different characterization of immunity that is boosted by exposure. The model characterizes the experience of a birth cohort based on: the asexual parasites density at age α, $p(\alpha)$; the immunity level geared against asexual parasite at age α, $r(\alpha)$; and gametocyte density at age α, $g(\alpha)$. The interaction between immunity and infection is modeled by assuming that the immunity against asexual parasitemia, r increases at a rate proportional to the asexual parasitemia whereas in the absence of parasitemia, it decreases. The density model is given as

$$\begin{aligned}\frac{dp}{d\alpha} &= \upsilon - (r + r_b)p, \\ \frac{dr}{d\alpha} &= ap - \beta r, \\ \frac{dg}{d\alpha} &= \gamma p e^{-(r+r_b)T} - \delta g,\end{aligned} \tag{6.B.2}$$

where υ is the influx rate of the asexual parasites (also called the force of infection) which declines at a clearance rate $r + r_b$ (see [146] for a robust formula for υ). The clearance rate is the sum of the rate that denotes the effect of acquired immunity r and the background rate r_b. T is the development period after which the gametocytes are produced by the asexual parasite, δ is the clearance rate of the gametocytes. Thus, the density of asexual parasites and gametocytes as a function of age, simulated from the above model is given in Figure 11. It can be seen from Figure 11 that the patterns for asexual parasites are different from that of gametocytes. It appears that compartmental model (Figure 6.2 a) characterize different levels of endemicity better than the density model (Figure 11 a).

However, the density model captures the repression of malaria as a result of reduced parasite densities, based on the levels of usage of antimalarial drug reflected in rates of recovery. In comparison with the compartmental model, the density model did not capture the potential of reduced transmission to increase malaria prevalence in older age groups, as predicted in the former model (see Equation 6.B.1). Thus, it is not wrong to expect that both models might have been created for different cases. Perhaps, the compartmental model was intended to be used for the study of prevalence whereas the density model

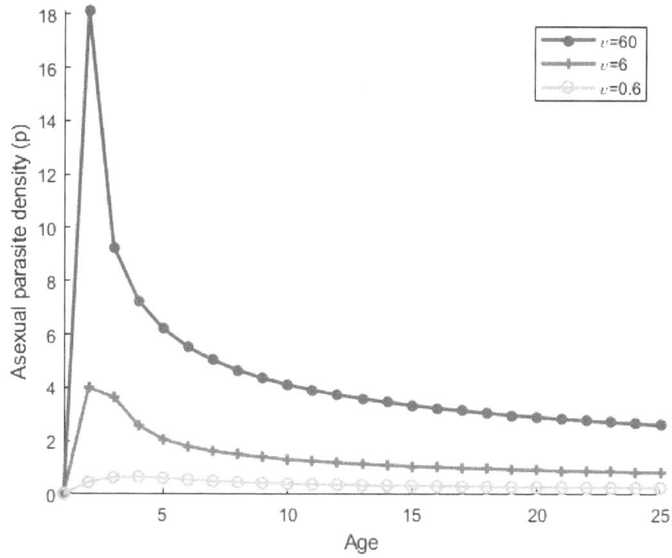

(a)

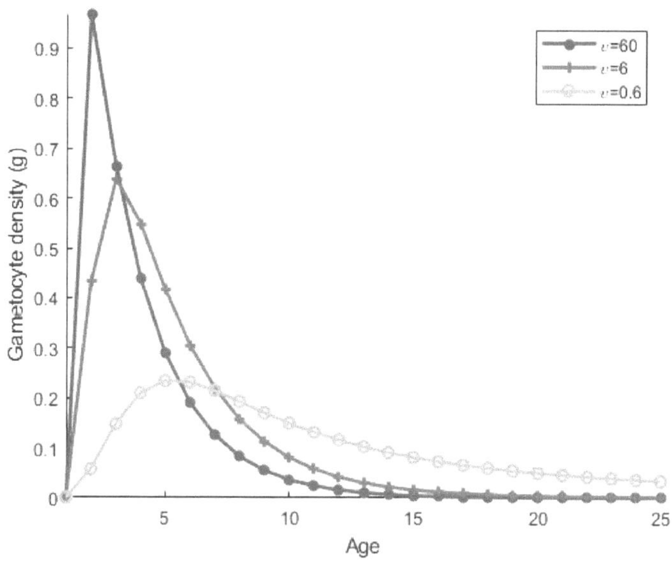

(b)

Figure 11: The density of (a) asexual parasites (b) gametocytes as a function of age simulated using the density model [43], for different parasite influx with $r_b = 0.7$, $a = 0.3$, $\beta = 0.005$, $\gamma = 0.5$, $T = 1$ and $\delta = 0.5$.

seemed to be better for studying parasite densities. As suggested by Aron [43], it could also be that each model is suitable for different ranges of infection rates. A density model could be appropriate when infection rates are so high in the sense that one does not have the whole time to clear infection before being reinfected, while the reverse is the case for a compartmental model. Obviously, these arguments are either not true or unconvincing because all prevalence indicators should be functions of density and diagnostic detection sensitivity rather than binary factors. This density model also models a collective behavior of a group and specific individual characteristics such as disease history, can not be tracked. The Aron models [43], [44] have in simplistically demonstrated what could happen if malaria transmission is reduced but did not address any factor that could lead to such reductions in transmission.

III

Mathematical Epidemiology including Mosquito Dynamics and Control Theory

CHAPTER 7

Multi-strain Host-vector Dengue Modelling: Dynamics and Control

Peter Rashkov*
Institute of Mathematics and Informatics, Bulgarian Academy of Sciences, Sofia, Bulgaria
** corresponding author, e-mail: p.rashkov@math.bas.bg*

Ezio Venturino
Dipartimento di Matematica "Giuseppe Peano", Università di Torino, Torino, Italy

Bob W. Kooi
Faculty of Science, VU University Amsterdam, Amsterdam, The Netherlands

CONTENTS

7.1 Introduction 118
7.2 Description of the models 119
7.2.1 Equilibria and basic reproduction number $\mathcal{R}_0$ 121
7.2.2 Time scale separation 122
7.2.3 Example: SIR-UV model 124
7.3 Two-strain dengue models 125
7.3.1 Host-only models 125
7.3.2 Host-vector models 128
7.4 Comparison of host-only and host-vector model 130
7.4.1 Results for autonomous systems 130
7.4.2 Results for seasonally-forced systems 131
7.5 Modeling and analysis of control measures for dengue fever 132
7.5.1 Description of a model with vaccination 132
7.5.1.1 Analysis of the SIRvUV model 133
7.5.1.2 Sensitivity analysis of the SIRvUV model 136
7.5.2 Model with vector control 137
7.5.2.1 Analysis of the SIRqVM model 139
7.5.2.2 Sensitivity analysis of the SIRqVM model 140
7.5.3 Viability analysis of vector control 141
7.6 Conclusions 142

DOI: 10.1201/9781003035992-7

7.A Time scale separation, example: SIR-UV model 147
7.B Parameter values 148

7.1 INTRODUCTION

Epidemiological models often must balance between accurate description of the disease dynamics, the different scales of modelling (within-host/micro scale, or population/macro scale), and the associated levels of complexity which allow for establishing tractable causal relationships in the health problems at hand. In the classical compartmental epidemiological models the human population is subdivided into two (susceptible and infected, SI, SIS-models), or three (susceptible, infected and removed/ recovered, SIR-models) compartments of individuals. This dichotomy is based on the importance of immunity against the disease in the situation of interest, and whether immunity is transient or permanent.

Ordinary differential equations describe the changes in the sizes of the different compartments. This means that with the analysis of these models use is made of analytical and numerical methods from nonlinear dynamical system theory. Epidemiological models have properties in common and as a result specific nomenclature is introduced, we mention the number $\mathcal{R}_0$, see for instance [18]. Continuous-time, deterministic compartmental mathematical models are most common tools to simulate and analyze epidemic outbreak, spread and course [5]. Stochastic models for epidemics also exist and they find application to emerging fields in mathematical epidemiology such as the study of epidemics on networks [6, 33].

However, in cases of vector-borne diseases such as dengue, malaria, yellow fever, zika, and so on, one must incorporate the presence of the vector population which plays a role as *carrier* or *vector* of the pathogen between the human hosts. Dengue fever (DF) causes a spectrum of diseases in humans ranging form clinically inapparent to severe and sometimes fatal hemorrhagic form and the associated dengue shock syndrome. Generally, dengue models are extensions of the classical models to account for multiple (two) serotypes of the virus and their interaction. An important characteristic observed from serological tests for dengue is that there are four different serotypes of the virus which can exist simultaneously and co-circulate in the human population (labelled in the literature as DENV-1 to DENV-4). Hence, in this case a model must reflect this variety in the types of dengue virus present both in the human and in the vector populations.

The main vectors of dengue transmission are the mosquitoes of the *Aedes* genus (*Ae. aegypti* and *Ae. albopictus*). These vectors are in the process of establishing themselves in the Europe due to multiple factors (climate patterns, increased travel and trade) and this has led to several dengue outbreaks in Southern Europe. Hence, study of the dengue epidemiology is important for health policymakers in Europe.

Since dengue is characterized by a multitude of specific mechanisms that drive the course of the disease (possibility of reinfection, antibody-dependent enhancement (ADE) [30, 28], and so on), the mathematical models often have many compartments and become high-dimensional. Dengue models without ADE but with or without temporary cross-immunity are proposed and studied in [22, 23, 24], with ADE in multiple strain host-only models [26, 12, 2, 1, 34], as well as host-vector models [25, 27, 44, 54, 42, 41]. By using different dimension reduction arguments to construct mathematically tractable models it is possible to focus on different aspects of the disease dynamics.

We shall discuss the *complexity reduction* by the means of time scale separation and singular perturbation analysis. These *model reduction* methods allow for the rigorous set-up of host-only models which represent the dynamics of a vector-borne disease, but without explicit inclusion of the vector population. We are interested in the role of vector modelling in models with multiple dengue virus serotypes and give an overview of the literature. Some models consider a single virus serotype/strain and model host-vector interactions [22]. Similar models are widely used in the modeling of other vector-borne diseases such as malaria. Many host-only models include implicitly the vector in their parameters [26, 12, 2, 43, 1, 34], whereas real world control measures (entomological surveillance, insecticide or larvicide spraying, fumigation, repellents for personal protection, long-lasting insecticidal nets) are usually aimed at altering the vector's demography, or host seeking behavior.

Those host-only models are not directly suited for studies of effects such as pest control or personal protection via repellents, which influence the mosquito dynamics, so such models require the explicit inclusion of vector dynamics. We provide an overview of host-vector models and approaches for complexity reduction based on time-scale separation. Finally, we touch upon simple dengue models incorporating control measures for dengue given by vaccination campaigns or control measures targeted at the vector (personal protection, use of repellents, and so on) that can be used to study efficacy of the measures undertaken to reduce the disease burden.

7.2 DESCRIPTION OF THE MODELS

Mechanisms included in epidemic models are transmission, i.e. contact either between susceptible and infected or, in the case of vector-borne diseases, between humans and vectors (mosquitoes), infection of susceptible hosts/vectors, recovery, development of temporary or lifelong immunity, development of cross-immunity, possibility of reinfection by a virus of a different serotype (strain). The basic models are the classical SI, SIS and SIR models where a (typically constant) population is subdivided in two or three compartments of individuals: susceptible, infected and recovered.

Demographic trends in the host and vector populations are usually neglected; hence, birth and death of the two populations is such that the total number of individuals in the populations remains constant over time. However, a seasonally varying vector population over time can be considered to account for seasonally changing climatic factors such as temperature or rainfall that affect the vector's breeding pattern, [51]. A common simplification in the modelling is to incorporate the seasonally changing vector population as a periodic forcing (often sinusoidal) onto the population size.

The earlier models were extensions of the epidemiological models used to model and simulate epidemics. Specific mechanisms for the dengue fever are modeled by adding other compartments. To reflect the epidemiological data we consider susceptible individuals without a previous dengue infection S_0, primary infected with i-th strain I_i, and recovered R_i from a primary infection respectively with strain $i = 1, 2, 3, 4$ depending on the total number of strains considered. After a period of a temporary cross immunity, recovered individuals in class R_i move to the class S_i of susceptible individuals with a history of a primary dengue infection with i-th strain $i = 1, 2, 3, 4$.

The underlying assumption of multi-strain dengue models is that infection with a given strain DENV-$i, i = 1, 2, 3, 4$ confers life-long strain-specific immunity. However, there are multiple approaches to modelling the transitions between the compartments depending on whether the model includes a period of cross-immunity. These will be described in detail in the following Section. In general multi-strain models assume that reinfection with a different strain is possible: the individuals in class S_i are then prone to reinfection and transition to the class I_{ij} with a history of a primary dengue infection with i-th strain and secondary infection with j-th strain, $i \neq j$. Because tertiary infections are rare, individuals from classes I_{ij} develop life-long immunity (global removed class R) and do not contribute to the force of infected thereafter. For vectors, we denote by U the susceptible and by V the infected individuals.

In a review paper on models and analysis for dengue [7] a systematic overview of all types of models is given with a "phylogenetic tree" of selected articles till 2012. We focus here on two-strain models only, but we mention that also multiple strain models with 1,2,3,4 or n serotypes are formulated and analyzed (see [32, Table 1]). Furthermore, we do not claim completeness and we focus on the most important mechanisms involved in modeling dengue fever: demographics (rate of birth and death), two-way vector-host transmission (and its respective approximation as host-to-host transmission), rate of infection or force of infection, anti-body-enhancement, (temporary) cross immunity, seasonal fluctuations and the import of infected individuals.

Transmission of the disease occurs when a diseased individual meets another host individual in the host-only model, or by an encounter with a individual vector in the host-vector model. The number of host individuals is denoted by N and the one of the vector population by M. We assume that the mosquitoes live in an environment of fixed size which is proportional to M. In this way the area-density of the vector-population remains constant when the size of the environment changes over time. Then, for host-only models [26, 12, 1, 34] the force of infection is $\beta I/N$ and for the host-vector models [42, 41] it is BV/M. This is based on the law of mass action, where I/N and V/M represent the probability of an susceptible human encountering an infected individual or a vector, respectively while β and B capture the respective encounter and pathogen transmission rates.

In the literature the formulation of the force of infection is discussed in many papers, we mention [20, 8]. Often the focus is on the comparison of density- (βI) versus frequency-dependency ($\beta I/N$) in the case of the single-strain SIR-model. Note that density is here a ratio of number of individuals and in this context different from the area-density mentioned above.

In the case of a vector-borne disease, such as dengue, the situation is more complex because contact between individuals belonging to different populations (host and vector) is involved which are not required to live in the same area, these areas only have to overlap. Here we used the same type of force of infection for both, namely frequency dependent. Recently in [11, 10] the authors use multi-patch formulations to model spatial-distributions of the dispersal of the individuals in the populations [11, 10] in order to take for instance spatial-heterogeneity within populations into account.

In [4, 45, 48, 46] the same host-vector vector-borne dengue system is modeled but the denominator of both force of infection terms is proportional to the human population numbers, N. In other words the force of infection of mosquitoes upon hosts is taken as density dependent, but the force of infection of host upon mosquitoes is frequency-dependent. Only when the sizes of the areas where host and vector live change proportionally, this model formulation is the same as model (7.4).

This work considers recent papers focusing on modeling of the epidemiological mechanisms specific for dengue fever and control measures such as vaccination campaigns and vector control.

7.2.1 Equilibria and basic reproduction number $\mathcal{R}_0$

In the study of disease dynamics described by a dynamical system one seeks to perform a qualitative analysis of the states where the system is at rest, namely the equilibria. At such equilibria the sizes of the compartments do not change over time. The equilibria analysis is useful for studying the *asymptotic behavior* of the model, which includes conditions under which the disease will be eliminated (the infected compartment will approach zero) or whether it will persist and become endemic (the infected compartment will be strictly positive). This fundamental question of determining existence and stability of disease-free versus endemic states pervades the mathematical epidemiology literature.

In the epidemiological literature one searches for a measure that tells whether an epidemic will occur or not. This purpose is served by the *basic reproduction number* $\mathcal{R}_0$ representing the number of secondary cases that one case generates on average over the course of the whole of its infectious period in an otherwise uninfected population [19, 18, 53]. It is a dimensionless quantity dependent on the parameters of the model equations. *The next-generation calculation* approach of $\mathcal{R}_0$ [19, 22, 18, 53, 27] has been used successfully in analyzing a whole class of compartmental models dealing with the transition from the disease-free to the endemic state or the reverse situation leading to the disease elimination. The number $\mathcal{R}_0$ is used frequently as a rule-of-thumb for determining the presence of an epidemic. The following threshold is established: whenever $\mathcal{R}_0 > 1$ the disease persists and there is an epidemic, and whenever $\mathcal{R}_0 < 1$ there is no epidemic and the disease fades away.

The transition between the elimination and endemic disease can also be studied by *bifurcation theory*: in which case the threshold is fixed by a so called transcritical bifurcation. That is $\mathcal{R}_0 = 1$ at the TC-point and therefore the associated threshold values are equal. The stable disease-free becomes unstable when a parameter is varied and there originates a stable (for a non-catastrophic or supercritical TC) or an unstable (for a catastrophic or subcritical TC) endemic equilibrium. In the second case, the second rule that $\mathcal{R}_0 < 1$ implying no epidemic is violated. Therein the transcritical bifurcation produces an unstable endemic equilibrium, and the term used in the epidemiology literature is a *backward bifurcation* [29, 53] instead of subcritical often used in the nonlinear dynamical system theory literature. Consequently, in the parameter region where $\mathcal{R}_0 < 1$ a bistable regime of another stable endemic equilibrium (or limit cycle) may coexist with the stable disease-free equilibrium and an epidemic can occur despite $\mathcal{R}_0$ being under the threshold value [27].

Coming back to a *multi-strain model*, the characteristic long-term dynamics, in addition to an equilibrium could exhibit several features such as limit cycles or chaotic behavior, because of the large number of equations and highly non-linear couplings among them. Besides the trivial disease-free equilibrium, endemic equilibria with a single strain (also known as *boundary* or *exclusion equilibria*) and endemic equilibria where multiple strains are present, are possible.

As an example, the presence of multiple strains in the model [25, 41] gives rise to multiple equilibria. Depending on the parameter values, their local asymptotic stability changes. In [25] the boundary equilibria are always locally asymptotically stable. While the general structure of these models is broadly similar, the presence of intermediate recovered host classes R_1, R_2 in the model [41] allows both boundary equilibria to be locally asymptotically unstable. This shows that the nonlinear interactions between the model compartments are an important factor in driving the asymptotic behavior of the model.

Furthermore, in realistic dengue models with infection/recovery rates above the $\mathcal{R}_0$ threshold the endemic equilibrium becomes unstable leading to more complex long-term dynamical behavior such as limit cycles and chaos. These types of dynamics can be studied using bifurcation analysis. Limit cycles describe periodic behaviour and typically arise from a *Hopf bifurcation*. For chaotic dynamics another tool for the study of non-linear dynamical systems, namely the calculation of Lyapunov exponents can be used [52]. Many of the multi-strain models show mathematical symmetry and this property governs specific types of bifurcations [2, 1, 34, 41].

7.2.2 Time scale separation

Mathematical models for vector-borne diseases are natural candidates for time scale separation analysis based on *singular perturbation theory*. Typically the vector epidemiology occurs at a much faster time scale due to the vector's much shorter life cycle relative to the host. The vector dynamics is, therefore, slaved by the host dynamics. This is an approach which allows model reduction, whereby the complexity of the model is reduced by considering the dynamics of some variables to be in a quasi-steady state, and transforming the original system of ordinary differential equations into a system of algebraic-differential equations.

Singular perturbation theory deals with systems whose solutions evolve on different time scales with a ratio characterized by a small parameter $0 < \varepsilon \ll 1$

$$\frac{d\mathbf{x}}{dt} = \mathbf{f}(\mathbf{x},\mathbf{y}), \quad \frac{d\mathbf{y}}{dt} = \epsilon \mathbf{g}(\mathbf{x},\mathbf{y}), \quad \mathbf{x} \in \mathbb{R}^m, \mathbf{y} \in \mathbb{R}^n . \tag{7.1}$$

In the context of vector-borne diseases, system (7.1) has the following interpretation: $\mathbf{x}$ describes the unknowns in the vector compartments (variables U, V_i denoting respectively, the susceptible and infected by DENV-i vectors), and $\mathbf{y}$ in the host compartments (variables S_i, I_i, R_i). The dynamics of the vector is given by $\mathbf{f}$, and the dynamics of the host by $\mathbf{g}$.

A change of time scale $\tau = \varepsilon t$ gives the *slow system* in the time scale of the host population:

$$\varepsilon \frac{d\mathbf{x}}{d\tau} = \mathbf{f}(\mathbf{x},\mathbf{y}), \quad \frac{d\mathbf{y}}{d\tau} = \mathbf{g}(\mathbf{x},\mathbf{y}) . \tag{7.2}$$

Systems (7.1) and (7.2) are equivalent if $\varepsilon \neq 0$. Letting $\varepsilon = 0$ in (7.2) leads to the *reduced system*:

$$0 = \mathbf{f}(\mathbf{x},\mathbf{y}), \quad \frac{d\mathbf{y}}{d\tau} = \mathbf{g}(\mathbf{x},\mathbf{y}) . \tag{7.3}$$

The differential-algebraic system (7.3) describes the evolution of the slow variable $\mathbf{y}(\tau)$ constrained to the set $\{(\mathbf{x},\mathbf{y}) \mid \mathbf{f}(\mathbf{x},\mathbf{y}) = 0\}$.

With a good Ansatz the relation $\mathbf{f}(\mathbf{x},\mathbf{y}) = 0$ can be rewritten as $\mathbf{x} = q(\mathbf{y})$, resulting in the *quasi-steady state approximation (QSSA)*:

$$\frac{d\mathbf{y}}{d\tau} = \mathbf{g}(q(\mathbf{y}),\mathbf{y}) .$$

The QSSA assumption is the approach followed by the host-only models for vector-borne diseases that take all fast variables representing classes of vector population to react instantaneously to changes in the slow variables, and hence assume them to be in a quasi-steady state.

In order to get a better approximation for $0 < \varepsilon \ll 1$, we follow the *geometric singular perturbation technique*. This approach has been exploited for single strain dengue [50, 44, 42] and for multi-strain dengue models [41]. In particular, it provides a rigorous framework for reducing the model complexity and deriving robust reduced-order approximations of the full host-vector model to a host-only model.

7.2.3 Example: SIR-UV model

We illustrate this approach for a simple single-strain host-vector SIR-UV model, reading

$$\frac{dS}{dt} = \varepsilon\left(\mu(N-S) - \frac{\beta}{M}SV\right), \quad \frac{dI}{dt} = \varepsilon\left(\frac{\beta}{M}SV - (\gamma+\mu)I\right), \quad \frac{dR}{dt} = \varepsilon(\gamma I - \mu R),$$
$$\frac{dU}{dt} = \nu(M-U) - \frac{\vartheta}{N}UI, \quad \frac{dV}{dt} = \frac{\vartheta}{N}UI - \nu V,$$

discussed in [44] and recently in [42]. Assuming the total host and vector populations N, M to be constant over time, we arrive to the ODE model

$$\frac{dS}{dt} = \varepsilon\left(\mu(N-S) - \frac{\beta}{M}SV\right), \quad \frac{dI}{dt} = \varepsilon\left(\frac{\beta}{M}SV - (\gamma+\mu)I\right), \tag{7.4a}$$
$$\frac{dV}{dt} = \frac{\vartheta}{N}(M-V)I - \nu V. \tag{7.4b}$$

The trajectory in (S,I)-plane of the system (7.4) is shown in Figure 7.1 (full model, blue curve) where the parameter values are given in Table 7.B.1. In [42] is was shown that with these parameter values the vector dynamics occurs at a much faster time-scale relative to the host's. This means that after a fast transient dynamics the slow dynamics occurs near a manifold that is a smooth surface in $\mathbb{R}^3$ given by the QSSA that reads:

$$V_{QSSA} = \frac{\vartheta MI}{\vartheta I + \nu N}, \quad V^S_{QSSA} = \frac{\vartheta M}{\nu N}I, \tag{7.5}$$

where V^S_{QSSA} denotes the value of the infected vector population under QSSA when the number of infected humans I is small. This plane is named $\mathcal{M}_0$ in App. 7.A. Starting with the same initial conditions as for the full model, the reduced system where V_{QSSA} is substituted in (7.4a), the trajectory is also shown in Figure 7.1 (left, QSSA green curve). Only after some transient dynamics this trajectory is close the that of the full model.

Here a mechanistic derivation is obtained for an infection mechanism with a saturated incidence rate where the force of infection is not linear in I but when the expression $V = V_{QSSA}$ is substituted in the infection rate terms in (7.4a), it is a hyperbolic relationship. In the epidemiological literature it has been used in [15, 21, 36]. In [15] the use of a saturated incidence rate is motivated because for large I the population may tend to reduce the number of contacts per unit of time. Below we will, in a host-only model formulation, use the simplified linearized expression V^S_{QSSA} which holds only for small I to get the unsaturated incidence rate back. This gives an "ordering" of nested models from a host-vector model to a host-only model with the QSSA-host-only model inbetween.

In Figure 7.1 also two approximations of V for terms up to $\mathcal{O}(\varepsilon)$ are shown (*left panel*, red curve) and up to $\mathcal{O}(\varepsilon^2)$ (*right panel*, red curve) where $\varepsilon = 1$. See also Appendix 7.A. For the first-order approximation the trajectory converges onto a so called spurious, stable equilibrium. This unexpected spurious equilibrium exists in addition to the expected endemic equilibrium in the full model. The spurious equilibrium exists with $S < N$ and $I > 0$

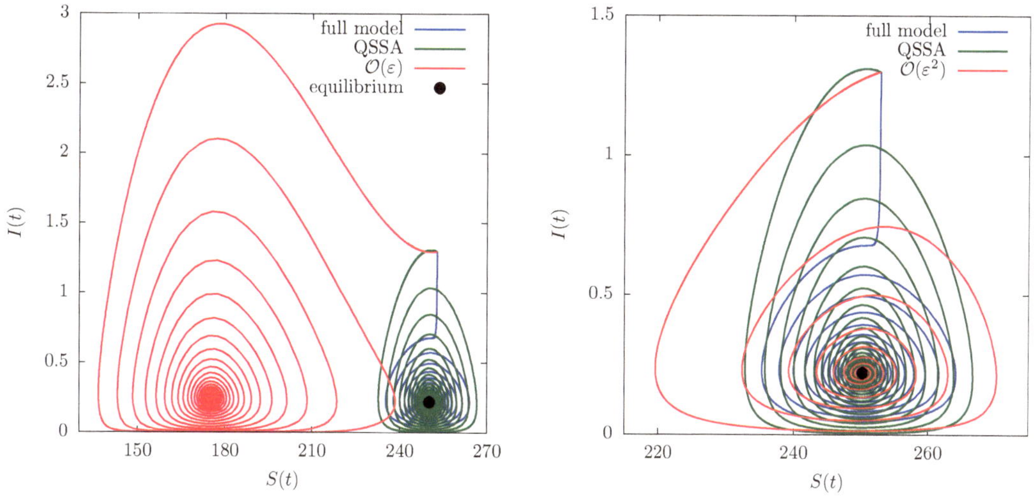

Figure 7.1: Trajectory in (S, I)-plane of (7.4) and trajectories with two approximations of V: the $\mathcal{O}(\varepsilon^0)$ or QSSA approximation and for terms up to $\mathcal{O}(\varepsilon)$ (left) and up to $\mathcal{O}(\varepsilon^2)$ (right).

only when $\varepsilon > 0.175482$. When $\varepsilon = 0.175482$ the spurious equilibrium equals $S = N$ and $I = 0$. Consequently the first order approximation approach can fail for $\varepsilon > 0.175482$ when the initial data of the trajectory is far from the expected endemic equilibrium close in the full model.

The second-order approximation does not have this shortcoming. However, for the initial condition used the calculated transient dynamics is also poor for the second-order approximation with $\varepsilon = 1$. The technique is applicable only when the starting point is sufficiently close to the equilibrium as in the case of the QSSA trajectory in Figure 7.1 (QSSA green curve). In (7.4) a value for ε was quantified by its interpretation as the ratio of the rates of changes of the state variables of the host and vector population near equilibrium. It was argued that $\varepsilon = 1/365$ is suitable value for the SIR-UV model. Simulations (not shown) for the first- and second-order approximations indicate that when starting close to the $\mathcal{M}_0$-plane defined in the Appendix 7.A, there are no spurious equilibria but higher-order approximations do not improve much the QSSA solutions when $\varepsilon = 1/365$.

7.3 TWO-STRAIN DENGUE MODELS

In this section we describe the two-strain dengue models, namely the Host-only and the host-vector model. The analysis of these models relies heavily on numerical techniques where the time dependency on parameter values is obtained by simulations and bifurcation analysis. Besides equilibria and limit cycles, both models show also chaotic dynamics.

7.3.1 Host-only models

In host-only models [2, 1, 12, 26, 34], the vector dynamics is considered implicitly in the parameters by assuming that the size of the infected vector population is proportional to that of the infected host population. In that respect this modeling approach closely resembles models of airborne diseases such as flu, measles, SARS. These models consider multiple virus strains and two characteristics of dengue fever which are important for the host epidemiology: antibody-dependent enhancement and temporary cross-immunity between the two strains.

In [43] models based on immunological serotype (strain) interactions are studied. They define two mechanisms: the increase in transmissibility during secondary infection (included as a factor in the force of infection terms for secondary infections) and enhancement of the susceptibility to secondary infection (included as an extra loss in the recovery rate terms by a factor for the force of infection). Figure 7.4 in [43] presents the analysis results by changing the two parameters presenting the two mechanisms show that both have qualitatively similar effects.

In this review, we only consider further the enhancement by increased transmissibility during secondary infection by a different strain. We also consider neutralization where the effect is a decrease of the transmissibility. In [26] a two-strain model with an antibody effect is proposed, where pre-existing immunity to dengue virus could be a factor for the development of severe dengue in a subsequent infection. The model includes a parameter ϕ representing the degree of antibody-dependent enhancement ($\phi > 1$) or neutralization ($\phi < 1$) caused by the presence of cross-reactive antibodies. The enhancement/neutralization is interpreted as an increase/decrease in the transmission probability of the dengue virus. The model structure is of the SEII-type (susceptible-exposed-infected-infected), because an immediate transition occurs between the compartments of exposed to one strain hosts to infected by a different strain hosts, in other words, there is no period of recovery after the primary infection. Thus, [26] implicitly assumes co-infection with both strains as there is no distinction between the compartments. If the antibody effect is strongly neutralizing ($\phi = 0$), the authors in [26] demonstrate that the strain with the higher basic reproduction number $\mathcal{R}_0$ will displace the other. However, the model exhibits periodic and chaotic behavior in large parameter ranges, under the assumption of strong ADE for one or both strains.

The models proposed in [49, 12, 43] including a compartment for the recovered from the primary or from both infections and can be thought of an extensions of the model [26]. The compartments of primary recovered hosts is susceptible to an infection with the different strain. These models are of the SIRIR-type (susceptible-infected-recovered-infected-recovered) type. The model equations [12, Eq.1] are easily generalized to a disease with n strains (serotypes).

In contrast to [26], the authors of [12] assume there is only antibody-dependent enhancement, so the compartments of hosts with secondary infection are more infectious. Analysis of the basic reproduction numbers $\mathcal{R}_0^i, i = 1, 2$ for each strain shows that if both $\mathcal{R}_0^i > 1$, the strain with the higher $\mathcal{R}_0^i$ will displace the other, and the boundary endemic equilibrium is asymptotically stable. In case $\mathcal{R}_0^1 = \mathcal{R}_0^2$, both boundary endemic equilibria are unstable, there is a coexistence equilibrium, and periodic or deterministic chaotic behavior near its vicinity is demonstrated by numerical bifurcation analysis.

The author of [49] studies the effect of ADE ($\phi > 1$) on the synchronization of infected by the different pathogen strains. They find that if seasonal forcing is included in the model, it tends to stabilise the dynamic patters by synchronising them. Thus, periodic or quasi-periodic cycles of each strain's prevalence are observed unless the parameter ϕ is large. In [43] the ADE is considered to act upon the force of infection via two pathways: enhancement of transmission during a secondary dengue infection and increased susceptibility due to presence of non-neutralising cross-reactive antibodies. The model exhibits chaotic dynamics, and the simulations can reproduce the time series of observed dengue fever outbreaks based on data from Vietnam.

The two-strain host-only model from [2] builds upon these previous works by adding temporary cross-immunity to the model. It is of the SIRSIR-type: the recovered from a primary infection hosts after a period of cross immunity become susceptible to infection with a different strain. The flow of individuals from compartment R_i of those already recovered from strain DENV-i enters an intermediate compartment S_i of susceptible individuals to the other strain. The individuals from S_1 transition to class I_{12} and from S_2 to class I_{21} during a secondary infection. The equations of [2] include a parameter α describing the average duration of temporary cross-immunity (the time before transitioning from R_i to S_i is $1/\alpha$). In more detail the model is

$$\dot{S}_0 = -\frac{\beta_1}{N} S_0(I_1 + I_2 + \phi(I_{12} + I_{21})) + \mu(N - S_0), \tag{7.6a}$$

$$\dot{I}_1 = \frac{\beta_1}{N} S_0(I_1 + \phi I_{21}) - (\gamma + \mu) I_1, \quad \dot{I}_2 = \frac{\beta_1}{N} S_0(I_2 + \phi I_{12}) - (\gamma + \mu) I_2, \tag{7.6b}$$

$$\dot{I}_{12} = \frac{\beta_2}{N} S_1(I_2 + \phi I_{12}) - (\gamma + \mu) I_{12}, \quad \dot{I}_{21} = \frac{\beta_2}{N} S_2(I_1 + \phi I_{21}) - (\gamma + \mu) I_{21}, \tag{7.6c}$$

$$\dot{S}_1 = \alpha R_1 - \mu S_1 - \frac{\beta_2}{N} S_1(I_2 + \phi I_{12}), \quad \dot{S}_2 = \alpha R_2 - \mu S_2 - \frac{\beta_2}{N} S_2(I_1 + \phi I_{21}), \tag{7.6d}$$

$$\dot{R}_1 = \gamma I_1 - (\alpha + \mu) R_1, \quad \dot{R}_2 = \gamma I_2 - (\alpha + \mu) R_2 \,. \tag{7.6e}$$

In particular, numerical bifurcation analysis shows that the ADE parameter ϕ could be less than 1, but the system still exhibits a rich dynamic structure (Hopf bifurcations and chaotic attractors) due to the presence of $\alpha > 0$. The assumption $\phi < 1$ is backed up by the observation that virus carriers with a secondary infection are more likely to be hospitalized and thus, less likely to contribute to the infectivity than carriers, with a primary infection who are often asymptomatic.

In [1] the model from [2] is equipped with additional assumptions: a seasonal variation in the force of infection and import of infected individuals from an external population. The seasonal variation has the form of a cosine function and mirrors the seasonal fluctuations in vector prevalence due to climate factors. Chaotic dynamics is also observed in this model. A common feature of the parameter sets employed in [12, 2, 1] is the epidemiological symmetry between the virus strains; that is, the type of strain does not alter the force of infection. A different approach is taken in [35] where asymmetry in the infectious between the two strains is introduced. The numerical results demonstrate that the chaotic dynamics is less profound in the asymmetric case.

An extension of the model with age-structure of the host population and introduction four dengue strains is analyzed in [3], where vaccination of different age groups is included and simulations reveal that the vaccine is most effective in reducing the prevalence if only individuals with a primary infection are vaccinated. A common feature of the host-only models is to provide a mathematical model with reduced complexity which is able to reproduce the observed irregular patterns of dengue seroprevalence and strain co-circulation in tropical countries. Thus, a model with relatively few variables exhibits complex dynamical behaviour ranging from limit cycles to chaotic trajectories.

7.3.2 Host-vector models

Host-vector models describe also the temporal dynamics of the vector population (in the case of dengue or yellow fever, mosquitoes *Ae. egypti* or *Ae. albopictus*) which transmits the pathogen to humans. In this regard their structure is closer to the epidemiology of the disease. However, as we have noted, because of the inherent difference in time scales which characterise the dynamics of the host and the vector populations, these models are described by stiff systems of ordinary differential equations. Thus, robust numerical methods must be used for their integration in time.

Model [22] considers a single strain dengue model of SIR type for the human host and of SI type for the vector. The authors demonstrate that whenever $\mathcal{R}_0 > 1$ any oscillatory dynamics is transient and the system converges to the endemic equilibrium. Optimal control is introduced into single-strain dengue models and publications analyze a multitude of strategies targeting both humans or vectors, based on educational campaigns and entomological surveillance [47], vector control via insecticides [46], use of bed nets [14] and vaccination [48].

Explicit inclusion of the mosquito dynamics in multi-strain models for dengue increases the model dimension by including susceptible and infected by DENV-i type vectors. That explains why they are less frequent in the modelling literature. Furthermore, care must be taken when interpreting the model parameters. In host-only models [26, 12, 1, 34], infection rate per infected host is used, while host-vector models [44, 42, 41] employ infection rate per infected vector. Thus, it is important to be able to compare the parameters used in each type of model and assess the differences.

In [25] the vector was modeled explicitly and furthermore the effects of primary and secondary infections was modeled with temporary cross-immunity. Similar to [26], the authors in [25] do not introduce a separate class of hosts recovered from a primary infection. Analysis of equilibria in [25] shows the existence of an unstable endemic steady state. Hence, the asymptotic behavior of the model shows a long transient of coexisting strains before one of the strains is displaced by the other.

In [24] the authors consider a model of the SISIR-type for the host and SI- type of the vector with 2 dengue strains with cross-immunity. Their results state that if both strains confer total cross-immunity, competitive exclusion is always the result and coexistence is possible under the assumption of increased susceptibility to the strain in a secondary infection. This model with optimal control has been studied in [54].

In [41] the authors extend the model of [2] by including a vector population. The model is of the SIRSIR-type for the host and SI for the vector. The authors propose a model for dengue fever with two strains and temporary cross-immunity (α) and different likelihood of transmission from hosts with primary or secondary infections to vectors (ϕ). The vector is included explicitly and furthermore the different effects of primary and secondary infections due to ADE are modeled.

The model equations of [41] for the host dynamics are recalled here:

$$\dot{S}_0 = -\frac{B_1}{M} S_0 (V_1 + V_2) + \mu(N - S) \,, \tag{7.7a}$$

$$\dot{I}_1 = \frac{B_1}{M} S_0 V_1 - (\gamma + \mu) I_1 \,, \quad \dot{I}_2 = \frac{B_1}{M} S_0 V_2 - (\gamma + \mu) I_2 \,, \tag{7.7b}$$

$$\dot{R}_1 = \gamma I_1 - (\alpha + \mu) R_1 \,, \quad \dot{R}_2 = \gamma I_2 - (\alpha + \mu) R_2 \,, \tag{7.7c}$$

$$\dot{S}_1 = -\frac{B_2}{M} S_1 V_2 + \alpha R_1 - \mu S_1 \,, \quad \dot{S}_2 = -\frac{B_2}{M} S_2 V_1 + \alpha R_2 - \mu S_2 \,, \tag{7.7d}$$

$$\dot{I}_{12} = \frac{B_2}{M} S_1 V_2 - (\gamma + \mu) I_{12} \,, \quad \dot{I}_{21} = \frac{B_2}{M} S_2 V_1 - (\gamma + \mu) I_{21} \tag{7.7e}$$

and for the vector dynamics:

$$\dot{V}_1 = \frac{\vartheta}{N} (M - V_1 - V_2)(I_1 + \phi I_{21}) - \nu V_1 \,, \tag{7.7f}$$

$$\dot{V}_2 - \frac{\vartheta}{N} (M - V_1 - V_2)(I_2 + \phi I_{12}) - \nu V_2 \,. \tag{7.7g}$$

Comparison with the host-only model shows that due to a different virus transmission mechanism the force of infection terms and the infection rates differ. The discussion in Sec. 7.2.2 of system with two time scales for the host and vector dynamics gives a possibility to connect the parameter β in Eq. (7.6b) with B in Eq. (7.7b). In [42] the following equation was derived using the linearized expression in (7.5) for the force of infection where $V = V^S_{QSSA}$:

$$\frac{B_i}{M} V = \frac{B_i}{M} \frac{\vartheta M}{\nu N} I = \frac{\beta_i}{N} I \quad \text{with} \quad \beta_i = \frac{\vartheta}{\nu} B_i \,. \tag{7.8}$$

Using the parameter values from [2, 34] yields $B_i = \beta_i / 2$ and makes it possible to compare the results of the host-vector model (7.7) from [41] with those from for the host-only model (7.6) in [34].

Temporary cross-immunity is considered alongside a parameter that quantifies the differences in likelihood for host-to-vector transmission between infected individuals in a primary and a secondary dengue infection. This is motivated by the fact that individuals in a secondary infection may develop a severe form of dengue and require hospitalization, thus reducing their contact with the vector in the daily routine. The surprising result from the numerical bifurcation analysis is that the introduction of a vector population tends to stabilise the chaotic dynamics, which has been noticed with model assumptions in several contexts of host-only models. Only by introducing an ecologically-motivated seasonal forcing of the vector population is the chaotic regime restored for a wide variety of parameters. A review of seasonality effects in epidemiological models is given in [13].

7.4 COMPARISON OF HOST-ONLY AND HOST-VECTOR MODEL

7.4.1 Results for autonomous systems

Here we discuss the model under the assumption of a constant vector population over time. All results for the autonomous system (7.7) use reference parameter values given in App. 7.B from [2, 34, 44]. The results are compared with those for earlier models in the literature: [12, 2, 34, 26]. Important is to recall that in [1] a realistic description of recorded disease incidents was produced for empirical data sets of dengue fever in Thailand.

In Figure 7.2 the two parameter diagrams are shown for the host-only model (7.6) from [34] (panel **a**) and host-vector model (7.7) (panel **b**). The bifurcation pattern for the host-only model in Figure 7.2a is dominated by two Hopf bifurcations: one supercritical H^+ and the other H^-. Furthermore, there is one Torus bifurcation TR also called a Neimark-Sacker bifurcation. These results have been discussed in [34] and the reader is referred to

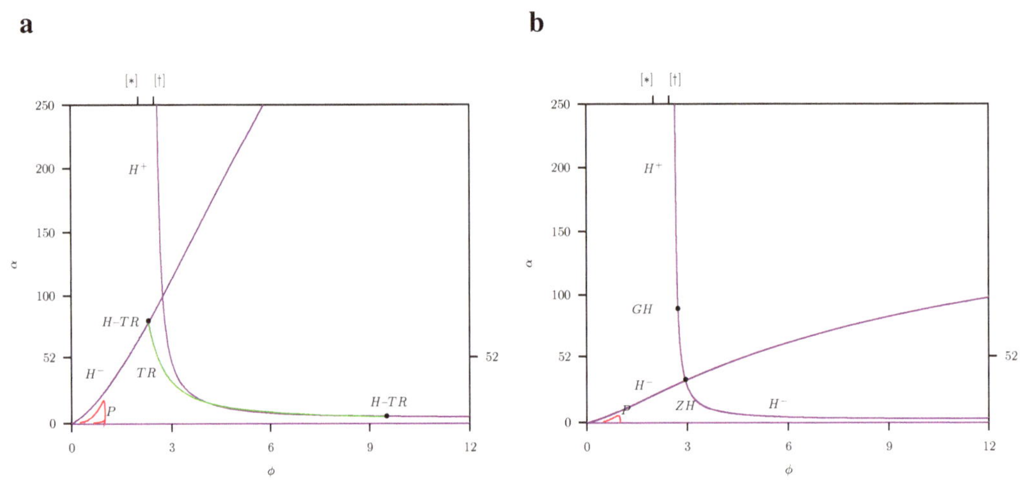

Figure 7.2: Two-parameter (ϕ, α) bifurcation diagram for the range $\phi \in [0, 12]$ and $\alpha \in [0, 250]$. **a** the host-only model (7.6) from [2] with $B(t)$ similar to (7.7) with $\eta = 0.1$ and **b** the host-vector model with $M(t)$ (7.7) with $\eta = 0.1$ in Eq. 7.9. For $\alpha \to \infty$ the Hopf bifurcation converges to the ϕ parameter value [†] for the model of [12] and [*] marks the value $\phi = 2.5$ in [26].

this paper for a detailed discussion. The Hopf bifurcations occur also for the host-vector model Figure 7.2b but there is no torus bifurcation TR.

7.4.2 Results for seasonally-forced systems

In [1, 41] dealing with dengue fever modelling, we considered a seasonally changing mosquito population due to climate factors such as temperature or rainfall. For the host-vector model the number of mosquitoes M is modeled as a seasonally-forced term and is given explicitly by a cosine function. For the host-only model in [1] the infection rate $\beta(t)$ was changed periodically:

$$M(t) = M_0(1+\eta\cos\omega(t+\varphi)) , \quad \beta(t) = \beta_0(1+\eta\cos\omega(t+\varphi)) . \tag{7.9}$$

Parameter M_0 is the mean vector population size in the host-vector model and β_0 the mean value for the host-only model. In the host-vector case the number of mosquitoes changes over time but because we assume a changing area size, the mosquito density remains the same. The results for the seasonally forced host-only model (parameter $\beta(t)$ with $\eta = 0.35$), and the host-vector model (parameter $M(t)$ with $\eta = 0.1$) are compared in Fig. 7.3 in the lower range of the ratio of likelihoods of transmission from hosts with secondary and hosts with primary infection to vectors, $\phi \in [0, 1.2]$.

In conclusion, these results indicate that the dynamics predicted by both models is qualitatively but not quantitatively the same.

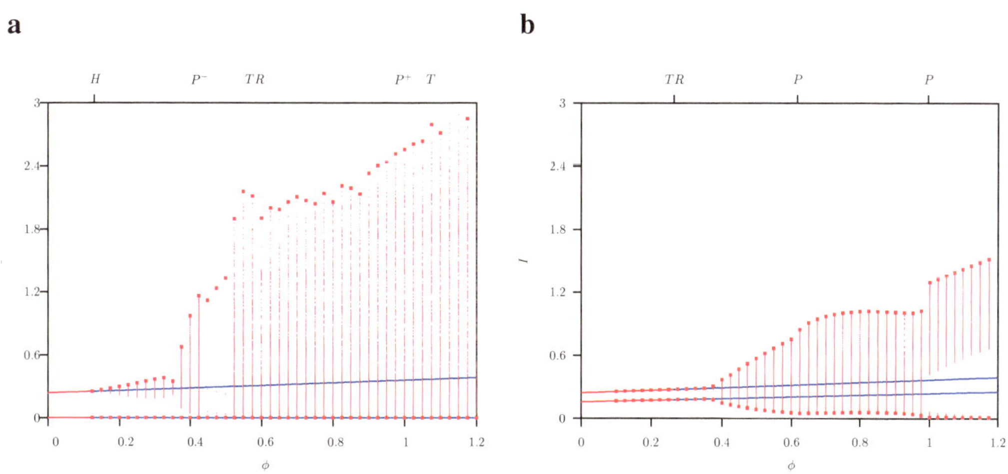

Figure 7.3: Two-strain non-autonomous **a** host-only model (7.6) and **b** host-vector model (7.7) with parameter $\alpha = 2$. The bullets mark the global maximum and minimum values for limit cycles for total infected I. Red indicates stable and blue unstable solutions.

7.5 MODELING AND ANALYSIS OF CONTROL MEASURES FOR DENGUE FEVER

The aim of vaccination is to protect the entire host population against dengue. Mathematical models for vaccination are reviewed in [32] with an overview of potential approaches. An important measure for the vaccination effectiveness, called *efficacy*, is the portion p of the population that acquires immunity. The threshold that assures eradication of dengue in the population is called the *critical vaccination threshold* p_c. In Fig. 2 of [32] the relationship between the basic reproduction number $\mathcal{R}_0 > 1$ and p_c is shown.

The basic reproduction number $\mathcal{R}_0$ (Section 7.2.1) for the vector-borne case is studied in [53] and in [16] for the analysis of a model very similar to the SIRvUV model (7.10). In [39] a simple example of a single-strain SIR-UV model is described and analyzed. In addition, the relationship between $\mathcal{R}_0$ and the critical vaccination proportion p_c is derived as $p_c > (1 - 1/\mathcal{R}_0)/p$, $0 \leq p \leq 1$ is the efficacy of the vaccination. That expression is only a rough estimate for the fraction of the population that must receive protection immunity especially due to the fact the dengue is a multi-serotype virus with cross-immunity effects. Exposure to a single serotype is generally assumed to give lifelong immunity to that serotype. However, the effect of immunity to one serotype on infections of the other serotype can lead to a more severe disease [32], ranging from clinically unapparent to the fatal hemorrhagic form and the associated dengue shock syndrome.

We model two control measures: vaccination and vector control. The model is the single-strain dengue model [44, 42] shown in (7.4). We use the parameter values given in Table 7.B.1 after [41]. The aim of vector control is again to protect the entire host population against dengue. Implementing a measure focusing on diminishing the number of mosquitoes one should not model the effectiveness of the change of their total number M like done in modelling seasonality (7.9) but a change of mosquitoes' death rate ν.

We analyze an extension of the single-strain host-vector model (7.4) by including control measures and therefore the focus is on changing parameter values that quantify the mechanisms enforcing the control, such as vaccination or mosquito control via insecticides, repellents, and other means.

7.5.1 Description of a model with vaccination

We use the simple model (7.4) and introduce new parameters to model vaccination, see also [16], namely: $0 \leq p_v \leq 1$ the fraction of newborns vaccinated and $0 \leq \alpha_v \leq 1$ the vaccine efficacy. Two new compartments for the vaccinated individuals are introduced: susceptible S_v and infected I_v. The model with vaccination, which we label SIRvUV, becomes

$$\dot{S} = -\frac{\beta}{M} SV + \mu((1-p_v)N - S)\,, \quad \dot{I} = \frac{\beta}{M} SV - (\gamma+\mu)I\,, \quad \dot{R} = \gamma(I+I_v) - \mu R\,, \tag{7.10a}$$

$$\dot{S}_v = -\frac{(1-\alpha_v)\beta}{M} S_v V + \mu(p_v N - S_v)\,, \quad \dot{I}_v = \frac{(1-\alpha_v)\beta}{M} S_v V - (\gamma+\mu)I_v \tag{7.10b}$$

$$\dot{U} = -\frac{\vartheta}{N} U(I+I_v) + \nu(M-U)\,, \quad \dot{V} = \frac{\vartheta}{N} U(I+I_v) - \nu V\,, \tag{7.10c}$$

$$N = S(t) + S_v(t) + I(t) + I_v(t) + R(t)\,, \quad M = U(t) + V(t)\,.$$

The human N and mosquito M population sizes are constant over time and therefore, the system can be reduced to a five dimensional system in the remaining state variables $S(t), I(t), V(t), S_v(t), I_v(t)$, $t \geq 0$.

7.5.1.1 *Analysis of the SIRvUV model*

When $p_v = 0$ and $\alpha_v = 0$ the vaccinated individuals behave just like the non-vaccinated and therefore the dynamics is the same as if no individuals were vaccinated. This is described by the SIR-UV model with $\varepsilon = 1$ in (7.4). If S vanishes in (7.10), the first equation implies either $N = 0$, which is of course senseless, or $p_v = 1$. In the extreme case $p_v = 1$ the system is effectively the SISUV-model [42] and becomes

$$\dot{S}_v = -\frac{(1-\alpha_v)\beta}{M} S_v V + \mu(N - S_v)\,, \quad \dot{I}_v = \frac{(1-\alpha_v)\beta}{M} S_v V - (\gamma+\mu)I_v\,, \quad \dot{R} = \gamma I_v - \mu R\,, \tag{7.11a}$$

$$\dot{U} = -\frac{\vartheta}{N} U I_v + \nu(M-U)\,, \quad \dot{V} = \frac{\vartheta}{N} U I_v - \nu V\,, \tag{7.11b}$$

$$N = S_v(t) + I_v(t) + R(t)\,, \quad M = U(t) + V(t)\,.$$

In [42] system (7.11) is studied with $\alpha_v = 0$. Using a reduction to a two-dimensional system, for the parameter values given in Table 7.B.1, the disease-free equilibrium is unstable and the endemic equilibrium is stable.

Note that in our case it is possible to introduce in (7.11) a compound parameter $\beta^* = (1-\alpha_v)\beta$. This means that the analysis of (7.11) is the same as the one performed in [42] where only the infection rate β is multiplied by a factor $1-\alpha_v$. Thus we can now safely assume in (7.10) that $S \neq 0$. There are two equilibria for system (7.10): the trivial, disease-free equilibrium $\mathcal{E}_0$ and the interior, endemic equilibrium $\mathcal{E}^*$. The trivial equilibrium equals

$$\mathcal{E}_0 = (S_0 = N(1-p_v),\ I_0 = 0,\ S_{v0} = p_v N,\ I_{v0} = 0,\ U_0 = M,\ V_0 = 0)\,, \tag{7.12}$$

and the Jacobian matrix evaluated at this point reads

$$J(\mathcal{E}_0) = \begin{pmatrix} -\mu & 0 & -\beta(1-p_v)\frac{N}{M} & 0 & 0 \\ 0 & -(\gamma+\mu) & \beta(1-p_v)\frac{N}{M} & 0 & 0 \\ 0 & \vartheta\frac{M}{N} & -\nu & 0 & \vartheta\frac{M}{N} \\ 0 & 0 & -(1-\alpha_v)\beta p_v\frac{N}{M} & -\mu & 0 \\ 0 & 0 & (1-\alpha_v)\beta p_v\frac{N}{M} & 0 & -(\gamma+\mu) \end{pmatrix}.$$

This matrix has two explicit eigenvalues, $-\mu$, that do not affect stability. In addition, the determinant of the remaining minor factorizes as follows,

$$\det(\mathcal{E}_0) = (\gamma+\mu)[\beta\vartheta(1-\alpha_v p_v) - (\gamma+\mu)\nu],$$

thereby indicating that another possible eigenvalue is $-(\gamma+\mu)$, a fact that is easily verified by direct substitution into the cubic characteristic equation. The remaining quadratic, after factoring out these known eigenvalues, is

$$\lambda^2 + \lambda(\gamma+\mu+\nu) + \nu(\gamma+\mu) - \beta\vartheta(1-\alpha_v p_v) = 0.$$

Note that the corresponding discriminant is

$$\Delta = (\gamma+\mu+\nu)^2 - 4[\nu(\gamma+\mu) - \beta\vartheta(1-\alpha_v p_v)] = (\gamma+\mu-\nu)^2 + 4\beta\vartheta(1-\alpha_v p_v) \geq 0.$$

Its roots are therefore real, and one eigenvalue is

$$\lambda_- = -\frac{1}{2}[(\gamma+\mu+\nu) + \sqrt{\Delta}] \leq 0.$$

On the other hand, we find the fifth eigenvalue

$$\lambda_+ = -\frac{1}{2}\frac{(\gamma+\mu+\nu)^2 - \Delta}{(\gamma+\mu+\nu) + \sqrt{\Delta}} = 2\frac{\beta\vartheta(1-\alpha_v p_v) - (\gamma+\mu)\nu}{(\gamma+\mu+\nu) + \sqrt{\Delta}}.$$

Thus to ensure stability, the following condition must hold:

$$\beta < \beta_{vTC} = \nu\frac{\gamma+\mu}{(1-\alpha_v p_v)\vartheta}. \tag{7.13}$$

We recall that in the reference case without control measures we have

$$\beta_{TC} = \frac{(\gamma+\mu)\nu}{\vartheta} \tag{7.14}$$

When β crosses from below the critical threshold β_{vTC}, a transcritical bifurcation occurs through which the endemic equilibrium is found. Further, since all eigenvalues are real, Hopf bifurcations will never occur.

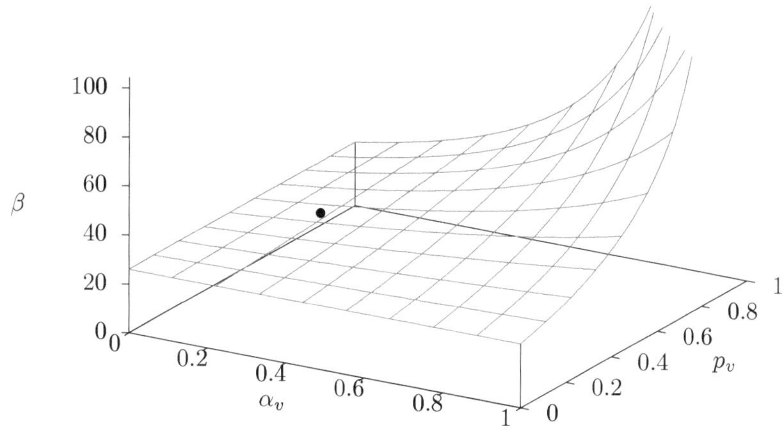

Figure 7.4: Bifurcation diagram for the transcritical bifurcation TC fixed by β_{vTC} ((7.13)) in the three-parameter (α_v, p_v, β)-space. The dot • marks the parameter values $\alpha_v = 0.2$, $p_v = 0.5$ used for Figure 7.5b.

Note that β_{vTC} (7.13) increases without bounds whenever α_v and p_v approach 1. This implies that when either the vaccine efficacy and the fraction of vaccinated newborns approach 100%, the endemic equilibrium is hard to attain, and the disease is essentially eradicated. But these percentages are difficult to attain in practical situations. In summary, knowing the infection rate β, vaccination is successful when the two control parameters are chosen below the TC-surface in Figure 7.4 where the values for all epidemiological and demographic parameter are from Table 7.B.1 in Appendix 7.B.

In order to evaluate the vaccination control measure, we compute the expression for the threshold parameter values. We give the expressions for these TC thresholds for the two control parameters p_v and α_v separately. These expressions can be used in a sensitivity analysis in order the judge the effectiveness of changing these parameters separately. For the proportion p_v of vaccinated immediately after birth it reads:

$$p_{vTC} = \frac{\beta\vartheta - (\gamma + \mu)\nu}{\alpha_v \beta\vartheta},$$

and for vaccine efficacy α_v

$$\alpha_{vTC} = \frac{\beta\vartheta + (\gamma + \mu)\nu}{p_v \beta\vartheta}.$$

Note that only the expressions at the occurrence of the TC, the infection rate parameters β and ϑ, the birth and death rates μ, ν respectively of host and vector, appear in these expressions, but not N and M.

In the next section we use the bifurcation plots where the measure parameters p_v and α_v vary to see the effects on the equilibrium values of the state variables. This information can be used as an analytic approach to predict the effects in disease-control campaigns.

7.5.1.2 Sensitivity analysis of the SIRvUV model

We start with a numerical bifurcation analysis where the infection rate β varies and we fix the control parameters p_v and α_v. In Figure 7.5 the bifurcation diagram is shown for the non-vaccinated where $\alpha_v = 0$ and $p_v = 0$ and the vaccinated case where $\alpha_v = 0.2$ and $p_v = 0.5$. When the parameter β increases past the transcritical bifurcation point TC, the disease-free equilibrium becomes unstable and the endemic equilibrium stable. Below the TC point the system is disease-free and above it the disease persists endemically. For the reference case where we have, using (7.14): $\beta_{TC} = 26.02$ in Figure 7.5a and in Figure 7.5b: $\beta_{vTC} = 28.90$.

The results in Figures 7.4 and 7.5 show that the TC threshold value β_{vTC} increases when both control parameters increase. Hence, there is complete eradication of the disease in a larger parameter range of infection rates β. For the reference value $\beta = 104$ the number of infected individuals $I + I_v$ is somewhat lower when $\alpha_v = 0.2$ and $p_v = 0.5$ and furthermore the number of infected mosquitoes V is much lower, see Figure 7.5b with respect to Figure 7.5a. For the sensitivity analysis with respect to the control parameters p_v and α_v we perform a numerical bifurcation analysis with the parameter values given in Table 7.B.1 after [42] and we fix the infection rate at $\beta = 104$. In Fig. 7.6a,b the effect of vaccination

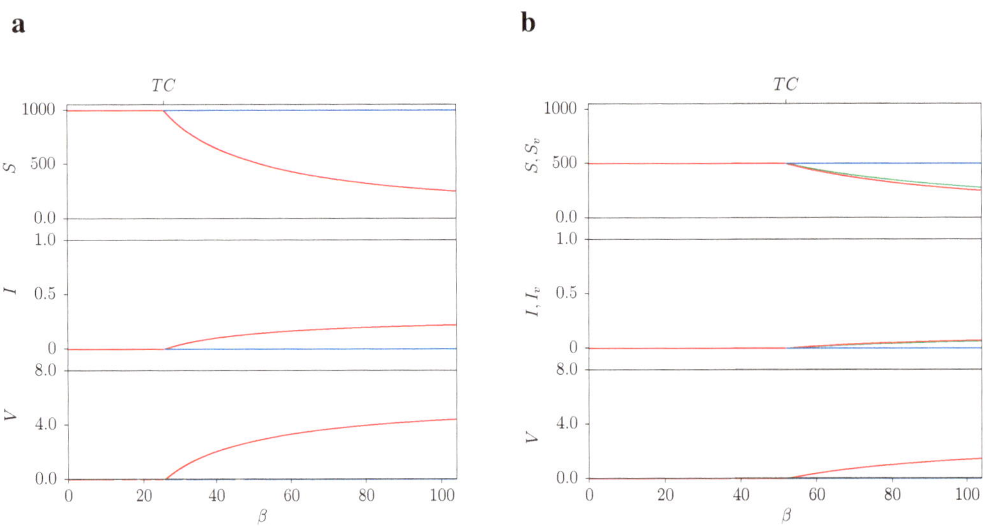

Figure 7.5: One-parameter diagram for the bifurcation parameter β for SIRvUV model. Stable equilibria for the state variables S, I, V are shown in red and unstable in blue. In panel **a** without vaccination ($\alpha_v = p_v = 0$) where $\beta_{TC} = 26.02$. In panel **b** with vaccination. Stable equilibria for the state variables S_v, I_v are shown in green and unstable in magenta). The vaccination parameters are $\alpha_v = 0.2$ and $p_v = 0.5$ and $\beta_{vTC} = 28.90$. All other parameter values are given in Table 7.B.1.

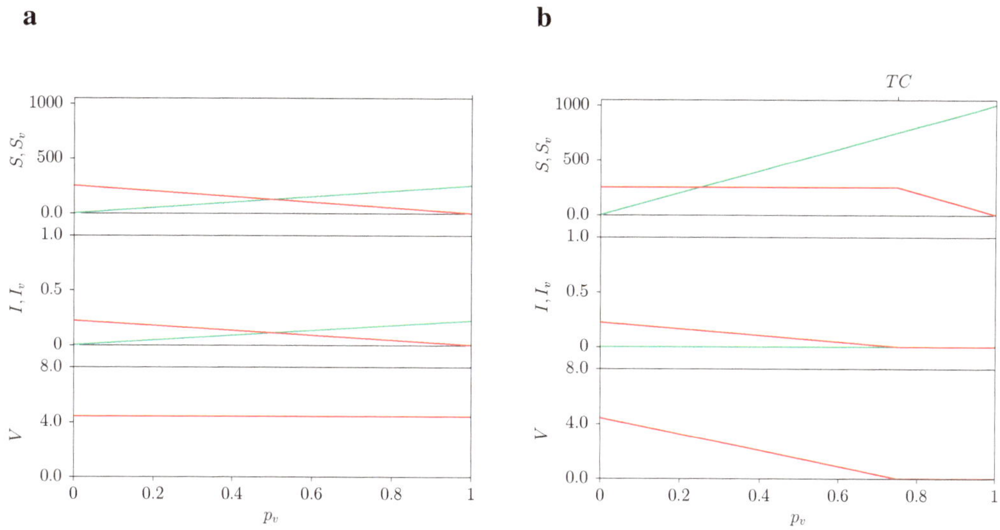

Figure 7.6: One-parameter diagram for the bifurcation parameter for SIRvUV model for p_v and $\beta = 104$. The curves are the stable equilibrium values. Red curves are for the host and vector compartments S, I, V and green curves for the vaccinated host compartments S_v, I_v. In panel **a**: $\alpha_v = 0$ and in panel **b**: $\alpha_v = 1$. In the latter case the transcritical bifurcation TC occurs for $p_{vTC} = 0.75$.

where $\alpha_v = 0$ and $\alpha_v = 1$ respectively, where p_v is increased from 0 to 1. For $\alpha_v = 0$ the vector population is constant while for the non-vaccinated population the susceptible S and infected I population deceases to zero while those S_v and I_v for the vaccinated population increase such that the sums are independent. Only for $p_v = 1$ the whole population is disease-free.

For $\alpha_v = 1$ and all p_v values there are no infected vaccinated individuals I_v while the susceptible vaccinated individuals S_v increase linearly. Below the transcritical bifurcation point TC the susceptible host population S remains the same and the number of infected individuals I decreases. With $\alpha_v = 1$ there is a TC at $p_{vTC} = 0.75$. Hence an disease-free population exists now for an interval above this TC. The vaccinated host population S_v increases linearly with p_v and equals M at $p_v = 1$. and the vaccinated infected host population I_v is extinct. Above the TC point the non-vaccinated susceptible host S population decreases and is extinct for $p_v = 1$. The infected vector population V is also extinct above the TC. This shows that there is a positive effect for the hosts $I = 0$ only above this TC threshold value.

7.5.2 Model with vector control

We study now vector control measures for the model (7.4) by introducing vector control population parameters that represent the effect of insecticides and personal protection targeting the mosquito (SIRqVM model). The equation for the host population remains

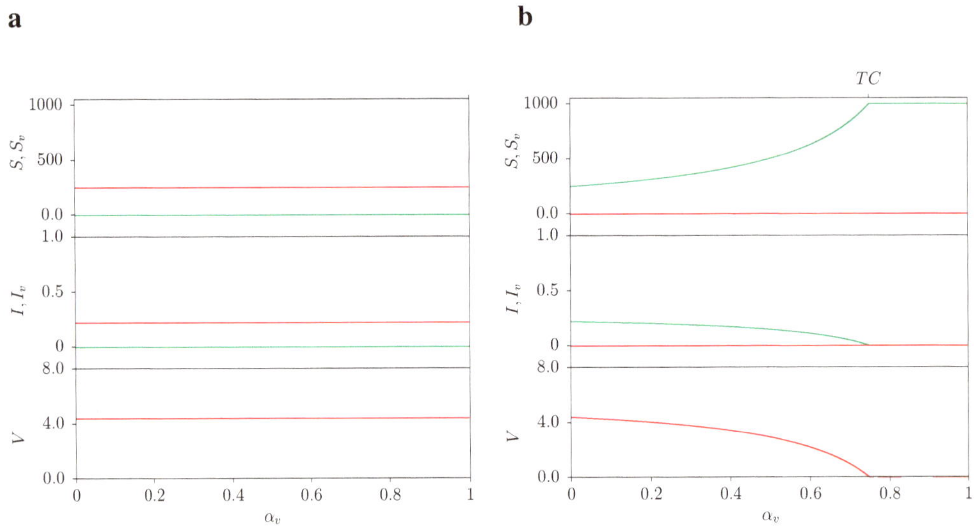

Figure 7.7: One-parameter diagram for the bifurcation parameter for SIRvUV model for α_v and $\beta = 104$. The curves show the stable equilibrium values. Red curves are for the host and vector compartments S, I, V and green for the vaccinated host compartments S_v, I_v. In panel **a**: $\alpha_v = 1$ and in panel **b**: $\alpha_v = 1$. In the latter case the transcritical bifurcation TC occurs for $\alpha_{vTC} = 0.75$.

the same as in (7.10a). The equations for the vector population (7.10c) are replaced by the following for V and M where two control parameters q_b and q_ν are introduced

$$\dot{S} = -\frac{\beta}{M} SV + \mu(N - S)\,, \quad \dot{I} = \frac{\beta}{M} SV - (\gamma + \mu) I\,, \quad \frac{dR}{dt} = \gamma I - \mu R\,, \tag{7.15a}$$

$$\dot{V} = q_b \frac{\vartheta}{N}(M - V) I - \nu(1 + q_\nu \frac{M}{M_\infty}) V\,, \quad \dot{M} = \nu(1 - q_\nu \frac{M}{M_\infty}) M\,. \tag{7.15b}$$

Note that the total number of mosquitoes $M(t) = U(t) + V(t)$ *does not need to be constant* in time. We consider two scenarios for disease control campaigns: the parameter q_b is a factor that reduces the force of infection rate of the vector, while q_ν is proportional to the demographic loss rate for the vector population where the number of mosquitoes changes as a logistic decay with a lower bound parameter $0 < M_\infty \leq M$. This represents a practical threshold value for the possibility of the vector population's extermination. The vector population's growth is again exponential with linear birth rate proportional to M, and the death rate is quadratic: proportional to M^2.

We remark that the density dependent force of infection formulation seems to give problems when the vector population is extinct: $M = 0$. However, for the host population it is possible to use the densities U/M and V/M instead of the numbers U and V where M is not used explicitly for the host population modelling. This also shows that the epidemiological and demographic mechanisms can be combined as well as strictly separated.

The bite efficiency ϑ is decreased by multiplication with a factor $0 \leq q_b \leq 1$. This is obtained by replacing ϑ by $q_b\vartheta$ in model (7.10). Scenario $q_b < 1$ models the use of personal household protection such as repellents, window screens or wearing long-sleeved clothes. The mosquito population size M is in this case constant. The model accounts also for an additional loss rate of the mosquitoes q_ν due to, for instance, the use of insecticides in water storage outdoor containers, or insecticide treated materials, coils and vaporizers.

7.5.2.1 Analysis of the SIRqVM model

There are two equilibria for system (7.15): the trivial, disease-free equilibrium $\mathcal{E}_0$ and the interior, endemic equilibrium $\mathcal{E}^*$. The trivial equilibrium equals

$$\mathcal{E}_0 = (S_0 = N,\ I_0 = 0,\ V_0 = 0,\ M_0 = \frac{M_\infty}{q_\nu})\,, \tag{7.16}$$

and the Jacobian matrix evaluated at this point reads

$$J(\mathcal{E}_0) = \begin{pmatrix} -\mu & 0 & -q_\nu\beta\dfrac{N}{M_\infty} & 0 \\ 0 & -(\gamma+\mu) & q_\nu\beta\dfrac{N}{M_\infty} & 0 \\ 0 & q_b\vartheta\dfrac{M_\infty}{q_\nu N} & -2\nu & 0 \\ 0 & 0 & 0 & -\nu \end{pmatrix}.$$

This matrix has two explicit real negative eigenvalues, $-\mu$ and $-\nu$ that do not affect stability.

The stability is fixed by the 2×2 internal block matrix of $J(\mathcal{E}_0)$. Indeed the trace of this matrix is $-(\gamma+\mu+2\nu)$ and therefore there cannot be a Hopf bifurcation for the disease-free equilibrium. The determinant of this matrix is zero at

$$\beta_{\nu TC} = \frac{2(\gamma+\mu)\nu}{q_b\vartheta}\,. \tag{7.17}$$

and this determines the position of the transcritical bifurcation TC when β is the bifurcation parameter. Note that this expression is independent of M_∞ as well as q_ν and therefore both parameters have no effect on the position of the extinction threshold. Therefore, we will not analyze their effects in detail. Figure 7.8 gives the surface in the three-parameter space for this function (7.17). When β crosses from below the threshold $\beta_{\nu TC}$, a transcritical bifurcation occurs. Note that $\beta_{\nu TC}$ (7.17) increases without bounds whenever q_b approaches 0. This situation shows that for all q_ν values the system converges to the disease-free equilibrium (7.16). However, this is hard to attain in practice.

From (7.17) and Figure 7.8 we see that reducing the biting rate q_b increases the critical threshold $\beta_{\nu TC}$. The same effect is obtained independently by increasing the mosquito mortality rate. The combined measures have of course a much stronger reinforcement of the increase in the threshold for attaining the endemic equilibrium, thereby increase the

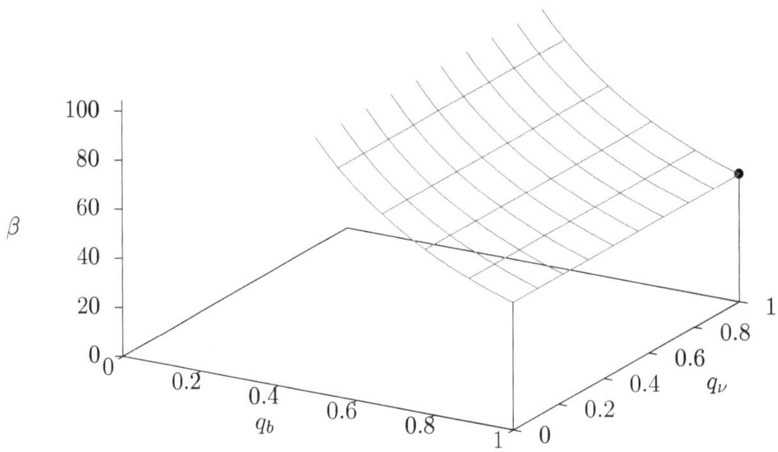

Figure 7.8: Bifurcation diagram of the SIRqVM model (7.15) for the transcritical bifurcation TC fixed by $\beta_{\nu TC}$ (7.17) in the three-parameter (q_b, p_ν, β)-space. The dot • marks the parameter values $q_b = 1.0$ and $q_\nu = 1.0$ used in Figure 7.9.

chances of disease eradication. The endemic equilibrium $\mathcal{E}^*$ reads:

$$S^* = \frac{N(\mu q_b \vartheta + 2\nu\gamma + 2\nu\mu)}{q_b \vartheta(\beta + \mu)}, \quad I^* = \frac{N\mu(\beta q_b \vartheta - 2\nu\gamma - 2\nu\mu)}{q_b \vartheta(\beta + \mu)(2\gamma + 2\mu)}, \tag{7.18a}$$

$$V^* = \frac{\mu M_\infty(\beta q_b \vartheta - 2\nu\gamma - 2\nu\mu)}{q_v \beta(\mu q_b \vartheta + 2\nu\gamma + 2\nu\mu)}, \quad M^* = \frac{M_\infty}{q_\nu}. \tag{7.18b}$$

7.5.2.2 Sensitivity analysis of the SIRqVM model

Similar to the analysis for vaccination controls, we give bifurcation diagrams for the two control parameters q_b and q_ν where (7.17) implies

$$q_{bTC} = \frac{2(\gamma + \mu)\nu}{\beta \vartheta}.$$

We start with an increase of the mortality of vector population modelled in (7.15) with $q_b = 1$ and $q_\nu = 1$ and whereby $0 \leq \beta \leq 104$ is varied. The bifurcation diagram for parameter β is shown in Figure 7.9. The transcritical bifurcation occurs at $\beta_{\nu TC} = 52.02$. This means that due to the control measures the system becomes endemic at a much higher rate of infection β than in the original case without any control shown in Figure 7.5 where $\beta_{TC} = 26.02$.

The numerical bifurcation results for the control parameter q_b in Figure 7.10 show that there is a critical vector control threshold value q_b equal to the threshold parameter value at the transcritical bifurcation TC.

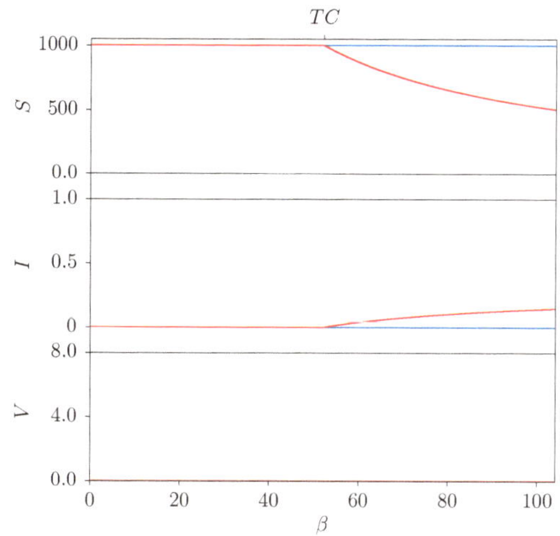

Figure 7.9: One-parameter diagram for the bifurcation parameter β for the SIRqVM model (7.15) with $q_b = 1$, $q_\nu = 1$ and $M_\infty = 1$ where using (7.17): $\beta_{TC} = 52.02$.

7.5.3 Viability analysis of vector control

In [40] the effect of introducing control through mosquito repellents used in textiles, paints and other household items (curtains, furniture) in a model for a vector-borne disease of a susceptible-infected-removed type for the host and susceptible-infected for the mosquito vector is investigated. Modeling of control measures in the context of vector-borne diseases has focused on optimal resource allocation [14, 37, 38, 47, 46, 54]. Stability analysis of epidemiological models investigates the asymptotic convergence of solutions to equilibria with specific properties, but does not answer the question of transient dynamic behavior.

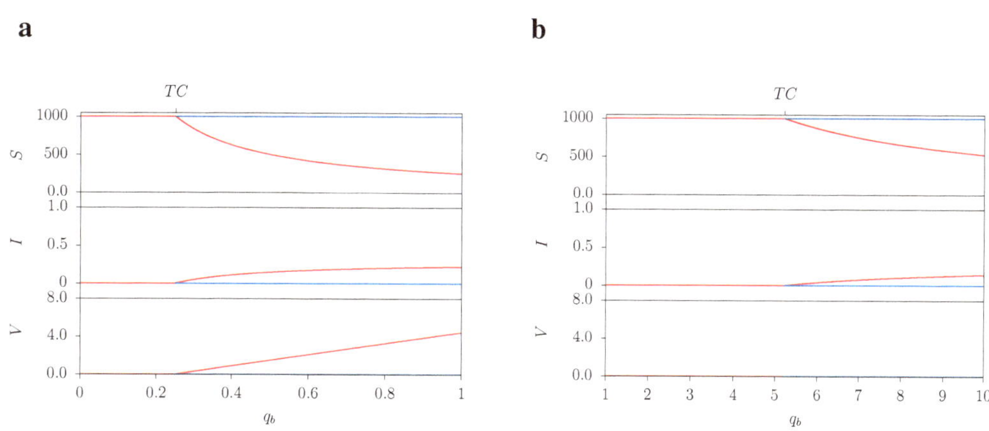

Figure 7.10: One-parameter diagram for the vector control parameter q_b for SIRqVM model (7.15), where $q_\nu = 1$ and $M_\infty = 1$. In panel **a** $\beta = 104$ where $q_{bTC} = 0.50$ and in panel **b** $\beta = 10$ where $q_{bTC} = 5.20$.

Viability analysis of controlled trajectories, on the other hand, is a novel problem in epidemiological models, especially in the case of vector-borne diseases. One example is the Ross-MacDonald model with control on the mosquito mortality by fumigation [17]. A possible motivation behind viability analysis is that policy-makers could be interested in maintaining prevalence of infection below a certain maximum level, which is linked to capacity constraints in the national or regional healthcare system, availability of medical workers, hospital beds, or medication.

The analysis in [40] establishes conditions for the existence of the initial points of solution trajectories meeting partial state constrains for all future times, in particular, initial conditions such that along the optimal controlled trajectory the proportion of infected individuals never exceeds a certain maximum level of infected individuals. The viability kernel, or the largest closed controlled forward-invariant subset which satisfies this constraint, is computed numerically using a variational approach leading to solution of an appropriate Hamilton-Jacobi-Bellman equation [9].

7.6 CONCLUSIONS

Due to the high model dimension, multi-strain models for vector-borne diseases often do not yield to theoretical analysis, and are dependent on numerical simulations. For models incorporating different types of controls aimed at reducing the disease burden, this complexity bears particular relevance for sensitivity and controllability analyses. In particular, one must use appropriate numerical methods for the time integration of stiff systems of ODEs, and robust methods for numerical bifurcation analysis.

In this work we combine epidemic modelling with model reduction techniques using time-scale separation for host-vector models, making them into host-only models based on QSSA. This approach provides a rigorous mechanism for checking that lower-dimensional models preserve features of the original model. Sensitivity analysis gives more insight into the effects of the different mechanisms included in the mathematical system or in the specific way they are modelled. This can be used for studying various scenarios for disease control in order to find regions in the parameter space corresponding to disease elimination, for example, and to study the effectiveness of varying those controls accordingly. However, as we have seen, introduction of control measures such as vaccination may rapidly introduce substantial complexity leading to large-dimensional systems that do not yield to theoretical analysis [3]. Hence, in the context of dengue simpler epidemiological models with just a single strain can be used as a starting point of the investigation. These models are useful in identifying transcritical bifurcation points which separate regions of disease elimination from endemic states via analytic relationships with the control variables as exemplified in Section 7.5. Furthermore, optimal control problems such as viability analysis of simple epidemiological models [40] require nontrivial transformations in order to apply theoretical results from the field of quasi-monotone dynamical systems.

This shows the importance of minimalistic models for the design and evaluation of scenarios for disease control campaigns until further theoretical advances in the field of dynamical systems are made.

ACKNOWLEDGMENT

This chapter is partly based on work performed within the framework of IMAAC (https://imaac.eu/) related to COST Action CA16227 (*Investigation & Mathematical Analysis of Avant-garde Disease Control via Mosquito Nano-Tech-Repellents*, https://cost.eu/actions/CA16227/), supported by COST Association (European Cooperation in Science and Technology). Peter Rashkov is partially supported by the National scientific program *Information and communication technologies for a single digital Market in science, education and security (IKTvNOS)* [Contract DO1-205/23.11.2018] financed by the Ministry of Education and Science in Bulgaria. Ezio Venturino is a member of the INdAM research group GNCS; he has been partially supported by the Research project "Modelli e metodi numerici in approssimazione, nelle scienze applicate e nelle scienze della vita" of the Dipartimento di Matematica "Giuseppe Peano", Università di Torino.

Appendices

7.A TIME SCALE SEPARATION, EXAMPLE: SIR-UV MODEL

The singular perturbation technique has been applied to the SIR-UV model [42, 41]. The slow (S,I)-flow in Eqn. (7.4) occurs near a manifold that is a smooth surface in $\mathbb{R}^3$. Letting $\varepsilon = 0$ in (7.2) determines the two-parameter nullspace for V in (7.4) consisting of the critical manifold in (7.5).

$$\mathcal{M}_0 = \left\{(S,I,V) \mid V = \frac{\vartheta MI}{\vartheta I + \nu N},\ 0 \le S \le N,\ 0 \le I \le N\right\},$$

and one can demonstrate $\mathcal{M}_0$ is normally hyperbolic. Using $\mathcal{M}_0$'s local invariance, V can be approximated by a power series

$$V = q_0(S,I) + q_1(S,I)\varepsilon + q_2(S,I)\varepsilon^2 + \ldots, \quad 0 < \varepsilon \ll 1\,.$$

$$\begin{aligned}
q_0(I) &= \frac{\vartheta MI}{\vartheta I + \nu N} \quad \text{(QSSA approximation)}\\
q_1(S,I) &= -\frac{\nu\vartheta MN^2}{(\vartheta I + \nu N)^3}\left(\frac{\beta}{M}Sq_0(I) - (\gamma+\mu)I\right)\\
q_2(S,I) &= \frac{\nu\vartheta^2 MN^3\beta I}{(\vartheta I + \nu N)^5}\left(\mu(N-S) - \frac{\beta}{M}Sq_0(I)\right) - \frac{\nu\vartheta MN^2}{(\vartheta I + \nu N)^3}q_1(S,I)\\
&\quad - \nu\vartheta MN^3\left(\frac{(\gamma+\mu)(\nu N - 2\vartheta I)}{(\vartheta I + \nu N)^5} - \frac{\vartheta\beta S(\nu N - 3\vartheta I)}{(\vartheta I + \nu N)^6}\right)\left(\frac{\beta}{M}Sq_0(I) - (\gamma+\mu)I\right)
\end{aligned}$$

The coefficients $q_i(S,I)$, $i = 0,1,2$ are computed from substitution of this equation invariance criterion. With $i = 0$ we get the QSSA expression Eqn. (7.5). For more details the reader is refered to [42, 41].

7.B PARAMETER VALUES

Table 7.B.1: Parameter values, most after [2, 34] for the host-only model (7.6) and [44] for the host-vector model. The units and values of the infection rate B in this study are different from those given: in the other references where the infection rate used is β. Remark: in previous papers N was equal to 100 but here it is taken as 1000. This means that in the comparison the results for the compartments of the previous papers have to multiplied by 10.

Parameter	**Description**	**Value**
Host		
N	Host population density	1000
B_i	Infection rate per infected vector	as indicated
β_i	Infection rate per infected host	$[0, 104]$ (or free)
μ	Susceptible birth rate	$1/65$
γ	Recovery rate	$365/7$
α	temporary cross-immunity rate	2, 52 or $[1, 250]$
Vector		
M	Vector population density	10000
ν	Susceptible birth rate	36.5
ϑ	Infection rate per host	73
η	Magnitude of sinusoidal fluctuation vectors	$0, 0.1, 0.35$
ϕ	Ratio of likelihoods of transmission from hosts with secondary and hosts with primary infection to vectors	$[0, 12]$
φ	Phase	0
Control parameters		
α_v	Vaccine efficacy	$[0, 1]$
p_v	Fraction of newborns vaccinated	$[0, 1]$
q_b	Decrease of bite efficiency	$[0, 10]$
q_ν	Control-based mosquito killing rate	$[0, 10]$

Mathematical Models and Optimal Control in Mosquito Transmitted Diseases

Peyman Ghaffari*

Chair of IMAAC (COST Action CA 16227) **&**
Center for Research and Development in Mathematics and Applications (CIDMA), Department of Mathematics, University of Aveiro, Aveiro, Portugal
** corresponding author, e-mail: pgsaid@fc.ul.pt*

Cristiana J. Silva

Center for Research and Development in Mathematics and Applications (CIDMA), Department of Mathematics, University of Aveiro, Aveiro, Portugal

Delfim F. M. Torres

Center for Research and Development in Mathematics and Applications (CIDMA), Department of Mathematics, University of Aveiro, Aveiro, Portugal

CONTENTS

8.1 Introduction 149
8.2 Controlled model 151
8.3 Optimal control problem 153
8.4 Numerical results and discussion 154
8.A Unique Optimal Solution 161

8.1 INTRODUCTION

Understanding, predicting, and mitigating the spread of mosquito-borne diseases, in diverse populations and geographies, poses several modeling challenges. In fact, despite centuries of enormous efforts, mosquito-borne diseases continue to cause significant public health burden and are widely re-emerging or emerging [27, 30]. Here our focus is on mathematical models in mosquito transmitted diseases. Such models can be classified in different classes, e.g., agent-based models [27]; networks [49]; models described by systems of ordinary differential equations [14, 35]; by fractional order differential equations [16, 43]; reaction–diffusion equations [4, 56]; or discrete systems [9, 24]. They also apply

DOI: 10.1201/9781003035992-8

to different diseases, e.g., Malaria [12, 32, 51], and Zika [14, 31] and Dengue [41, 43] viruses, which are infections transmitted primarily by *Aedes* mosquitoes.

Optimal control theory is an area of mathematical optimization that deals with finding a control for a dynamical system over a period of time such that an objective function is optimized [10, 34]. While classical applications are essentially found in engineering, physics, economy and business [19, 23, 29, 50], more recent applications are found in medicine, infectious diseases and epidemiology [15, 21, 26, 28]. For example, optimal control has shown to be very useful with respect to human respiratory infections [42], cholera [20, 21], tuberculosis [44], HIV [5, 37, 38], Ebola [8, 36], malaria [33, 45], Zika [6, 48], and dengue epidemics [39, 40]. Here we focus on optimal control to Malaria prevention via insecticide-treated nets [45].

Malaria is a life threatening disease caused by *Plasmodium* parasites and transmitted from one individual to another by the bite of infected female *anopheline* mosquitoes [3, 51]. In the human body, the parasites multiply in the liver, and then infect red blood cells. Following World Health Organization (WHO) 2019 report, an estimated 228 million cases of malaria occurred worldwide (95% confidence interval [CI]: 206–258 million), with most malaria cases from WHO African Region (213 million or 93%), followed by the WHO South-East Asia Region with 3.4% of the cases and the WHO Eastern Mediterranean Region with 2.1% [55]. Malaria is an entirely preventable and treatable disease, provided the currently recommended interventions are properly implemented. Following WHO, these interventions include (i) vector control through the use of insecticide-treated nets (ITNs), indoor residual spraying and, in some specific settings, larval control, (ii) chemoprevention for the most vulnerable populations, particularly pregnant women and infants, (iii) confirmation of malaria diagnosis through microscopy or rapid diagnostic tests for every suspected case, and (iv) timely treatment with appropriate antimalarial medicines [55]. An ITN is a mosquito net that repels, disables and/or kills mosquitoes coming into contact with insecticide on the netting material. ITNs are considered one of the most effective interventions against malaria [22]. In 2007, WHO recommended full ITN coverage of all people at risk of malaria, even in high-transmission settings [54]. By 2011, 32 countries in the African region and 78 other countries worldwide, had adopted the WHO recommendation. A total of 89 countries, including 39 in Africa, distribute ITNs free of charge. Between 2004 and 2010, the number of ITNs delivered annually by manufacturers to malaria-endemic countries in sub-Saharan Africa increased from 6 million to 145 million. Between 2016 and 2018, a total of 578 million ITNs were reported by manufacturers as having been delivered globally, with 50% going to Côte d'Ivoire, the Democratic Republic of the Congo, Ethiopia, Ghana, India, Nigeria, Uganda and the United Republic of Tanzania. In 2018, about 197 million ITNs were delivered by manufacturers, of which more than 87% were delivered to countries in sub-Saharan Africa. Globally, 80% of ITNs were distributed through mass distribution campaigns, 10% in antenatal care facilities and 6% as part of immunization programmes [55]. However, there is still an urgent need to identify new funding sources to maintain and expand coverage levels of interventions so that outbreaks of disease can be avoided and international targets for reducing malaria cases and deaths can be attained.

A number of studies reported that ITN possession does not necessarily translate into use. Human behavior change interventions, including information, education, communication (IEC) campaigns and post-distribution hang-up campaigns are strongly recommended, especially where there is evidence of their effectiveness in improving ITN usage [1, 25, 55]. Here we consider the model from [2] for the effects of ITNs on the transmission dynamics of malaria infection. Other articles considered the impact of intervention strategies using ITN (see, e.g., [18, 47]). However, only in [2] the human behavior is incorporated into the model. We follow [45], introducing in the model of [2] a *supervision* control, u, which represents IEC campaigns for improving the ITN usage. In Section 8.2, we present the mathematical model for malaria transmission with one control function u. In Section 8.3, we propose an optimal control problem for the minimization of the number of infectious humans while controlling the cost of control interventions. Finally, in Section 8.4, some numerical results are analyzed and interpreted from the epidemiological point of view. Future research aims to expand the developed model to include the effects of mosquito repellency incorporated in paints and textiles to reduce mosquito transmission of infectious diseases.

8.2 CONTROLLED MODEL

We consider a mathematical model presented in [2] for the effects of ITN on the transmission of malaria infection and introduce a time-dependent *supervision* control u. The model considers transmission of malaria infection of mosquito (also referred as vector) and human (also referred as host) population. The host population is divided into two compartments, susceptible (S_h) and infectious (I_h), with a total population (N_h) given by $N_h = S_h + I_h$. Analogously, the vector population is divided into two compartments, susceptible (S_v) and infectious (I_v), with a total population (N_v) given by $N_v = S_v + I_v$. The model is constructed under the following assumptions: all newborns individuals are assumed to be susceptible and no infected individuals are assumed to come from outside the community.

The human and mosquito recruitment rates are denoted by Λ_h and Λ_v, respectively. The disease is fast progressing, thus the exposed stage is minimal and is not considered. Infectious individuals can die from the disease or become susceptible after recovery while the mosquito population does not recover from infection. ITNs contribute for the mortality of mosquitoes. The average number of bites per mosquito, per unit of time (mosquito-human contact rate), is given by

$$\beta = \beta_{max}(1-b),$$

where β_{max} denotes the maximum transmission rate and b the proportion of ITN usage. It is assumed that the minimum transmission rate is zero. The value of β is the same for human and mosquito population, so the average number of bites per human per unit of time is $\beta N_v/N_h$ (see [2] and the references cited therein). Thus, the force of infection for susceptible humans (λ_h) and susceptible vectors (λ_v) are given by

$$\lambda_h = \frac{p_1 \beta I_v}{N_h} \quad \text{and} \quad \lambda_v = \frac{p_2 \beta I_h}{N_h},$$

Table 8.1: Parameter values.

Symbol	Description	Value
Λ_h	Recruitment rate in humans	$10^3/(70 \times 365)$
Λ_v	Recruitment rate in mosquitoes	$10^4/21$
μ_h	Natural mortality rate in humans	$1/(70 \times 365)$
δ_h	Disease induced mortality rate in humans	10^{-3}
b	Proportion of treated net usage	0.25; 0.3; 0.4; 0.5; 0.6; 0.7; 0.75
γ_h	Recovery rate of infectious humans to be susceptible	1/4
μ_{v1}	Natural mortality rate of mosquitoes	1/21
$\mu_{max}b$	Mortality rate of mosquitoes due to treated net	1/21
β_{max}	Maximum mosquito-human contact rate	0.1
p_1	Probability of disease transmission from mosquito	1
p_2	Probability of disease transmission from human to mosquito	1
A_1	Weight constant on infectious humans	25
C	Weight constant on control	50
$S_h(0)$	Susceptible individuals initial value	800
$I_h(0)$	Infectious individuals initial value	200
$S_v(0)$	Susceptible vectors initial value	4,000
$I_v(0)$	Infectious vectors initial value	900

where p_1 and p_2 are the transmission probability per bite from infectious mosquitoes to humans, and from infectious humans to mosquitoes, respectively. The death rate of the mosquitoes is modeled by $\mu_{vb} = \mu_{v1} + \mu_{max}b$, where μ_{v1} is the natural death rate and $\mu_{max}b$ is the death rate due to pesticide on ITNs.

The coefficient $1-u$ represents the effort of susceptible humans that become infected by infectious mosquitoes bites, such as educational programs/campaigns for the correct use of ITNs, supervision teams that visit every house in a certain region and assure that every person has access to an ITN, know how to use it correctly, and recognize its importance on the reduction of malaria disease transmission. The values of the parameters Λ_h, Λ_v, μ_h, δ_h, γ_h, μ_{v1}, $\mu_{max}b$, β_{max}, p_1 and p_2 are taken from [2] (see Table 8.1). The state system of the controlled malaria model is given by

$$\begin{cases} \dot{S}_h(t) = \Lambda_h - (1-u(t))\lambda_h S_h(t) + \gamma_h I_h(t) - \mu_h S_h(t), \\ \dot{I}_h(t) = (1-u(t))\lambda_h S_h(t) - (\mu_h + \gamma_h + \delta_h) I_h(t), \\ \dot{S}_v(t) = \Lambda_v - \lambda_v S_v(t) - \mu_{vb} S_v(t), \\ \dot{I}_v(t) = p_2 \lambda_v S_v(t) - \mu_{vb} I_v(t). \end{cases} \tag{8.1}$$

The rate of change of the total human and mosquito populations is given by

$$\dot{N}_h(t) = \Lambda_h - \mu_h N_h(t) - \delta_h I_h(t),$$
$$\dot{N}_v(t) = \Lambda_v - \mu_{vb} N_v(t).$$

8.3 OPTIMAL CONTROL PROBLEM

We formulate an optimal control problem that describes the goal and restrictions of the epidemic. In [2] it is found that the ITN usage must attain 75% ($b = 0.75$) of the host population in order to extinct malaria. Therefore, educational campaigns must continue encouraging the population to use ITNs. Moreover, it is very important to assure that ITNs are in good conditions and each individual knows how to use them properly. Having this in mind, we introduce a *supervision* control function, u, where the coefficient $1-u$ represents the effort to reduce the number of susceptible humans that become infected by infectious mosquitoes bites, assuring that ITNs are correctly used by the fraction b of the host population.

We consider the state system (8.1) of ordinary differential equations in $\mathbb{R}^4$ with the set of admissible control functions given by

$$\Omega = \{u(\cdot) \in L^{\infty}(0,t_f) \,|\, 0 \leqslant u(t) \leqslant 1, \ \forall t \in [0,t_f]\} .$$

The objective functional is given by

$$J_1(u) = \int_0^{t_f} A_1 I_h(t) + \frac{C}{2} u^2(t)\, dt , \tag{8.2}$$

where the weight coefficient, C, is a measure of the relative cost of the interventions associated to the control u and A_1 is the weight coefficient for the class I_h. The aim is to minimize the infectious humans while keeping the cost low. More precisely, we propose the optimal control problem of determining $(S_h^*, I_h^*, S_v^*, I_v^*)$ associated to an admissible control $u^*(\cdot) \in \Omega$ on the time interval $[0,t_f]$, satisfying (8.1), the initial conditions $S_h(0)$, $I_h(0)$, $S_v(0)$ and $I_v(0)$ (see Table 8.1) and minimizing the cost function (8.2), i.e.,

$$J_1(u^*(\cdot)) = \min_{\Omega} J_1(u(\cdot)) . \tag{8.3}$$

The existence of an optimal control $u^*(\cdot)$ comes from the convexity of the Lagrangian of (8.2) with respect to the control and the regularity of the system (8.1) (see, e.g., [11, 13] for existence results of optimal solutions). Applying the Pontryagin maximum principle [34], we derive the optimal solution $(u^*, S_h^*, I_h^*, S_v^*, I_v^*)$ of the proposed optimal control problem (see Appendix 8.A).

More generally, one could take the following cost function:

$$J_2(u) = \int_0^{t_f} A_1 I_h(t) + A_2 I_v(t) + \frac{C}{2} u^2(t)\, dt,$$

where A_2 is the weight constant on infectious mosquitoes (for numerical simulations we considered $A_2 = 25$). It turns out that when we include in the objective function the number of infectious mosquitoes, the distribution of the total host population N_h and vector population N_v by the categories S_h, I_h and S_v, I_v, respectively, is the same for both cost functions J_1 and J_2 (see Figures 8.1 and 8.2). On the other hand, the effort on the control is higher for the cost function J_2 (see Figure 8.3). Therefore, we choose to use the cost function J_1 in our numerical simulations (Section 8.4).

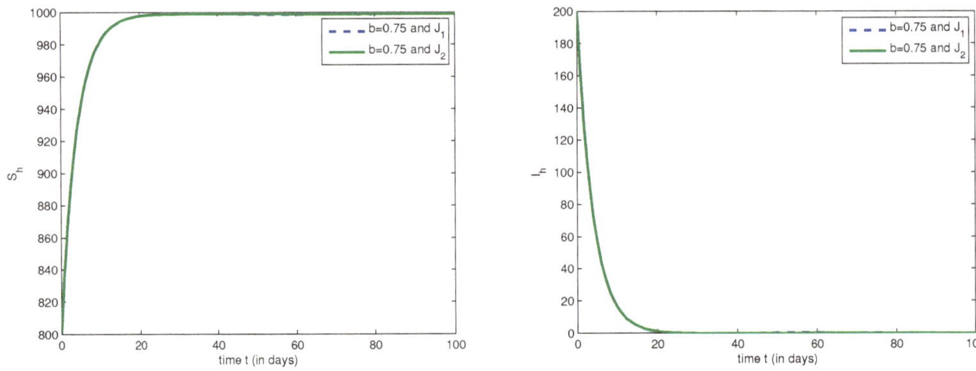

(a) Susceptible humans for J_1 and J_2. (b) Infectious humans for J_1 and J_2.

Figure 8.1: Susceptible and infectious individuals for different cost functions J_1 and J_2 (parameter/constant values from Table 8.1 and $b = 0.75$).

8.4 NUMERICAL RESULTS AND DISCUSSION

Our numerical results were obtained and confirmed following different approaches. The first approach consisted in using IPOPT [53] and the algebraic modeling language AMPL [7].

In a second approach, we used the PROPT Matlab Optimal Control Software [52]. The results were coincident and are easily confirmed by the ones obtained using an iterative method that consists in solving the system of eight ODEs given by (8.1) and (8.A.5) in Appendix 8.A. For that, one first solves system (8.1) with a guess for the control over the time interval $[0, t_f]$ using a forward fourth-order Runge–Kutta scheme and the transversality conditions (8.A.4) in Appendix 8.A.

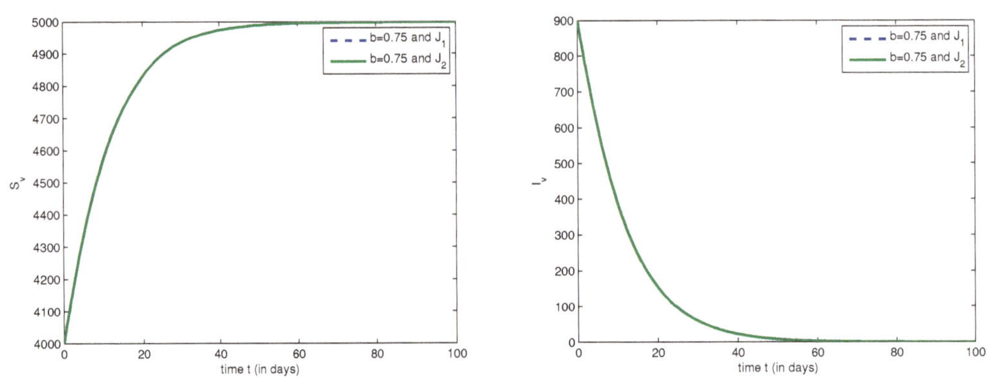

(a) Susceptible mosquitoes for J_1 and J_2. (b) Infectious mosquitoes for J_1 and J_2.

Figure 8.2: Susceptible and infectious mosquitoes for different cost functions J_1 and J_2 (parameter/constant values from Table 8.1 and $b = 0.75$).

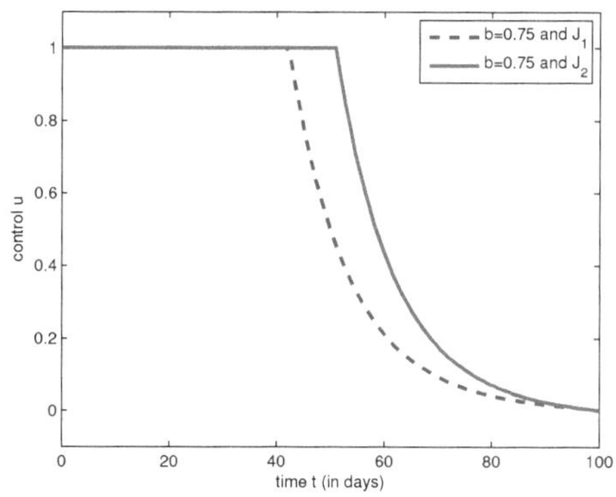

Figure 8.3: Optimal control u for different cost functions J_1 and J_2 (parameter/constant values from Table 8.1 and $b = 0.75$).

Then, system (8.A.5) is solved by a backward fourth-order Runge–Kutta scheme using the current iteration solution of (8.1). The controls are updated by using a convex combination of the previous controls and the values from (8.A.6) (see Appendix 8.A). The iterative method ends when the values of the approximations at the previous iteration are close to the ones at the present iteration. For details see [10, 17, 46].

First of all we consider $b = 0.75$ and show that when we apply the *supervision* control u, better results are obtained, that is, the number of infected humans vanishes faster when compared to the case where no controls are used. If the control intervention u is applied, then the number of infectious individuals vanishes after approximately 30 days. If no control is considered, then it takes approximately 70 days to assure that there are no infectious humans (see Figure 8.4 for the fraction of susceptible and infectious humans and Figure 8.5 for the optimal control).

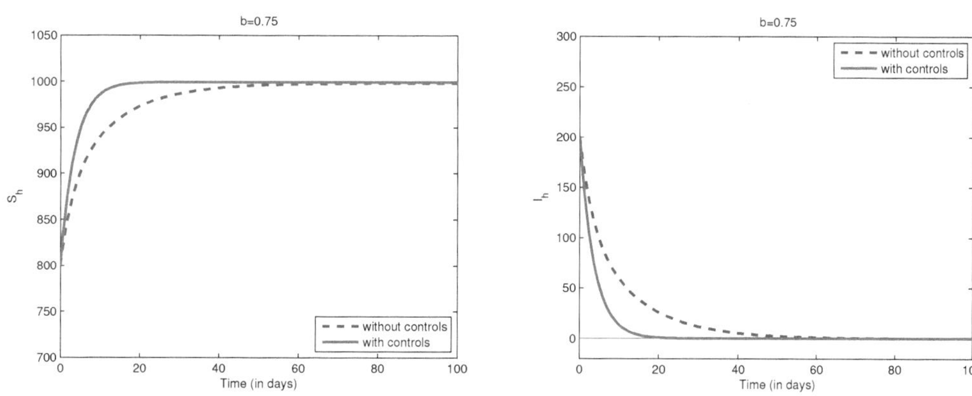

(a) Susceptible humans (b) Infectious humans

Figure 8.4: Susceptible and infectious humans for $b = 0.75$ with and without control.

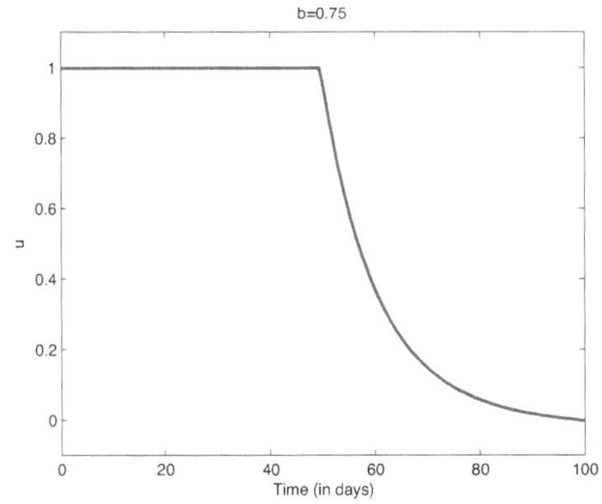

Figure 8.5: Optimal control u for $b = 0.75$.

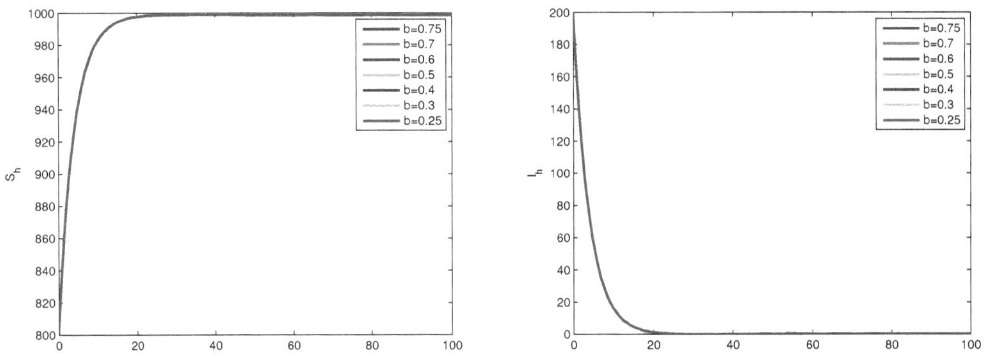

(a) Susceptible humans

(b) Infectious humans

Figure 8.6: Susceptible and infectious humans for $b = 0.25; 0.3; 0.4; 0.5; 0.6; 0.7; 0.75$.

For smaller proportions of ITN usage than $b = 0.75$, similar results on the reduction of infectious humans are attained when we consider the optimal *supervision* control u (see Figures 8.6 and 8.7). We note that the control u does not contribute significantly for the decrease of I_v (see Figure 8.8).

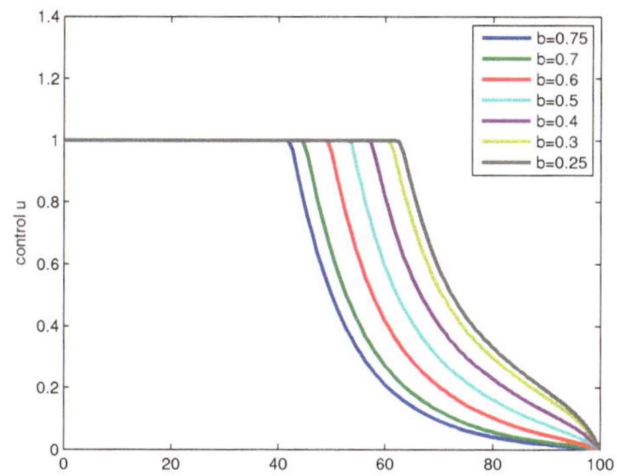

Figure 8.7: Optimal control u for $b = 0.25; 0.3; 0.4; 0.5; 0.6; 0.7; 0.75$.

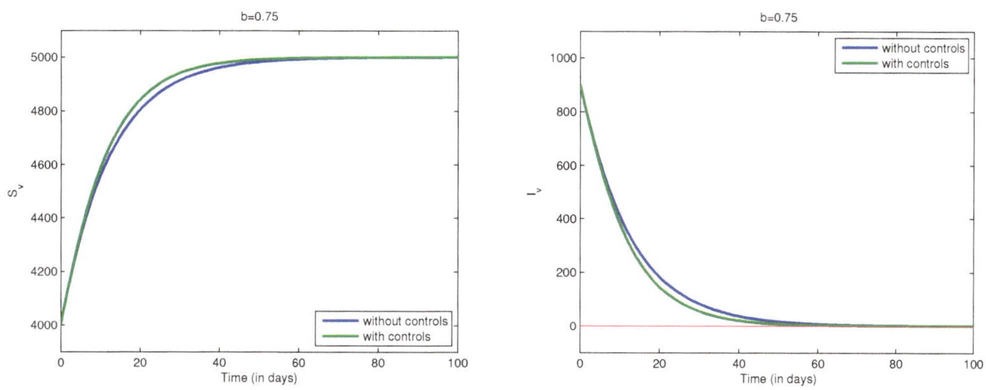

(a) Susceptible mosquitoes

(b) Infectious mosquitoes

Figure 8.8: Susceptible and infectious mosquitoes for $b = 0.75$ with and without control.

ACKNOWLEDGMENTS

This work was supported by the Portuguese Foundation for Science and Technology (FCT) within project UIDB/04106/2020 (CIDMA). This chapter is partly based on work performed within the framework of IMAAC (`https://imaac.eu/`) related to COST Action CA16227 (*Investigation & Mathematical Analysis of Avant-garde Disease Control via Mosquito Nano-Tech-Repellents*, `https://cost.eu/actions/CA16227/`), supported by COST Association (European Cooperation in Science and Technology).

Appendices

8.A UNIQUE OPTIMAL SOLUTION

According to the Pontryagin Maximum Principle [34], if $u^*(\cdot) \in \Omega$ is optimal for the problem (8.1), (8.3) with the initial conditions given in Table 8.1 and fixed final time t_f, then there exists a nontrivial absolutely continuous mapping $\lambda : [0, t_f] \to \mathbb{R}^4$, $\lambda(t) = (\lambda_1(t), \lambda_2(t), \lambda_3(t), \lambda_4(t))$, called *adjoint vector*, such that

$$\dot{S}_h = \frac{\partial H}{\partial \lambda_1}, \quad \dot{I}_h = \frac{\partial H}{\partial \lambda_2}, \quad \dot{S}_v = \frac{\partial H}{\partial \lambda_3}, \quad \dot{I}_v = \frac{\partial H}{\partial \lambda_4} \tag{8.A.1}$$

and

$$\dot{\lambda}_1 = -\frac{\partial H}{\partial S_h}, \quad \dot{\lambda}_2 = -\frac{\partial H}{\partial I_h}, \quad \dot{\lambda}_3 = -\frac{\partial H}{\partial S_v}, \quad \dot{\lambda}_4 = -\frac{\partial H}{\partial I_v}, \tag{8.A.2}$$

where function H defined by

$$\begin{aligned} H &= H(S_h, I_h, S_v, I_v, \lambda, u) \\ &= A_1 I_h + \frac{C}{2} u^2 \\ &\quad + \lambda_1 \left(\Lambda_h - (1-u)\lambda_h S_h + \gamma_h I_h - \mu_h S_h\right) \\ &\quad + \lambda_2 \left((1-u)\lambda_h S_h - (\mu_h + \gamma_h + \delta_h) I_h\right) \\ &\quad + \lambda_3 \left(\Lambda_v - \lambda_v S_v - \mu_{vb} S_v\right) \\ &\quad + \lambda_4 \left(p_2 \lambda_v S_v - \mu_{vb} I_v\right) \end{aligned}$$

is called the *Hamiltonian*, and the minimization condition

$$\begin{aligned} &H(S_h^*(t), I_h^*(t), S_v^*(t), I_v^*(t), \lambda^*(t), u^*(t)) \\ &\quad = \min_{0 \leqslant u \leqslant 1} H(S_h^*(t), I_h^*(t), S_v^*(t), I_v^*(t), \lambda^*(t), u) \end{aligned} \tag{8.A.3}$$

holds almost everywhere on $[0, t_f]$. Moreover, the transversality conditions

$$\lambda_i(t_f) - 0, \quad i = 1, \ldots, 4, \tag{8.A.4}$$

hold.

Theorem 8.A.1 *Problem* (8.1), (8.3) *with fixed initial conditions* $S_h(0)$, $I_h(0)$, $S_v(0)$ *and* $I_v(0)$ *and fixed final time* t_f, *admits an unique optimal solution* $(S_h^*(\cdot), I_h^*(\cdot), S_v^*(\cdot), I_v^*(\cdot))$ *associated to an optimal control* $u^*(\cdot)$ *on* $[0, t_f]$. *Moreover, there exists adjoint functions* $\lambda_1^*(\cdot)$, $\lambda_2^*(\cdot)$, $\lambda_3^*(\cdot)$ *and* $\lambda_4^*(\cdot)$ *such that*

$$\begin{cases} \dot{\lambda_1^*}(t) = \lambda_1^*(t)\left((1 - u^*(t))\lambda_h + \mu_h\right) - \lambda_2^*(t)\lambda_h(1 - u^*(t)) \\ \dot{\lambda_2^*}(t) = -A_1 - \lambda_1^*(t)\gamma_h + \lambda_2^*(t)(\mu_h + \gamma_h + \delta_h) \\ \dot{\lambda_3^*}(t) = \lambda_3^*(t)(\lambda_v + \mu_{vb}) - \lambda_4^*(t)(\lambda_v)) \\ \dot{\lambda_4^*}(t) = \lambda_4^*(t)\mu_{vb}, \end{cases} \tag{8.A.5}$$

with transversality conditions

$$\lambda_i^*(t_f) = 0, \quad i = 1, \ldots, 4.$$

Furthermore,

$$u^*(t) = \min\left\{\max\left\{0, \frac{\lambda_h(b)S_h^*(t)}{C}(\lambda_2^*(t) - \lambda_1^*(t))\right\}, 1\right\}. \tag{8.A.6}$$

Proof 8.A.1 *Existence of an optimal solution* $(S_h^*, I_h^*, S_v^*, I_v^*)$ *associated to an optimal control* u^* *comes from the convexity of the integrand of the cost function* J *with respect to the control* u *and the Lipschitz property of the state system with respect to state variables* (S_h, I_h, S_v, I_v) *(see, e.g., [11, 13]). System* (8.A.5) *is derived from the Pontryagin maximum principle (see* (8.A.2), *[34]) and the optimal controls* (8.A.6) *come from the minimization condition* (8.A.3). *The optimal control pair given by* (8.A.6) *is unique due to the boundedness of the state and adjoint functions and the Lipschitz property of systems* (8.1) *and* (8.A.5) *(see, e.g., [17] and references cited therein).*

IV

Topological Studies: Topology Meets Mosquito Control

CHAPTER 9

On the Shape and Design of Mosquito Abatement Districts

James R. Bozeman*

Department of Mathematics, American University of Malta (AUM), Triq Dom Mintoff, Bormla, Malta

** corresponding author, e-mail: james.bozeman@aum.edu.mt*

CONTENTS

9.1 Introduction 165
9.2 Designs of Current Mosquito Abatement Regions 166
9.2.1 Rhode Island, USA [3] 166
9.2.1.1 Mosquito Control Measures: 2019 Pesticide Applications 166
9.2.1.2 Mosquito Control Measures: 2019 Pesticide Applications 167
9.2.2 Winnipeg, Canada [4] 168
9.3 Flight distances, patterns and times of varied mosquitoes and disease agents 168
9.4 Creation of districts 169
9.5 Analysis and Conclusions 171

9.1 INTRODUCTION

The control of mosquito populations to tamp down disease outbreaks is an ongoing operation in much of the world. Some of these vector-borne diseases include dengue (DG), Eastern Equine Encephalitis (EEE), malaria (M), West Nile virus (WNV), yellow fever (YF), etc. Methods used to eradicate the mosquitoes that carry these diseases include fogging and spraying of insecticides and the ground placement of same. Larvaciding and the introduction of infertile males are also applied. Other techniques include addition of additives to paints and textiles, the use of mosquito nets, and other amelioration steps. In this chapter we only deal with those operations that include the need to define a certain area for the application of the method.

DOI: 10.1201/9781003035992-9

When designing the regions for spraying or fogging or ground placement of insecticides, for example, many considerations must be taken into account. These include the type of mosquito being eradicated, their flight ranges, and flight patterns. Also of concern are the demographics of the region to be sprayed, including vulnerable populations, and its topography. Often political issues must be taken into account, e.g. public opposition to spraying, which is very similar to the matters of concern when designing voting districts.

The author and colleagues developed the convexity ratio [1] to measure the shape of voting districts. A district is *nicely shaped* if it is *nearly convex*, i.e. $\mathrm{CR}(\mathrm{D}) > 0.5$, where D is the district being measured and CR is its convexity ratio. Otherwise it is *poorly shaped*. The convexity ratio is a measure of how close a planar region D is to being *convex*, meaning any two points lying in D can be connected by a straight line lying entirely in D. CR(D) equals the area of the largest convex set within D, the *endogon*, divided by the area of the *convex hull* of D, i.e. the smallest convex set containing D, or the *exogon*. The author and colleagues applied this to the redistricting problem in [2] and indicated applications to other areas of Business and Industry. In [2] the entire State of Texas in the USA was completely redistricted with the goal of having each district as close to convex as possible. In this paper we apply the same techniques, which utilized ArcGIS amongst other methods, to design mosquito control districts which are also as close to convex as possible. This will enhance the eradication of the mosquitoes in question as they can fly in any direction from a given starting point, creating a convex area of possible paths.

This chapter is organized as follows: In Section 9.2 we look at different designs of mosquito abatement districts from varying countries and regions. In Section 9.3 the flight patterns of different types of mosquitoes are examined. Section 9.4 includes a description of the redistricting mentioned above. The methodology used in that application is then applied to the design of mosquito control districts. We conclude with an analysis of our results in Section 9.5.

9.2 DESIGNS OF CURRENT MOSQUITO ABATEMENT REGIONS

What follows are descriptions of regions in the United States and Canada where spraying or fogging was applied:

9.2.1 Rhode Island, USA [3]

9.2.1.1 Mosquito Control Measures: 2019 Pesticide Applications

In 2019, aerial spraying occurred in four areas of Rhode Island that state officials assessed to be at critical risk for the Eastern Equine Encephalitis (EEE) virus.

- **September 8 - 10, 2019**
  In all, the state treated parts of 21 communities over three nights, from September 8 to 10, with a pesticide formulated to kill adult mosquitoes. The flight crew used the pesticide, called Anvil $10+10$, at an extremely low concentration, dispersing

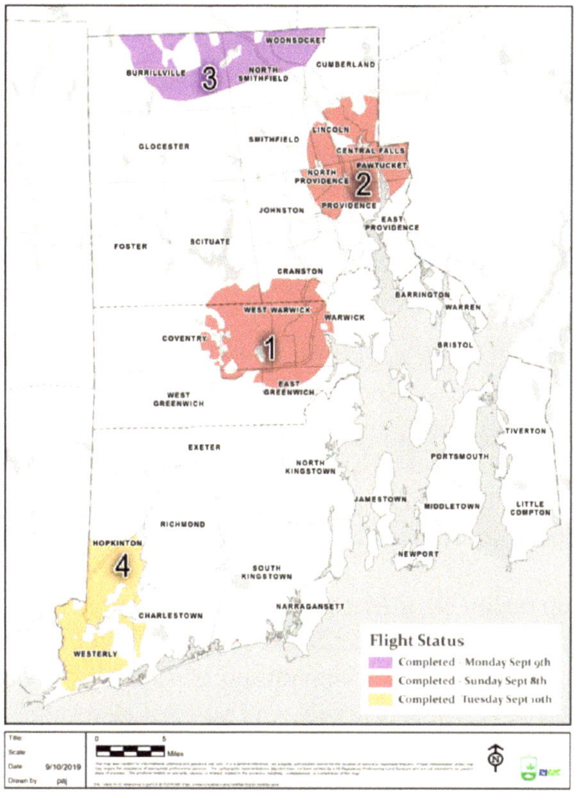

Figure 9.1: Aerial spraying occurred in four areas of Rhode Island [3].

a total of 556 gallons across 115,179 total acres – meaning that 6/10 of an ounce, aerosolized, was used to treat an acre. That's the equivalent of slightly less than four teaspoons per acre. In Figure 9.1 notes that Regions 1 and 2 are nearly convex, whereas Regions 3 and 4 are not.

- **Wednesday, September 25, 2019**
  A second aerial spraying application was held on September 25 to control adult mosquitoes in two areas of Rhode Island assessed at a critical risk for the EEE virus. The areas were identified using several factors, including information about new human cases of EEE, cases of EEE in non-human mammals, positive mosquito samples in Rhode Island and in neighboring states, and information about the habitats in which mosquitoes most readily breed.

9.2.1.2 Mosquito Control Measures: 2019 Pesticide Applications

In 2019, aerial spraying occurred in four areas of Rhode Island that state officials assessed to be at critical risk for the Eastern Equine Encephalitis (EEE) virus.

- **September 8 - 10, 2019**
  In all, the state treated parts of 21 communities over three nights, from September 8 to 10, with a pesticide formulated to kill adult mosquitoes. The flight crew used the pesticide, called Anvil $10+10$, at an extremely low concentration, dispersing a total of 556 gallons across 115,179 total acres – meaning that $6/10$ of an ounce, aerosolized, was used to treat an acre. That's the equivalent of slightly less than four teaspoons per acre. In Figure 9.1 notes that Regions 1 and 2 are nearly convex, whereas Regions 3 and 4 are not.

- **Wednesday, September 25, 2019**
  A second aerial spraying application was held on September 25 to control adult mosquitoes in two areas of Rhode Island assessed at a critical risk for the EEE virus. The areas were identified using several factors, including information about new human cases of EEE, cases of EEE in non-human mammals, positive mosquito samples in Rhode Island and in neighboring states, and information about the habitats in which mosquitoes most readily breed.

In Figure 9.2, the top region is nearly convex while the bottom region is quite non-convex. It is likely the re-spraying occurred because of this, as not all areas were treated. Parts of 12 communities were aerially treated with mosquito pesticide. The spray area surrounding West Warwick included all West Warwick and parts of Cranston, Warwick, East Greenwich, West Greenwich, Coventry, and Scituate. Some of this area was previously sprayed on September 9, but officials expanded this zone westward to Route 102 in Coventry and both westward and southward in West Greenwich. The southwest area included much of Westerly and parts of Hopkinton and Charlestown that were already sprayed on September 10. This expanded area of critical risk encompassed new swaths of Hopkinton, Richmond, and Charlestown as well as the southwestern section of South Kingstown.

9.2.2 Winnipeg, Canada [4]

The fogging program (Figure 9.3) meandered throughout the city, a clear indication of non-convexity.

9.3 FLIGHT DISTANCES, PATTERNS AND TIMES OF VARIED MOSQUITOES AND DISEASE AGENTS

The flight distance data in Table 9.1 below comes from [5] and only includes a few mosquito species that can spread the diseases mentioned above. Nonetheless, the ranges vary from less than half a mile up to 40 miles (there are a few examples of longer flights). The flight patterns are largely downwind, but wind directions are quite variable from day to day. Female mosquitoes (the ones that bite) fly from 1 to 1.5 miles per hour and in a zig-zag pattern when they detect the presence of a likely target [6]. Note that there is no constraint on the direction of flight. Hence the convex set of all possible routes is possible.

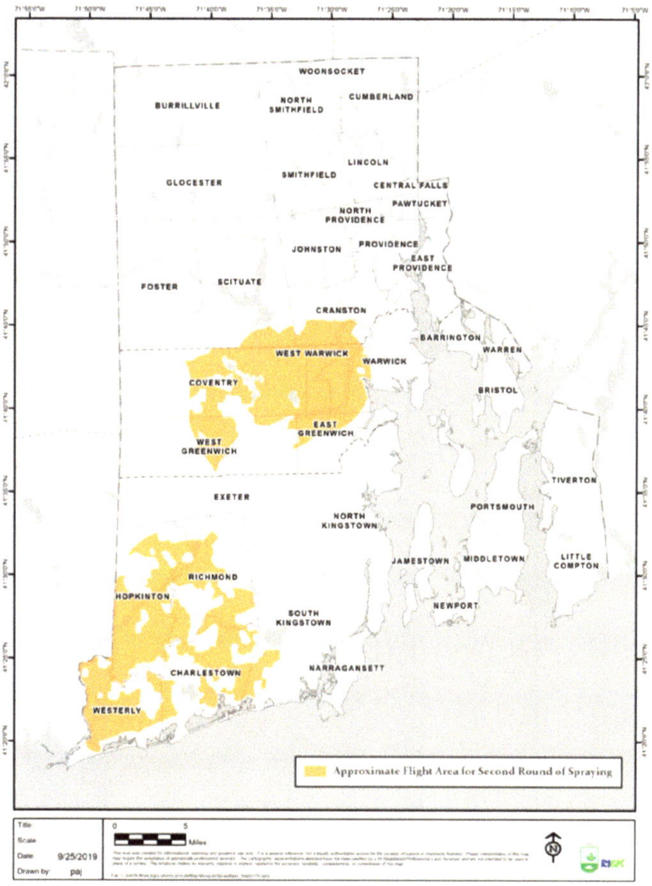

Figure 9.2: Second aerial spraying application held to control adult mosquitoes in two areas of Rhode Island.

9.4 CREATION OF DISTRICTS

Figure 9.5 below shows the US State of Delaware decomposed into a grid of 216 convex rectangles [7]. A user may then click on the rectangle in which they are located in order to see if any mosquito amelioration method is about to be utilized. These include the techniques described in Figure 9.5. While the entire convex region may not be sprayed,

Table 9.1: Flight distance data.

Mosquito Species	Flight Range	Disease Agent
Aedes aegypti	< 0.5 mile	DG, YF
Aedes albopictus	< 0.5 mile	DG, YF, WNV
Anopheles crucians	1 to 2 miles	M, EEE
Aedes vexans	1 to 5 miles	EEE, WNV
Culex salinarius	1/4 to 5 miles	EEE, WNV
Ochlerotatus sollicitans	5 to 40 miles	EEE, WNV

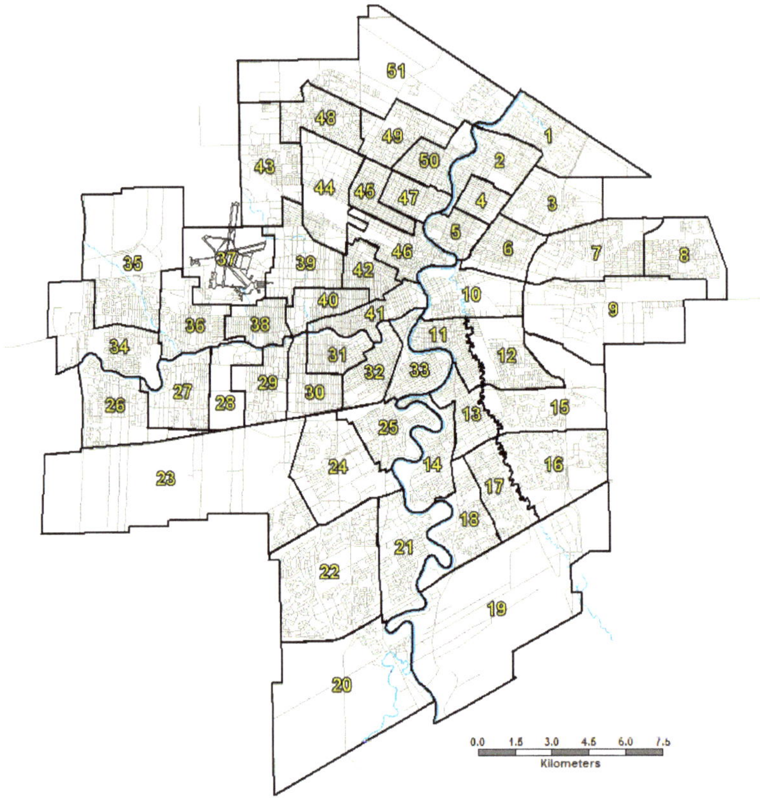

Figure 9.3: Nuisance Mosquito Fogging Program 2021, Winnipeg, Canada.

this is possible and will cover all potential flight paths of the mosquitoes in question. This map was formed using the ArcGIS Web AppBuilder which has a Mosquito Spray Area function [7]. The author and colleagues in [2] used ArcGIS to entirely redistrict the State of Texas for voting purposes (in this case for the US House of Representatives). We took a districting plan which had been found to be *gerrymandered*, that is to favour one political

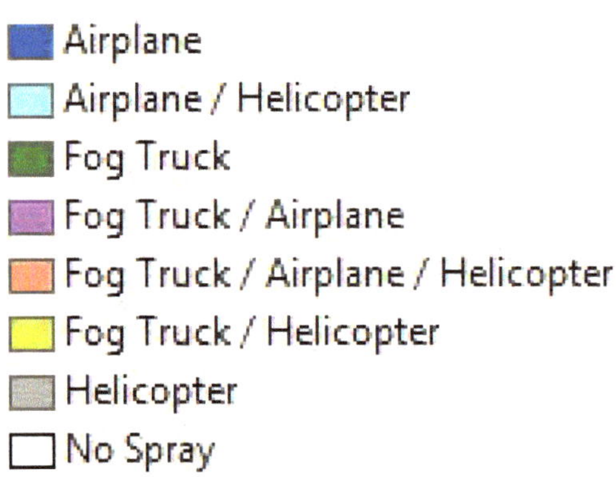

Figure 9.4: Spray activity within Zone.

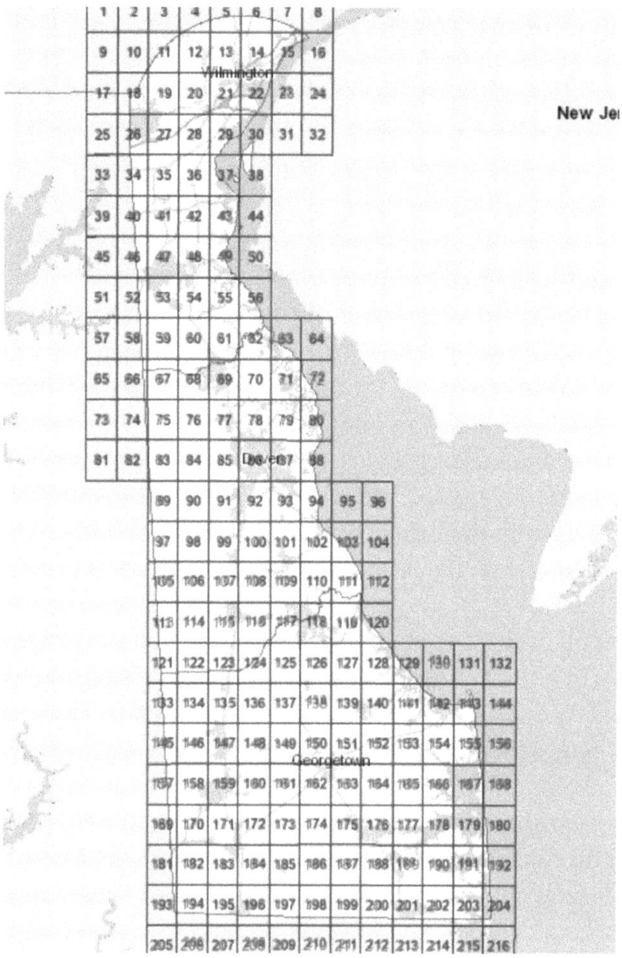

Figure 9.5: The US State of Delaware decomposed into a grid of 216 convex rectangles.

party (in this case the Republicans), because most districts were poorly shaped. In our plan almost all districts were nicely shaped, i.e. nearly convex. We propose applying the same methodology when designing mosquito abatement districts.

9.5 ANALYSIS AND CONCLUSIONS

The following steps when designing mosquito abatement regions are recommended in [5].

Survey Develop and maintain a map system that includes the following information:

- The area under your protection
- Access routes into the area
- Mosquito production zones

Develop and Plan Control Strategies for Each Type of Production Zone:

- Analyze each zone individually to determine which control strategy will provide the most sound and effective control – prevention, larvicide or adulticide controls.
- Plan ground treatment routes that are based on providing service to the citizens of the community while incorporating mosquito hot spots.

Precautions:
KEEP THE PUBLIC INFORMED about mosquito control operations. Whenever possible, notify the public of the date and time of applications before any applications for larval or adult mosquito control are made. In the case of applications directed to control adult mosquitoes, individuals with severe allergy conditions and persons with asthmatic problems may wish to stay indoors or plan to be away from the community during the treatment hours. Car finishes may be spotted with certain adulticidal insecticide sprays, and owners may wish to house them in the garage during the treatment hours. The understanding and cooperation of the general public is necessary if the program is to be successful.

We agree with all of these recommendations. Note that in the applications of our convexity techniques in [2] we dealt with the problem of finding ground access routes in different scenarios (snow-removal, solid waste pick-up, etc.). These can be applied to the ground treatment routes mentioned above.

We advocate following a model similar to the one used by Delaware when designing mosquito control districts. This model meets the requirements listed above and deals with the problem of covering all potential flight paths, a convex set. Tarrant County and North-Richland Hills in Texas, the USA, use a similar method, just not with ArcGIS [8]. But as is clear from the first examples in this paper, not every locale may follow this conclusion. In that case we recommend that each mosquito abatement district is at a minimum nearly convex. We would actually suggest a stronger version, with $\mathbf{CR}(\mathbf{D}) > \mathbf{0.6}$. This was true of most of the districts in our plan for Texas.

ACKNOWLEDGMENTS

This chapter is partly based on work performed within the framework of IMAAC (`https://imaac.eu/`) related to COST Action CA16227 (*Investigation & Mathematical Analysis of Avant-garde Disease Control via Mosquito Nano-Tech-Repellents*, `https://cost.eu/actions/CA16227/`), supported by COST Association (European Cooperation in Science and Technology). The study was performed by the author James R. Bozeman at The American University of Malta (AUM), who is thankful for its support.

GLOSSARY

Mosquito Abatement Region: An area in which spraying or fogging or ground placement of insecticides occur, e.g. [7].

Convexity: In this context, an area in which any 2 points within the region may be connected by a straight line lying entirely within the region [2].

Convexity Ratio: The ratio of the largest convex set inside a planar region to the area of the smallest convex set containing the region. This is a number between 0 and 1 inclusive [1].

Nearly Convex: A region whose convexity ratio is > 0.5 [1].

Vector-borne Diseases: In this context, diseases, e.g. malaria, spread by mosquitoes, the vector.

FURTHER READING

Vector Disease Control International: `www.vdci.net`

Center for Disease Control: `wwwn.cdc.gov/arbonet/Maps/ADB.Diseases.Map/index.html`

North Richland Hills, Texas: `nrhtx.com/994/Mosquito-Spraying`

ArcGIS: `solutions.arcgis.com/local-government/help/mosquito-spray-areas/`

World Health Organization: `apps.who.int/iris/bitstream/handle/10665/37329/9241700661_eng.pdf;sequence=1`

V

Chemometric and Mathematical Approach for Modelling and Designing Mosquito Repellents

A Multiplatform Chemometric Approach to Molecular and Mathematical Modeling of Mosquito Repellents

Milica Z. Karadzic Banjac*
University of Novi Sad, Faculty of Technology Novi Sad, Department of Applied and Engineering Chemistry, Novi Sad, Serbia
** corresponding author, e-mail: mkaradza@uns.ac.rs*

Strahinja Z. Kovacevic
University of Novi Sad, Faculty of Technology Novi Sad, Department of Applied and Engineering Chemistry, Novi Sad, Serbia

Sanja O. Podunavac-Kuzmanovic
University of Novi Sad, Faculty of Technology Novi Sad, Department of Applied and Engineering Chemistry, Novi Sad, Serbia

CONTENTS

10.1 Introduction 178
10.2 Repelling compounds in the spotlight 179
10.3 The importance of chemometric modeling in design, classification and selection of repelling compounds 182
10.3.1 QSAR platform for modeling of repellent activity 182
10.3.2 Linear chemometric regression modeling of repellence index 182
10.3.3 Non-linear chemometric regression modeling of repellence index ... 184
10.3.4 Mathematical validation of QSAR models 186
10.3.5 Chemometric classification methods as a platform for repellents selection 187
10.3.5.1 Cluster analysis 187

DOI: 10.1201/9781003035992-10

10.3.5.2 Principal component analysis 188
10.3.5.3 Sum of ranking differences 189
10.4 Concluding remarks and further research 191

10.1 INTRODUCTION

Today, the vector-borne diseases (VBD) present a severe public health issue worldwide. Spreading of VBD is conditioned by a joint action of different demographic, environmental and social factors. The vectors for the VBD transmission are various: mosquitoes, ticks, blackflies, fleas, lice, bugs, etc. Still, mosquitoes are the most important since they are a primary vectors for transmitting the wide range of the VBD. Transmission of different VBD can be mechanical, sexual, maternal, fetal and through blood transfusion (Abushouk et al. 2016). Three mosquito genus are responsible for the VBD transmission via viruses or parasites as pathogens (10.1). VBD such as dengue, Zika, chikungunya and yellow fever are viral infections while malaria is a parasite infection. According to World Health Organization (WHO 2021) VBD cause more than 700,000 deaths per year, accounting malaria with more than 400,000 deaths per year and dengue with estimated 40,000 deaths per year. A great effort is being invested through financial assets to control and eliminate VBD. For example, funding for malaria control and elimination reached an estimated 3 billion dollars in year 2019 (WHO 2021).

Majority of the efficient repellents, insecticides and pesticides are the chemical compounds with biological activity (Tsikolia et al. 2018; Jiang et al. 2017). Beside new chemical compounds, still the major interest and influence for VBD control is held by natural plant products, manly essential oils (Aungtikun and Soonwera 2021; Li et al. 2020) and acids (Gurunathan et al. 2016; Moreira et al. 2016). In the field of vaccines, new discoveries have occurred so in recent years new vaccines have been tested such as vaccines for malaria (Datoo et al. 2021), Zika (Poland et al. 2019), West Nile (Ulbert 2019), dengue (Aguiar et al. 2016), etc. New discoveries in the field of novel biologically active compounds are largely potentiated by computational, mathematical and molecular modeling.

Table 10.1: Summary of VBD with their pathogens and mosquito genus.

Vector-borne diseases	**Type of pathogen**	**Mosquito genus**
Zika	virus	*Aedes*
dengue	virus	*Aedes*
malaria	parasite	*Anopheles*
chikungunya	virus	*Aedes*
yellow fever	virus	*Aedes*
West Nile fever	virus	*Culex*
lymphatic filariasis	parasite	*Aedes, Anopheles, Culex*
Japanese encephalitis	virus	*Culex*
Rift Valley fever	virus	*Aedes*

A multiplatform chemometric approach has an outstanding roll in pharmacology and chemistry for characterization and design of biologically active compounds (Kovačević et al. 2019; Vukić et al. 2019; Kovačević et al. 2018a; Kovačević et al. 2018b; Jevrić et al. 2017; Karadžić et al. 2017a; Karadžić et al. 2017b; Kovačević et al. 2016a; Kovačević et al. 2016b; Karadžić et al. 2015a; Karadžić et al. 2015b). Nowadays, chemometrics, mathematical modeling and molecular docking are essential and valuable tools in the initial stages of the repelling compounds development. Since mosquitoes rapidly develop resistance to repelling compounds, it is necessary to involve various chemometric techniques in order to shorten the time for laboratory experiments and to save resources in the search for new highly-effective repelling compounds. Multiple linear regression (MLR), principal component regression (PCR), partial least squares (PLS) and artificial neural networks (ANN), together with pattern recognition techniques such as principal component analysis (PCA) and hierarchical cluster analysis (HCA) as well as molecular docking approach (Kovačević et al. 2020a; Kovačević et al. 2020b; Karadžić Banjac et al. 2019) can be used for virtual screening of a large number of compounds with potential repelling properties and prediction of biological activity or different physicochemical properties of novel or not yet synthesized or tested repellents or pesticides for prevention of VBD.

All of these methods form a powerful multiplatform for design, selection, testing and application of novel safe and effective compounds with desired repellent activity. A significant attention is also paid to the vector modeling (Rashkov 2021; Rashkov et al. 2019). The epidemiological models have an important role in understanding the spread pattern of the infectious diseases and evaluating different control treatments such as vector control or vaccination.

10.2 REPELLING COMPOUNDS IN THE SPOTLIGHT

The use of mosquito repellents is an important tactic worldwide considering that mosquitoes transmit pathogens that cause various VBD (Zika, dengue, malaria, chikungunya, West Nile yellow fever, etc). Repellents are a chemical-based vector control designed to act locally or at the appointed distance to deter insects from biting humans or animals. In the market, there are various kinds of repellent products: textiles (clothes), sprays, lotions, aerosols, stickers, wristbands, nets and vaccines. Repellents should be designed to match with specific mosquito species sensitivity for selected repellent, biting time, host and habitat preferences. Although there are many commercially available products, scientists all over the world are making great efforts to discover new repelling compounds that are both effective and safe for use. Until today, *N,N*-diethyl-3-methylbenzamide (DEET) is observed as a "golden standard" used for repellent candidates comparison in research activities to obtain long-lasting repellency (Bohbot et al. 2014).

Chemically-based repellents can be on natural or synthetic basis. Many studies report that different plant extracts and essential oils express larvicidal, adulticidal and repellent activities (Ghosh et al. 2021; Sharma et al. 2021; Wu et al. 2019; Zhu et al. 2018; Costa et al. 2017; Das et al. 2015). Recent research of the larvicidal, adulticidal and repellent activities of *Origanum vulgare* L. and *Thymus vulgaris* L. essential oils against *Aedes aegypti* were reported by de Oliveira et al. (2021). The authors concluded that these two essential oils with 4-terpineol, carvacrol and thymol have larvicidal and adulticidal potential for the control of *Ae. aegypti* and, therefore, can be considered eco-friendly source for development of new insecticides. The essential oil from Dai medicinal plant *Zingiber cassumunar*, containing 4-terpineol, is used in traditional medicine and also express larvicidal, adulticidal and repellent activities against *Aedes albopictus* (Ming-Xiang et al. 2020). The field efficacy of the smoke repellency of ethnomedicinal plant (*Azadirachta indica*, *Eucalyptus camaldulensis* and *Ocimum forskolin*) against *Anopheles arabiensis* and *Ae. aegypti* was analyzed in Ethiopia (Wendimu and Tekalign 2021). Tested powders shown significant protection ($> 90\%$) against both mosquito species and have the potential to be used for the mosquito control. Additionally, these repellents are reported to be safe, eco-friendly, cheap and easy to use while providing the maximum area repellency against mosquitoes. Benelli et al. (2020) have tested the essential oils from the stem wood, fresh and dry bark of *Hazomalania voyronii* against *Ae. aegypti* and *Culex quinquefasciatus* in Madagascar. They reported that essential oils from *H. voyronii* can be used in the fabrication of green repellents and insecticides for the mosquito control.

The synergistic effect of the essential oils from *Cinnamomum* plants were tested against *Ae. aegypti* and *Ae. albopictus* (Aungtikun and Soonwera 2021). A high insecticidal efficacy against *Aedes* population has been observed. A mosquito repellent activity of isolated oleic acid, eicosyl ester from *Thalictrum javanicum* was evaluated against *Ae. aegypti* and *C. quinquefasciatus* (Gurunathan et al. 2016). Results from this research suggest that these substances express larvicidal activity. A type of lichen (*Ramalina usnea*) was tested for larvicidal activity against *Ae. aegypti* (Moreira et al. 2016). Compounds 2-hydroxy-4-methoxy-6-propyl-methyl benzoate and usnic acid demonstrated the potential for the development of new synthetic molecules with larvicidal activity. Recent researches from Kajla et al. (2019) and Kajla (2020) revealed bacteria as a novel source for potent mosquito control. Fabclavines, compounds isolated from Gram-negative bacteria *Xenorhabdus budapestensis*, manifest a potent feeding-deterrent activity against important mosquito vectors *Ae. aegypti*, *Anopheles gambiae* and *Culex pipiens* (Kajla et al. 2019). Authors reported that the mosquito feeding-deterrent activity is comparable to or better than repellents currently available on the market, such as DEET or picaridin. Article published by Kajla (2020) pointed out that Gram-negative bacteria from *Xenorhabdus* and *Photorhabdus* species produce insecticidal compounds that can be used as a feeding-deterrents. Singh and Sheikh (2021) focused their research on the synthesis of novel mosquito repellent dyes from a combination of mosquito repellents. They pointed out that novel disperse dyes can be used as a tool for the multifunctional modification of polyester-based textile substrates.

A great influence in the field of mosquito repellents discovery holds odorant-binding protein (OBP)-based molecular docking, ligand-based screening and molecular simulation. Balachandran et al. (2021) conducted a molecular docking study of natural alkaloids that represent an acetylcholinesterase (AChE1) inhibitors in *Ae. aegypti*. Twenty-five alkaloids served as ligands and their docking ability with an AChE1 receptor was tested. According to the minimum energy results and the best fit into the binding pocket the alpha-solanine was chosen as the best inhibitor of AChE1 in *Ae. aegypti*. A novel bioinspired synthetic

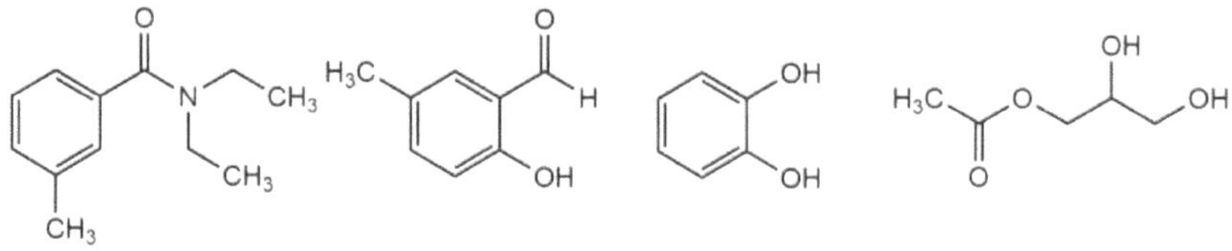

1 2 3 4

Figure 10.1: Some synthetic (**1**) and natural (**2** - **4**) compounds with repellent activity: (**1**) DEET, (**2**) 2-hydroxy-6-methylbenzaldehyde, (**3**) catechol, (**4**) monoacetin; The compounds **2** - **4** have been studied in the paper by Gaddaguti et al. (2016).

mosquito repellents were identified by Thireou et al. (2018). The authors used ligand-based screening and odorant-binding protein-structure-based molecular docking. A set of 16 compounds was tested for their affinity to AgamOBP1 *in vitro* and repellence against *A. gambiae*. Kröber et al. (2018) used an odorant-binding protein-based identification of natural spatial repellents against *A. gambiae*. This study gave an insight into approach for the identification of the biologically active molecules of natural origin that can be used as mosquito repellents. In a research of Gaddaguti et al. (2016) repelling potential of the *Ocimum* compounds (Figure 10.1) was tested against 3Q8I and 3N7H of *A. gambiae*.

If at least two compounds with best docking score are applied together, there is enhanced protection involved. So *Ocimum* compounds can be used further for eco-friendly and safe repellents production. Molecular docking and molecular dynamics simulations were utilized in a research by Mourão et al. (2021). They identified molecular scaffolds from Caatinga Brazilian biome as potential inhibitors of the sterol carrier protein-2 from *Ae. aegypti*. The biflavonoid loniflavone from leaves of Brazilian plant called catingueira was the most promising regarding the interaction with target protein.

The attention should also be paid to the unexpected and adverse effects of different repellents and pesticides on the human health. Roy et al. (2017) and Legeay et al. (2018) published overviews of the unexpected and adverse effects of different repellents (DEET, diethyl phthalate, permethrin, picaridin, DEPA, pyrethroid, tetramethrin and IR3535). Recent chapter published by Khater et al. (2019) gathered a variety of commercial repellents and gave an overview regarding safety concerns. The climate variability, primarily temperature and rainfall, is an important geographic factor since climate changes have resulted in the VBC increase (Rocklöv and Dubrow 2020; Fouque and Reeder 2019; Dhimal et al. 2015; Parham et al. 2015). Some studies indicate that temperature in Europe has increased for $0.8°C$ over the last 100 years (Githeko et al., 2000). Overall, the most important prevention and control measures regarding VBD is vector control: reduction of the mosquito populations and elimination of the breeding sites since “No mosquito – no VBD”.

10.3 THE IMPORTANCE OF CHEMOMETRIC MODELING IN DESIGN, CLASSIFICATION AND SELECTION OF REPELLING COMPOUNDS

10.3.1 QSAR platform for modeling of repellent activity

The new repellent discovery and development process is very similar to the drug discovery. The main dissimilarity in these two processes is financial side. In both of these processes chemometric approach based on the quantitative structure-activity relationship (QSAR) methodology stands as one of the crucial steps (Figure) symbolically illustrates the selection of target compounds through so-called Computer-Aided (Assisted) Drug Design (CADD) funnel where initially huge number of compounds is significantly reduced to several hits applying defined filters based on desirable molecular properties. QSAR modeling correlates chemical structure with biological properties by using various linear and non-linear methods (Natarajan et al. 2008).

10.3.2 Linear chemometric regression modeling of repellence index

Linear chemometric modeling is usually based on univariate linear regression (ULR), multiple linear regression (MLR), principal component regression (PCR) and partial least squares (PLS) regression. ULR is the simplest regression method that correlates an independent variable with one dependent variable, while in MLR two or more independent variables are correlated with one dependent variable. PCR is used when multicollinearity among the independent variables is present so the utilization of MLR method is limited. In this case it is necessary to normalize (scale) the variables. When multicollinearity occurs, PLS regression method can also be used. This technique reduces the set of independent

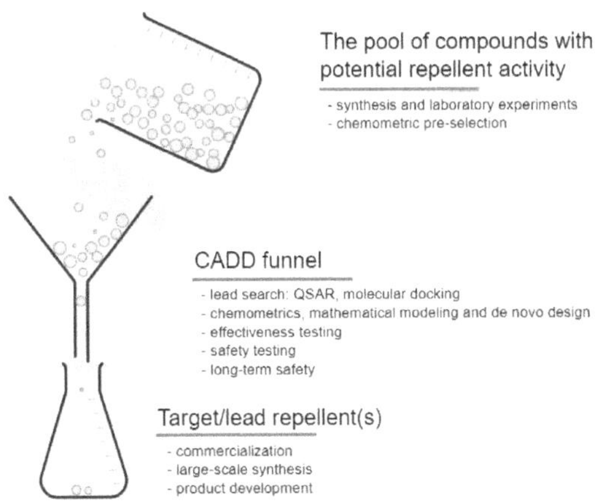

Figure 10.2: Computer-aided drug design (CADD) with chemometrics and mathematical modeling as crucial part of the process of selection of target or lead compounds and discovery and development of new repellents (*Created with Chemix (https://chemix.org)*).

variables to a smaller set of uncorrelated components. Then least squares regression is performed on these new components, instead of the original data. ULR, as the simplest method, is usually the first step in the regression modeling.

The linear modeling can be illustrated on the example of the QSAR modeling of repellence index (R_{index}) of the set containing several natural compounds (carvacrol, thymol, cuminic acid, *n*-butyl cinnamate, ethyl cinnamate, benzyl benzoate, lauric acid) and some newly synthesized compounds (Syn1 – KO5, Syn2 – KO10, Syn3 – KO2, Syn4 – KO3, Syn5 – KO9, Syn6 – KO6, Syn7 – KO4, Syn8 – KO7, Syn9 – KO11, Syn10 – KO13, Syn11 – KO12, Syn12 – KO8, Syn13 – KO16) (Thireou et al. 2018). The repellence indices toward *A. gambiae* females of these compound was published in the study by Thireou et al. 2018. The simplest model is the ULR model. It correlates R_{index} with boiling point (BP) of the compounds.

$$ULR : R_{index} = 252.8713(\pm 38.36695) - 0.3041248(\pm 0.05775952)\mathbf{BP} \tag{10.1}$$

The MLR models correlate R_{index} of the same group of the compounds with more than one molecular descriptor. The MLR1 model predicts the R_{index} based on critical pressure (CP) and calculated molar refractivity (CMR):

$$\begin{aligned} MLR1 : R_{index} &= 404.7651(\pm 56.47803) - 4.499053(\pm 1.119779)\mathbf{CP} - \\ &- 36.69531(\pm 5.468419)\mathbf{CMR} \end{aligned} \tag{10.2}$$

This model can be presented as 3D surface plot as it is given in Figure 10.3 so it can be easily noticed what values of CP and CMR a compound should have to express desirable R_{index}.

The MLR2 model presents the relationship between R_{index} and three independent variables: BP, total polar surface area (tPSA) and calculated lipophilicity descriptor (ClogP):

$$\begin{aligned} MLR2 : R_{index} &= 248.8165(\pm 37.2906) - 0.480915(\pm 0.06351143)\mathbf{BP} + \\ &+ 1.853831(\pm 0.4399472)\mathbf{tPSA} + 16.48189(\pm 5.434551)\mathbf{ClogP} \end{aligned} \tag{10.3}$$

This model implies the significance of three molecular features that affect the repellence ability of the studied series of compounds. Considering the highest value of the regression coefficient in this model, the lipophilicity parameter (ClogP) has the greatest influence on R_{index}. The selection of the most suitable descriptors for the MLR models was carried out by NCSS 2007 program by *all possible regression* routine from the set of the descriptors that contained boiling point (BP), melting point (MP), critical temperature (CT), critical pressure (CP), critical volume (CV), Gibbs energy (GE), lipophilicity (logP), molar refractivity (MR), total polar surface area (tPSA), calculated lipophilicity descriptor (ClogP) and calculated molar refractivity (CMR). All the descriptors were calculated by ChemBioDraw Ultra 13.0 program (PerkinElmer Inc.).

Although mathematically the simplest and easiest to interpret, ULR models often cannot fully describe the dependence of the biological response on the molecular structure,

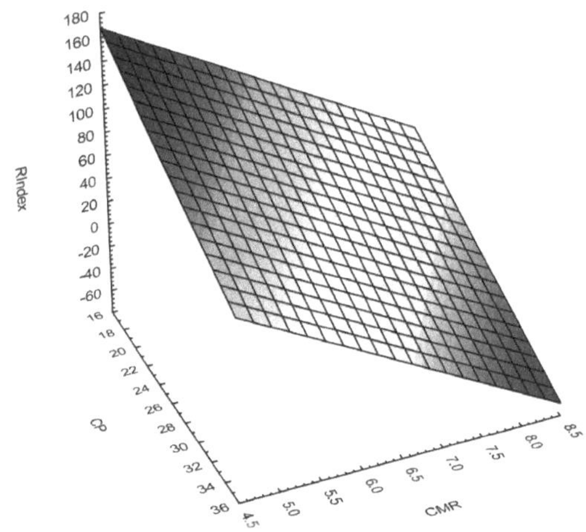

Figure 10.3: 3D model of QSAR MLR1 equation that correlates R_{index} with critical pressure (CP) and calculated molar refractivity (CMR).

since this dependence is often very complex. Therefore, MLR modeling is more often used in linear QSAR modeling than the ULR. The number of independent variables in MLR models is limited according to the Topliss-Costello rule which says that the ratio between the number of the samples and the number of independent variables should be greater than five. It is worth stressing that in MLR modeling, multicollinearity is one of limiting factors and must be examined. This is usually done based on the value of variance inflation factor (VIF; if VIF > 5, the multicollinearity is significant). If multicollinearity is significant, it is better to apply PCR or PLS regression methods where the multicollinearity is one of the conditions for their application. The application of ridge regression (RR), PCR and PLS methods in modeling of repellent activity of a set of compounds toward females of *A. aegypti* mosquitoes was demonstrated in the study by Natarajan et al. 2008. MLR and various machine learning approaches in the modeling of repellent activity to *A. aegypti* of a series of carboxamides was done by Doucet et al. 2019. In the study by De et al. 2018, the MLR modeling, stepwise regression (SR) and PLS regression methods were successfully applied in QSAR modeling of larvicidal activity of plant derived compounds against Zika virus vector *A. aegypti* based on *in silico* molecular descriptors.

10.3.3 Non-linear chemometric regression modeling of repellence index

The modeling based on the application of artificial neural networks (ANNs) has become one of the most used non-linear regression methods in chemometric modeling of biological activity (Kovačević et al. 2018b). The ANNs are the structures composed of densely connected adaptive process elements. They have the ability to mimic the basic characteristics of the human brain because each neural network consists of artificial neurons that have a task to mimic biological neurons. The efficiency of this technique is reflected in the ability to recognize complex relationships between input and output variables without prior information related to the very nature of the problem. The modeling of R_{index} of the aforementioned set of natural and synthesized compounds based on BP, tPSA and ClogP molecular descriptors (the same inputs as in MLR2 model) was carried out applying ANN approach as well.

The modeling was done applying multi-layer perceptron (MLP) feedforward neural networks with Broyden-Fletcher-Goldfarb-Shanno (BFGS) algorithm with different hidden and activation functions. The main set of the compounds was divided into three sets: Eq. 10.1 training set for the networks' training, Eq.10.2 test set for determination of generalization error and Eq.10.3 validation set for finding the best ANN architecture and training parameters. The architectures of the obtained networks are presented in Table 10.1.

The networks' architecture is described in the form of number of input variables – number of hidden neurons – number of output variables. The results indicate a good quality of the obtained networks considering high correlation coefficients (*R*) of the training, validation and test sets, as well as acceptable room mean square error (*RMSE*) values. The predictive ability of the established ANNs was estimated based on the comparison of experimental and predicted values of R_{index} and, as it can be seen on Figure 10.4, there is quite good concurrence between the experimental data and data predicted by the established ANNs. The best concurrence between the data was achieved by the network MLP 3-8-1. One of the main flaws of the ANN approach is that there is no the exact mathematical equation that describes the relationship between input and output variables. This is the reason that some researchers consider neural networks to be a "black box".

Another application of the non-linear modeling of mosquito repellency of acylpiperidines, carried out by using the ANN modeling approach, was presented in the study by Katritzky

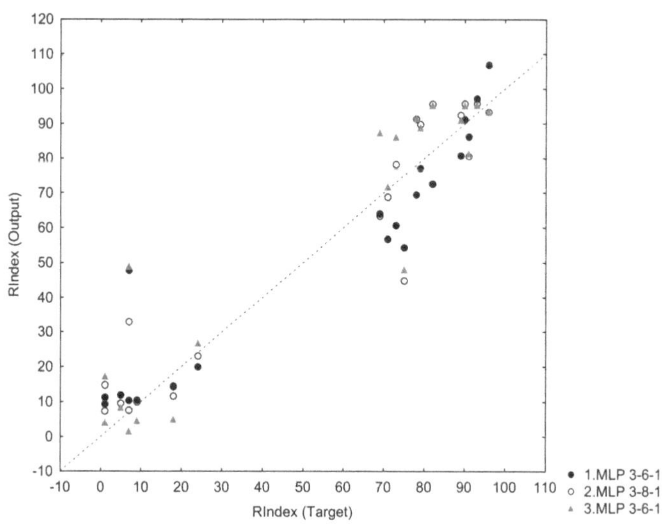

Figure 10.4: The comparison between the experimental (target) R_{index} values and R_{index} values (output) predicted by the established ANNs.

Table 10.2: The architecture of ANN models aimed for prediction of R_{index} based on physicochemical properties and some statistical parameters of the networks.

Network Architecture	R_{train}	R_{test}	R_{valid}	$RMSE_{train}$	$RMSE_{test}$	$RMSE_{valid}$	Training Algorithm	Hidden Activation Function	Output Activation Function
MLP 3-6-1	0.9183	0.9116	0.9998	100.7	12.8	38.6	BFGS 24*	Tanh	Exponential
MLP 3-8-1	0.9396	0.8294	0.9989	75.6	10.4	67.3	BFGS 24*	Logistic	Logistic
MLP 3-6-1	0.9103	0.6379	0.9990	117.5	31.3	104.7	BFGS 10*	Exponential	Logistic

**the number of training cycles after which the best network architecture is reached*

et al. 2008. The obtained high-quality model is aimed for prediction of repellent activity of novel compounds structurally similar to the compounds used in the ANN modeling.

10.3.4 Mathematical validation of QSAR models

A formed mathematical model is not applicable and cannot be considered reliable if it is not statistically validated by using a proper validation approach (Gramatica and Sangion, 2016; Chirico and Gramatica, 2012; Chirico and Gramatica, 2011). Some of the standard validation parameters are Pearson correlation coefficient (R), determination coefficient (R^2), adjusted determination coefficient (R^2_{adj}), Fisher test (F-value), root mean square error (*RMSE*) and probability (p-value). As a part of internal validation of the models, cross-validation (also known as out-of-sample testing) is often applied. This heuristic validation method is based on the omitting one or more objects from the set and the modeling is than based on the remaining compounds in the training set and the activity of the removed compounds is then estimated based on the newly established QSAR model (Gramatica and Sangion 2016; Chirico and Gramatica 2012; Chirico and Gramatica 2011). These cycles are repeated for all the compounds from the training set. Eventually, the predictivity of the QSAR model is judged based on the following parameters: cross-validation determination coefficient ($R^2{}_{cv}$), total sum of squares (*TSS*), predicted residual error sum of squares (*PRESS*), *PRESS/TSS* ratio and predicted standard deviation (SD_{PRESS}).

One of the most reliable validation approaches of the QSAR models is the external validation when the external test set is kept out of the training set and then after the modeling is used for the testing of real predictivity of the QSAR model. The parameters of the external validation are determination coefficient of the prediction of the external set ($R^2{}_{ext}$), mathematically different determination coefficient for the external validation including $Q^2{}_{F1}$, $Q^2{}_{F2}$, $Q^2{}_{F3}$ and $r^2{}_m$, as well as concordance correlation coefficient (*CCC*). Detailed explanation of the validation of QSAR models can be found elsewhere (Gramatica and Sangion 2016; Chirico and Gramatica 2012; Chirico and Gramatica 2011).

The statistical parameters of the established linear models from the subsection 3.1.1. are presented in Table 2. The results indicate that the model MLR2 has the highest predictivity according to the highest $R^2{}_{cv}$ coefficient and the lowest error (the lowest *RMSE* parameter), while the ULR model makes the biggest error in prediction and may be used for approximate estimation of R_{index} of the compounds structurally similar to the compounds used in model's calibration. According to the values of $R^2{}_{adj}$ it can be concluded

Table 10.3: Statistical parameters of the established linear QSAR models for prediction of R_{index} of the set of natural and synthesized compounds

Regression model	R^2	R^2_{adj}	R^2_{cv}	*RMSE*	*F*
ULR	0.6063	0.5845	0.5306	24.3495	27.7
MLR1	0.7289	0.6971	0.6552	20.7907	22.9
MLR2	0.8150	0.7804	0.7192	17.7024	23.5

that the introduction of additional predictor (increase in the number of variables) variable improves the model's quality more than it would be expected by chance.

Another confirmation of the quality of QSAR models is comparison between experimental and predicted values, as well as the analysis of amplitude and randomness of residuals (absolute differences between the experimental and predicted values). In an ideal case, the relationship between experimental and predicted values is described by $R^2 = 1$, while the absolute values of the residuals are equal to zero. Quite extensive validation approaches, including the cross-validation, have been applied in the studies by De et al. 2018, Natarajan et al. 2008 and Wang et al. 2017.

10.3.5 Chemometric classification methods as a platform for repellents selection

10.3.5.1 Cluster analysis

Cluster analysis is one of the most favored chemometric pattern recognition techniques. In the modeling of the compounds with repellent activity it can be applied for the purpose of grouping of the compounds based on their molecular of bioactivity properties. The clustering can be carried out as agglomerative clustering (each object observed individually then gradually objects are merged into one group) or as division clustering (two groups are being formed from one and then the next two from them). Since there is a building of hierarchy of clusters, this analysis is also known as hierarchical cluster analysis (HCA). The results of HCA are usually presented in a visual form known as dendrogram (Figure 10.5).

The dendrogram presented in Fig. 10.5 shows the grouping of natural repellents and novel compounds synthesized by Thireou et al. 2018 in the space of their calculated physicochemical descriptors, including: boiling point (BP), melting point (MP), critical temperature (CT), critical pressure (CP), critical volume (CV), Gibbs energy (GE), lipophilicity (logP), molar refractivity (MR), total polar surface area (tPSA), calculated lipophilicity descriptor (ClogP) and calculated molar refractivity (CMR). All the descriptors were calculated by ChemBioDraw Ultra 13.0 program (PerkinElmer Inc.). The dendrogram indicates that some of the synthesized compounds are quite similar in the space of the calculated molecular features with the natural repellents. The closest similarity is between *n*-butyl cinnamate and Syn7 compound, as well as ethyl cinnamate and Syn4 compound, whose structures are presented in Figure 10.6. Also, on the basis of the presented results of HCA analysis in Figure 10.5 it can be seen that there are two main clusters: one with the group of seven synthetic compounds together with lauric acid, and other one with the rest of the compounds.

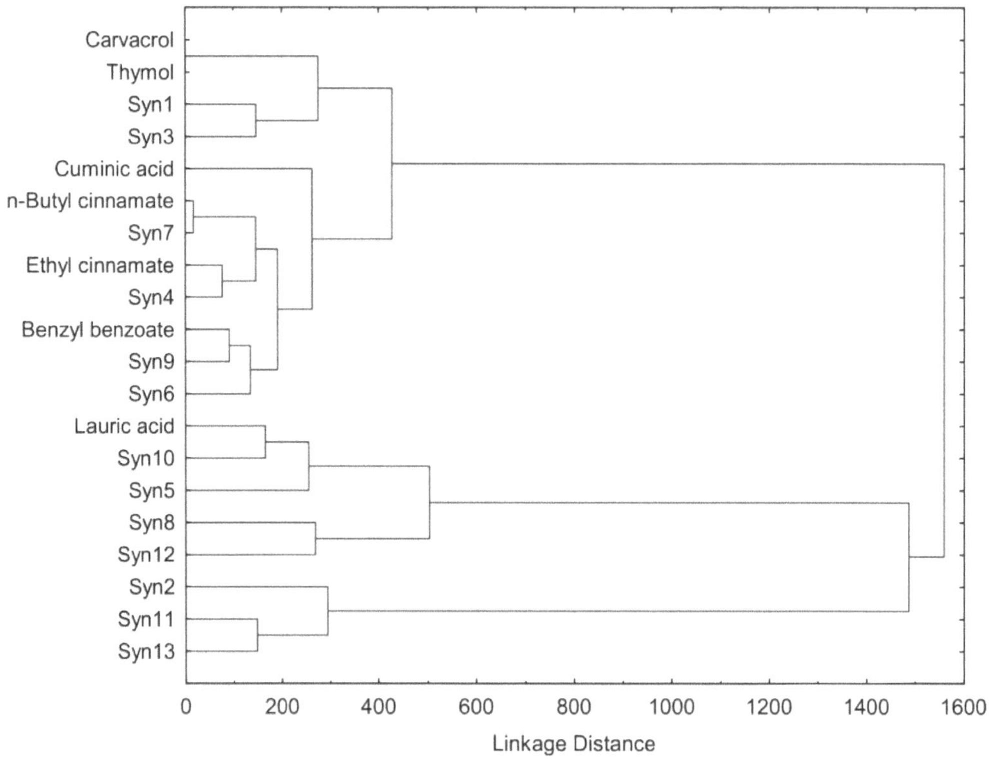

Figure 10.5: The clustering of natural and synthesized compounds (Syn1 – Syn13) with repellent activity toward *A. gambiae* females (Thireou et al. 2018) based on calculated physicochemical descriptors.

10.3.5.2 Principal component analysis

Along with cluster analysis, principal component analysis (PCA) is one of the most often exploited pattern recognition method. If multicollinearity among the studied variables occurs, it is meaningful to apply PCA in order to reduce the data set and define new principle variables. Scores plot and loadings plot are used to present the result of analysis and they serve for the observation of the similar variables. The score plot of the PCA that presents the distribution of the same set of compounds that was analyzed by HCA on the basis of the same set of molecular descriptors is presented in Figure 10.7. The score plot shown in Figure 10.7 indicates significant separation of the majority of synthesized compounds along the PC1 axis that takes into account 47.34% of total variance. Most of the natural repellent compounds are placed on the positive end on the PC1 axis. The distribution of the compounds along the PC2 axis, that covers 34.46% of total variability, is mostly based on their lipophilicity that has the strongest influence on PC2 axis. The influence of the descriptors on the compounds distribution is determined on the basis of the loadings plot (not shown).

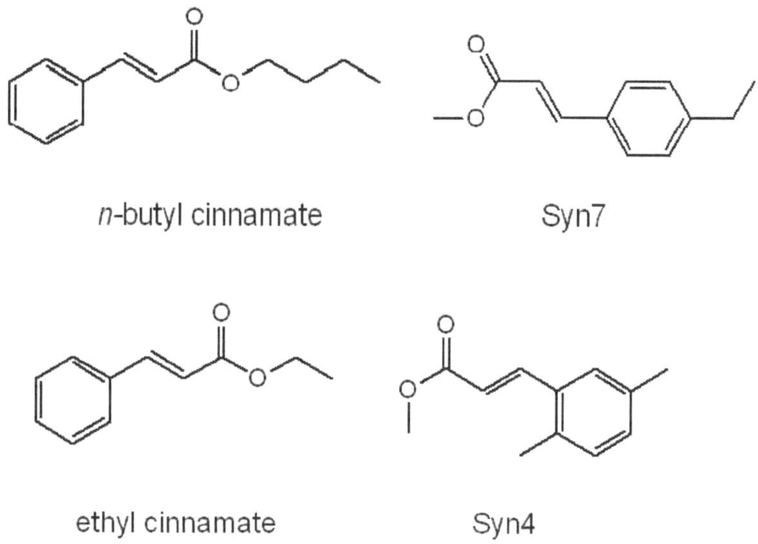

Figure 10.6: The molecular structures of the pairs of compounds classified as the most similar according to the results of HCA.

The number of principal components is determined based on Eigenvalues. If Eigenvalue of a PC is greater than 1, it can be considered in further analysis. If there is more than two PCs that fulfill this rule, the distribution of the compounds can be studied in all possible combinations of chosen PCs. Practical application of PCA in the analysis of repellence activity or structural properties of the compounds with repellence activity is actually in their possibility to point out which sub-group of the compounds from the original group is possibly separated and based on which feature. This can be important for further selection of target compounds. Compared to simple HCA, the PCA has significant advantage since it provides the information which variables are actually responsible for the grouping of compounds in the space of the chosen PCs, while in a simple HCA this cannot be seen. However, the double dendrograms that in one graph take into account both the clustering of compounds and clustering of variables can provide this answer.

10.3.5.3 Sum of ranking differences

Sum of ranking differences (SRD) is a non-parametric method used for comparison of different samples, techniques or models. This methods is introduced by Héberger (Héberger, 2010) and it has become much utilized in many QSAR studied (Kovačević et al., 2018a). Briefly, the SRD analysis is based on calculation of the rank differences between the rank of the model and the rank of the reference (Kollár-Hunek and Héberger, 2011). It is crucial to set the "golden standard" correctly in order to have realistic referent ranking. SRD can be validated by the comparison of ranks by random numbers (CRRN) procedure. Detailed theoretical background and working principles of SRD method were introduced

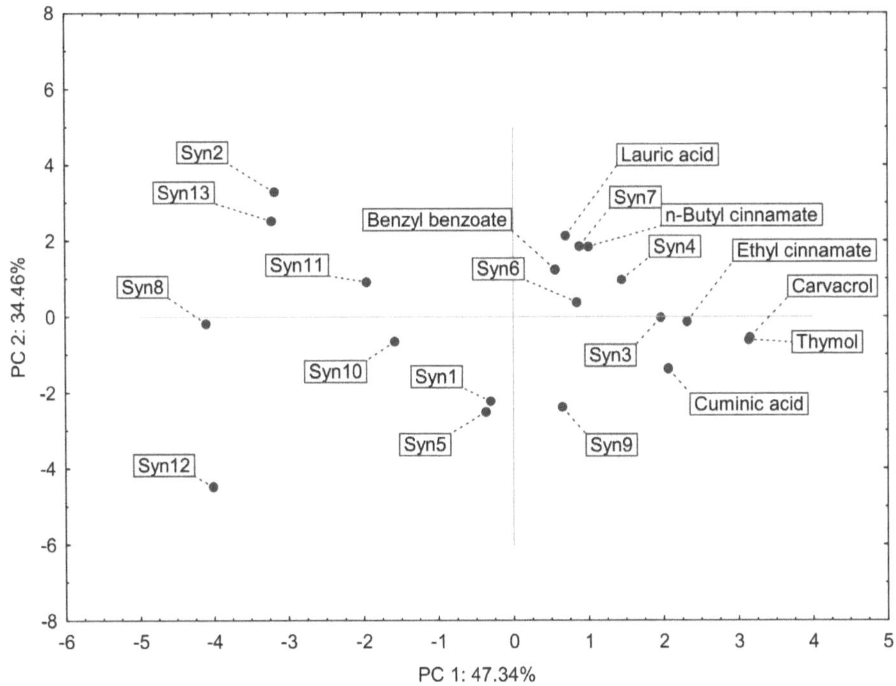

Figure 10.7: The distribution of the compounds on the score plot based on their physicochemical properties.

in the literature (Héberger, 2010; Kollár-Hunek and Héberger, 2011; Kollár-Hunek and Héberger, 2013). The practical application of SRD method in the ranking of compounds based on their physicochemical descriptors is demonstrated on the aforementioned set of natural and synthetic compounds with repellent activity towards *A. gambiae* females.

The results of the SRD analysis are presented in Figure 10.8. The reference ranking was the row average of the normalized values of molecular descriptors. The results indicate that ethyl cinnamate and benzyl benzoate are the closest to the average ranking, while the compound Syn12 is placed furthest from it. This means that Syn12 may have significantly different molecular features than other compounds from the same set. This does not necessarily mean that the Syn12 compound has the weakest repellent activity but it possess extreme lipophilicity, boiling point, melting point, critical temperature and other molecular features. The SRD approach is quite useful in quick detection of compounds with extreme molecular properties based on the established reference ranking.

Considering the similarities between the ranking numbers of different compounds, the SRD approach can be used for the analysis of the grouping of similar compounds in the space of selected molecular properties. For example, in Figure 10.8 it can be seen that

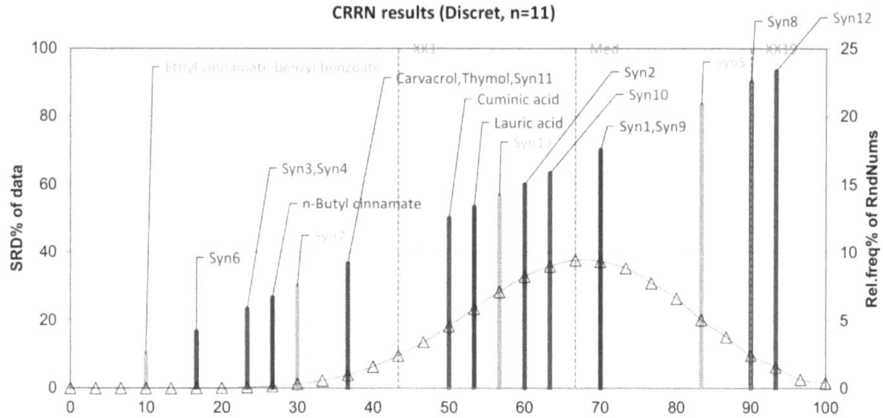

Figure 10.8: The ranking of the analyzed natural and synthesized compounds with repellence activity towards *A. gambiae* females based on their normalized physicochemical properties and row average as the reference ranking. The statistical characteristics of Gaussian fit are the following: first icosaile (5%), XX1 = 26; first quartile, Q1 = 34; median, Mediana (Med) = 40; last quartile, Q3 = 46; last icosaile (95%), XX19 = 54.

carvacrol, thymol and Syn13 have the same ranking number meaning that they have the same ranking with regard to the reference ranking. The grouping of the compounds can be evaluated on the basis of the proximity of the ranking numbers as well: close SRD values mean a close ranking position.

10.4 CONCLUDING REMARKS AND FURTHER RESEARCH

"No mosquito – no VBD" remains the most important parole regarding VBD since the most effective vector control strategy is reduction of the mosquito populations and elimination of the breeding sites. The modeling platform based on chemometrics and all its modeling tools provides quick answers by the means of the selection of the most potent but safe compounds with significant repellent activity toward mosquitoes. Both regression and pattern recognition chemometric methods have found a significant place in the modern design and selection of the repellents reducing the time and costs of this complex task. Also, it should be borne in mind that the application of these methods implies excellent knowledge of the issues related to the selection of new repellents, as well as the expertise in interpretation of the data resulting from the application of sophisticated and complex chemometric methods.

ACKNOWLEDGMENTS

This chapter is partly based on work performed within the framework of IMAAC (`https://imaac.eu/`) related to COST Action CA16227 (*Investigation & Mathe-*

matical Analysis of Avant-garde Disease Control via Mosquito Nano-Tech-Repellents, `https://cost.eu/actions/CA16227/`), supported by COST Association (European Cooperation in Science and Technology).

GLOSSARY

ANN: artificial neural networks,

CRRN: comparison of ranks by random numbers,

DEET: N,N-diethyl-3-methylbenzamide,

DEPA: N,N-diethyl phenylacetamide,

HCA: hierarchical cluster analysis,

IR3535: 3-[*N*-butyl-*N*-acetyl]-aminopropionic acid,

MLR: multiple linear regression,

LR: linear regression,

OBP: odorant binding protein,

PCA: principal component analysis,

PCR: principal component regression,

PLS: partial least squares,

QSAR: quantitative structure–activity relationship,

RR: ridge regression,

SRD: sum of ranking differences,

VBD: vector-borne diseases.

FURTHER READING

Becskei, A. and Serrano, L. (2000). Engineering stability in gene networks by autoregulation. *Nature,* 405: 590–593.

VI

Pharmacy Meets Mosquito Control: Using Pharmacological Tools Combating Mosquito Transmitted VBDs

CHAPTER 11

Pharmacological Approach to Combat Mosquito Transmitted Malaria

Ellen Kalesi Gondwe Mhango

Faculty of Pharmaceutical Sciences, School of Health Sciences, University of Iceland, Reykjavik, Iceland &
Department of Pharmacy, Kamuzu University of Health Sciences, Blantyre, Malawi

Baxter Hepburn Kachingwe

Department of Pharmacy, Kamuzu University of Health Sciences, Blantyre, Malawi

Peter E. Olumese

Diagnosis Medicines and Resistance, Global Malaria Programme, World Health Organization (WHO), Geneve, Switzerland

Precious Ngwalero Katundu

Department of Pharmacy, Kamuzu University of Health Sciences, Blantyre, Malawi &
Division of Clinical Pharmacology, University of Cape Town, Cape Town, South Africa

Kamunkhwala Gausi

Division of Clinical Pharmacology, University of Cape Town, Cape Town, South Africa

Sveinbjorn Gizurarson*

Faculty of Pharmaceutical Sciences, School of Health Sciences, University of Iceland, Reykjavik, Iceland &
Department of Pharmacy, Kamuzu University of Health Sciences, Blantyre, Malawi &
Hananja plc, Reykjavik, Iceland
** corresponding author, e-mail: sveinbj@hi.is*

CONTENTS

11.1 Introduction 196
11.2 Pharmacological treatment of malaria 197

DOI: 10.1201/9781003035992-11

11.3 Resistance to antimalarial treatment, a global threat 198
11.4 Clinical pharmacokinetics of antimalarial drugs 200
11.5 Treatment of pregnant women 203
11.6 Treatment of infants and young children 205
11.7 Conclusion 209

11.1 INTRODUCTION

Malaria is a parasitic disease transmitted mainly by the bite of an infected female *Anopheles* mosquitoes. Although more than 120 *plasmodium* species exist, only five of them cause malaria in humans viz: *Plasmodium falciparum*, *Plasmodium vivax*, *Plasmodium ovale*, *Plasmodium malariae* and *Plasmodium knowlesi*. *P. falciparum* and *P. vivax* are the most infectious parasites in Africa and in many countries outside Sub-Saharan Africa (SSA), respectively. *P. falciparum* has been reported to be responsible for most of the deaths, accounting for more than 99% of the entire malaria related mortalities worldwide. Though *P. vivax* is largely associated with uncomplicated malaria, evidence exists of its possibility to trigger severe malaria [1]. Although *P. malariae* and *P. ovale* are usually associated with uncomplicated malaria, they can hardly cause other complications [1, 2, 3]. *P. knowlesi* cause malaria in both humans and some primates. Upon the bite of the mosquito, the parasite goes to the liver for maturation; and after some days, it migrates to the bloodstream where it infects red blood cells (RBCs). While inside the RBCs, it takes $48 - 72\,h$ for the parasites to multiply, and therefore, causing rupturing of RBCs. Then the RBCs continue getting infected by the parasite with subsequent symptoms that follow in $48 - 72\,h$ [1].

Almost 50 % of the earth's population are at risk of getting malaria, which is presently widespread in tropical and subtropical countries, including all of SSA together with huge areas of South East Asia, Eastern Mediterranean, Western Pacific, and the Americas [2]. According to the 2019 world malaria report, over 400,000 deaths in 2019 were due to malaria [3]. Malaria caused 405,000 mortalities worldwide in 2018, and 94 % of all mortalities happened in Sub Saharan Africa. Global mortalities caused an overwhelming US $\$ \, 3.1$ billion financial burden [1, 2].

Worldwide, *a child perishes every two minutes as a result of malaria*. Africa bears about 90% of all malaria mortalities especially among children [4, 5, 6]. Children below 5 years of age suffer the greatest burden of the disease representing more than 50% of worldwide deaths. In Africa, the risk of severe anemia linked to malaria is greatest in children under the age of five and is a cause of an elevated risk of perishing from severe malaria especially when hemoglobin levels drop below $1.86\ mmol/L\ \ (3g/dL)$ [2, 7, 8, 9].

In pregnancy, malaria is detrimental to both the pregnant woman and the fetus. Out of ten maternal mortalities in malaria regions, one is likely to be caused by *P. falciparum*.

Malaria in pregnancy causes anemia, miscarriage in the first trimester, stillbirths, premature births (birth prior to 37 weeks of gestation), and low birthweight (i.e. less than 2.5 kg). In Africa, up to 100,000 infant mortalities per annum are due to low birthweight because of maternal infection with *P. falciparum* whilst pregnant. Low birthweight is the main cause of the diseases and deaths in neonates and early childhood and cardiac diseases late in life [7, 10, 11, 12, 13]. In extreme transmission regions, notwithstanding the hostile effects on fetal growth, malaria is generally asymptomatic in pregnancy or is coupled with symptoms that are non-specific and mild. Inadequate data exists on the safety, efficacy, and pharmacokinetics of most antimalarial drugs, especially in the first trimester.

11.2 PHARMACOLOGICAL TREATMENT OF MALARIA

The principal objective of treatment[11.1] is to necessitate the quick and complete removal of the *Plasmodium* parasites from a patient's circulation to prevent an uncomplicated malaria from progressing to severe infection or mortality. Effective malaria management also decreases transmission of the disease to other people by decreasing the disease reservoir and by preventing the emergence and spread of resistance to antimalarial drugs.

World health organization (WHO) recommended the use of artemisinin based combination therapy (ACT) as first line treatment for uncomplicated malaria [14]. ACT is a combination of a fast-acting artemisinin derivative with a slower acting partner drug. This combination is based on the fact that the fast, short acting artemisinin derivative decreases the number of parasites quickly while the slower, prolonged acting partner drug clears the residual parasites from the blood and protects artemisinin derivatives form developing resistance. Regardless of whether the patient is semi immune or not, a complete treatment course of a greatly efficacious ACT must be administered. Effective ACT regimens must be provided as a 72 *h* treatment with an artemisinin derivative. The following five ACTs on Table (11.1)[11.2] have been recommended for use in children and adults with the exception of pregnant women in the first trimester.

Table 11.1: The five recommended ACTs for treating uncomplicated *P. falciparum* malaria.

Artemisinin derivative / drug	**Partner drug**
Artemether	Lumefantrine
Artesunate	Amodiaquine
Artesunate	Mefloquine
Dihydroartemisinin	Piperaquine
Artesunate	Sulphadoxine – pyrimethamine

[11.1] Kindly note, as described in the introduction of this book, the Editor is not responsible for any suggestion for treatments or therapies described in this chapter or other chapters. For detailed information, please get in touch with the authors or the corresponding author directly.

[11.2] Adapted from WHO 2015. Guidelines for treatment of malaria 3rd Ed. [15].

A different ACT with known efficacy in the area can be used as the second line of treatment when failure happens within 28 days. However, a treatment after 28 days of the first treatment ought to be regarded as new diseases and should be treated using the first line ACT, except for mefloquine that cannot be reused within 60 days of initial treatment, as it is known to elevate the risk of neuropsychiatric reactions.

The antimalarial action of artemether is dependent on its peroxide bridge. When it interacts with hemoglobin-iron in the food vacuole of the parasite, its endoperoxide bridge rupture with resultant formation of free radicals. These free radicals will trigger delay of protein growth throughout development of trophozoites [16]. Artemether also works by disrupting the mitochondria in the parasite, hindering formation of new blood vessels, and by modulating the immune role of the host [17, 18].

Lumefantrine acts by blocking the detoxification of hemoglobin, inside the parasite. When that happens, toxic hemoglobin and free radicals will cause the parasite to die [17]. Patients who are unable to swallow or take oral ACTs are recommended to be given parenteral or rectal medication for $24 - 48\ h$ until they can swallow or take oral medicine.

11.3 RESISTANCE TO ANTIMALARIAL TREATMENT, A GLOBAL THREAT

Antimalarial drug resistance is defined as the ability of a parasite strain to survive or multiply despite the proper administration and absorption of an antimalarial drug at the recommended dose. Drug resistance to an antimalarial compound reflects a right-hand shift in the concentration–effect (dose–response) relation Figure (11.1).

Resistance is a right-hand shift in the concentration–effect relation for a particular malaria parasite population. It may be a parallel shift (red) from the "normal" profile

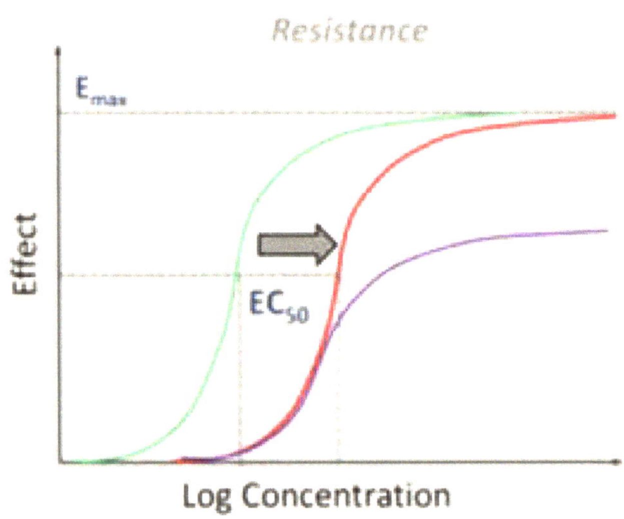

Figure 11.1: The concentration–effect relationship. E_{max} is the maximal effect of the drug, where EC50 is the concentration required to induce 50% efficacy.

(green), or, in some circumstances, the slope changes or the maximum achievable effect (E_{max}) is reduced (purple). The effect measured in vivo is parasite killing (reflected by reduction in parasite density), and that in vitro is usually a measure of parasite development [15].

Resistance to antimalarial agents arises because of the selection of parasites with genetic changes (mutations or gene amplifications) that confer reduced susceptibility. To date, parasite resistance to antimalarial medicines has been documented in 3 of the 5 malaria species known to affect humans: *P. falciparum*, *P. vivax* and *P. malariae*. Resistance has also been documented to all classes of antimalarial medicines, including the artemisinin derivatives, and it is a major threat to malaria control. The main consequence of antimalarial drug resistance is treatment failure [19].

Widespread inappropriate use of antimalarial drugs exerts a strong selective pressure on malaria parasites to develop high levels of resistance. Resistance can be prevented, or its onset slowed considerably by combining antimalarial drugs with different mechanisms of action and ensuring high cure rates through full adherence to correct dose regimens. If different drugs with different mechanisms of resistance are used together, the emergence and spread of resistance should be slowed.

Artemisinin based combination therapies (ACTs) are a combination of an artemisinin component and a partner drug which is currently the main strategy to combat resistance to antimalarial medicines. However, in the WHO Western Pacific Region and in the WHO South-East Asia Region, partial resistance to artemisinin and resistance to a number of the ACT partner drugs has been confirmed in Cambodia, Lao People's Democratic Republic, Myanmar, Thailand, and Viet Nam through studies conducted between 2001 and 2019. In Africa, evidence has recently been published showing emergence of mutations linked to partial artemisinin resistance in Rwanda. A summary of worldwide data on antimalarial drug efficacy and drug resistance is available on GMP website.[11.3]

In 2015, the WHO World Health Assembly endorsed a global plan of action against antimicrobial resistance. The goal of the draft global action plan is to ensure, for as long as possible, continuity of successful treatment and prevention of infectious diseases with effective and safe medicines that are quality-assured, used in a responsible way, and accessible to all who need them [20]. To achieve this goal, the global action plan sets out five strategic objectives:

- to improve awareness and understanding of antimicrobial resistance;
- to strengthen knowledge through surveillance and research;
- to reduce the incidence of infection;
- to optimize the use of antimicrobial agents; and

[11.3] https://www.who.int/malaria/areas/drug_resistance/drug_efficacy_database/en/

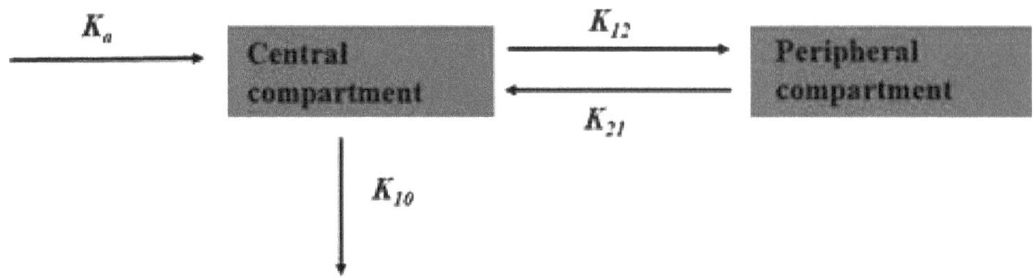

Figure 11.2: Illustrating a pharmacokinetic two-compartment model and associated rate constants.

- develop the economic case for sustainable investment that takes account of the needs of all countries, and increase investment in new medicines, diagnostic tools, vaccines and other interventions.

So far, ACTs that have been tested remain highly efficacious. However, further spread of resistance to artemisinin and ACT partner drugs could pose a major public health challenge and jeopardize important gains in malaria control. Regular monitoring of drug efficacy is needed to inform treatment policies in malaria-endemic countries, and to ensure early detection of, and response to, drug resistance.

11.4 CLINICAL PHARMACOKINETICS OF ANTIMALARIAL DRUGS

The two-compartment pharmacokinetic model fit for artemether and lumefantrine, demonstrated by a few studies for both drugs administered through the extravascular (mostly oral) route [21, 22, 23, 24]. The two-compartment model has is made up of a central compartment representing plasma and highly perfused tissues and a peripheral compartment which represents all the tissues and organs of the human body. There is bidirectional movement of the antimalarial drug between the central and peripheral compartments with drug input and elimination occurring from the central compartment (Figure 11.3). The two-compartment model pharmacokinetics describes three main phases of absorption, distribution, and elimination with rate constants $\alpha, \beta(K_{10})$, respectively with assumptions that absorption, distribution, metabolism and elimination processes follow first order kinetics and the movement of drugs between compartments is through passive diffusion. In addition, it assumes that the antimalarial concentration measurements are from blood and the organ of elimination is in the central compartment.

The parameters of a two-compartment model extravascular administration include: the absorption rate constant (K_a), the rate constant from central to the peripheral compartment (K_{12}), and reverse (K_{21}), the distribution coefficient (A) and rate constant (α), the volume of distribution (V_c, V_{ss}, V_z), the elimination coefficient (β) and rate constant (K_{10}), the elimination half-life ($t_{1/2}$), the area under the concentration-time curve (AUC) and clearance (Cl).

The distribution of the free fraction between central and peripheral compartment is dependent on the rate constants of movement of drug molecules in and out of the two compartments. The elimination rate constant (K_{10}) describes the rate of removal or elimi-

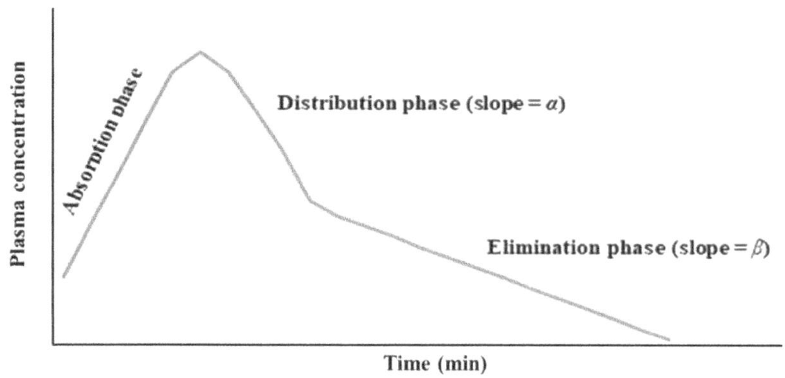

Figure 11.3: A graph Illustrating the phases of a plasma concentration-time curve of a two-compartment model of an orally administered drug.

nation of drug from central compartment in relation to the distribution and elimination rate constants and the inter-compartmental constant K_{21} as follows:

$$K_{10} = \frac{\alpha\beta}{K_{21}} \tag{11.1}$$

The rate constant for the movement of the antimalarial drug from peripheral compartment to the central compartment (K_{21}):

$$K_{21} = A\alpha + \frac{B\beta}{(A+B)} \tag{11.2}$$

and the rate constant from movement from central compartment to peripheral compartment (K_{12}) :

$$K_{12} = \alpha + \beta - K_{21} - K_{10} \tag{11.3}$$

The estimation of volumes of distribution, in two-compartment model are as follows:

- The volume of distribution in the central compartment (V_c) of an intravenously administered antimalarial is given by,

$$V_c = \frac{X_0}{C_0} \tag{11.4}$$

- For the extravascular route the X_0 is replaced by FX_0, where F is the bioavailability of the drug. Therefore, the apparent volume of distribution (V_b) of drug in the body is used (V_b) and given by (for intravenous route):

$$V_b = \frac{X_0}{\beta(AUC_{0-\infty})} \tag{11.5}$$

- For extravascular administration, the bioavailability is added as described above. The volume of distribution at steady state (V_{ss}) is described below:

$$V_{ss} = V_c \frac{(K_{12} + K_{21})}{K_{21}}, \tag{11.6}$$

  or where the denominator K_{21} is replaced with α.

The V_c and the V_{ss} are the most useful volumes, they can be used in calculation of initial concentration and the loading dose, respectively.

The absorption phase has three processes: absorption, distribution and elimination occurring simultaneously with absorption being dominant leading to the overall transfer of drug from absorption site into the central compartment. The absorption rate constant for a two-compartment model is determined by feathering or by using the Loo-Reigelman method that requires intravenous administration of the drug in addition to the extravascular route, the equation for fraction of drug absorbed at a time point (F_t) is as follows:

$$F_t = \frac{(C_p)_t + \frac{K_{10} AUC_{0-\infty} (X_{peri})_t}{V_c}}{K_{10} AUC_{0-\infty}} \tag{11.7}$$

X_{peri} represent the amount of drug in the peripheral compartment.

The absorption of lumefantrine is first order with a lag time and a time to maximum concentration (t_{max}) of 6 hours. The fraction of dose absorbed increases with increased fat content in food with factor of 16. In the fasted state, absorption decreases by approximately 10 percent. These differences due to diet content can be one of the contributory factors to the individual variability in bioavailability [23, 25] with significant improvements in model data description with the incorporation of inter-individual variability in K_a.

In malaria, the disease itself, affects food intake and thus causing variations in the absorption of lumefantrine with parasite count, leading to decrease in bioavailability seen with high counts, and high bioavailability achieved with clinical recovery from Malaria. The increase in bioavailability with treatment progression is attributable to a return to normal food intake that comes with clinical improvement after the first dose. Various drugs may affect the bioavailability of malarial drugs, such as efavirenz that reduces the bioavailability of lumefantrine. Artemether is absorbed more rapidly with a t_{max} of approximately 2 hours. The bioavailability of artemether increases two-fold with an increase in dietary fat content. There is marked variability in the absorption of artemether in malaria patients. There is no evidence of clinically significant effects on the bioavailability of artemether caused by concomitantly administered drugs. However, grapefruit juice may increase plasma levels of artemether in plasma and the extent of interaction is dependent on volume of juice consumed.

Following oral administration lumefantrine and artemether are extensively distributed into body tissues and highly protein bound with over 90% of the two being bound to plasma proteins. The contribution of malaria to the volume of distribution of lumefantrine and artemether is still an area for research.

There is significant first pass metabolism of orally administered lumefantrine and artemether. Lumefantrine is excreted unchanged through the bile as well as desbutylated metabolite, that is rapidly excreted. The elimination of artemether is through metabolism mainly by CYP3A4 and CYP3A5 liver enzymes, that also catalyzes the metabolism of lumefantrine. The main metabolite of artemether is dihydroartemether (DHA) and it is an active metabolite with antimalarial activity. DHA is further glucuronidated and excreted through bile. The role of CYP3A4 in the metabolism of both lumefantrine and artemether means there is potential for drug interactions with inhibitors and inducers of CYP3A4, such as ketoconazole and antiretrovirals. Lumefantrine is also an inhibitor of CYP2D6.

Finally, the clearance (Cl) is estimated by using the formula:

$$Cl = K_{10} \times V_c \tag{11.8}$$

Since both lumefantrine and artemether are eliminated predominantly by the liver, which is part of the central compartment, Cl is related to elimination half-life ($t_{1/2}$) as follows:

$$t_{1/2} = \frac{0,693V_c}{Cl} \tag{11.9}$$

The elimination half-life for of lumefantrine is 3 to 4 days and artemether is between 1 to 3 hours [25] thus lumefantrine easily accumulates to higher levels in the body and persists longer than artemether producing effect for longer time after administration. The inhibition of CYP3A4 has been associated with a decrease in the clearance of lumefantrine and artemether. Inhibitors of CYP3A4 significantly decrease the clearance (Cl) of artemether by 70 percent. There interindividual variations in Cl are seen with body weight, age and height. The potential for clinically significant interaction is always there, therefore caution is emphasized when using drugs that are known to be metabolized by CYP2D6 and induce or inhibit CYP3A4 [21].

11.5 TREATMENT OF PREGNANT WOMEN

When a woman becomes pregnant, her physiology start to adjust to the new condition. These factors will affect the pharmacokinetics of the drugs. This can be shown graphically in (11.4), with the appearance of a new compartments. Among these physiological changes, that are affected by pregnancies and will impact the pharmacokinetics of drugs, are the cardiovascular system, the liver and the renal excretion, just to mention few examples. The portal vein blood flow is increased from 1.25 L/min to 1.92 L/min and the hepatic artery blood flow is increased from 0.57 L/min to 1.06 L/min [26]. Similarly, glomerular filtration rate is increased from 97 mL/min to 144 mL/min [27]. Plasma volume is also increased from 2.6 L to about 3.5 L [28]. The ratio of liver enzymes is also changed across gestation, such as CYP3A4, that goes from 73% in non-pregnant women, to 75%, 80% and 83% in weeks 10, 20 and 30, respectively. Other enzymes may decrease such as CYP2B6 that are found in 9%, 8%, 6% and 6% in weeks 0, 10, 20 and 30, respectively [29].

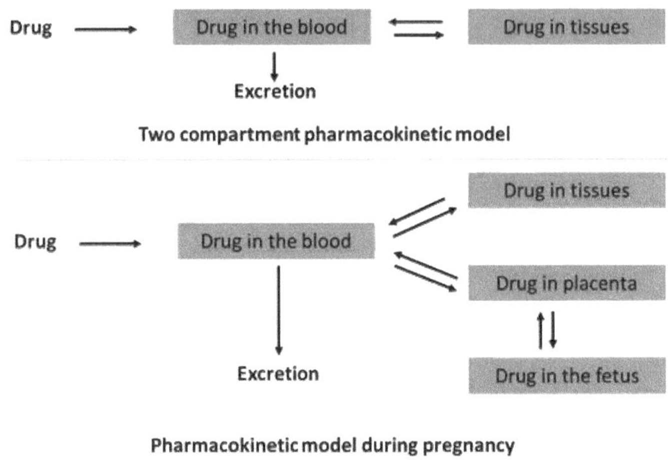

Figure 11.4: Two models, one showing a simple two compartment pharmacokinetic model, the other show how the model changes during pregnancy.

Treatment of pregnant women is never an easy task, especially during organogenesis in the first trimester. Therefore, the safety and effectivity of many antimalarial drugs is of concern, in pregnancy. It is recommended by WHO to give quinine plus clindamycin for 7 days to pregnant women having uncomplicated *P. falciparum* malaria during the *first trimester.* In situations where access to clindamycin is limited, quinine alone can be given [15]. However, in situations where the adherence to quinine cannot be assured, ACTs can be used in the first trimester of pregnancy. Also, recently more evidence have become available on the safety of ACTs in the first trimester of pregnancy [13] and WHO is presently reviewing the recommendations on the use of ACTs in the first trimester of pregnancy.

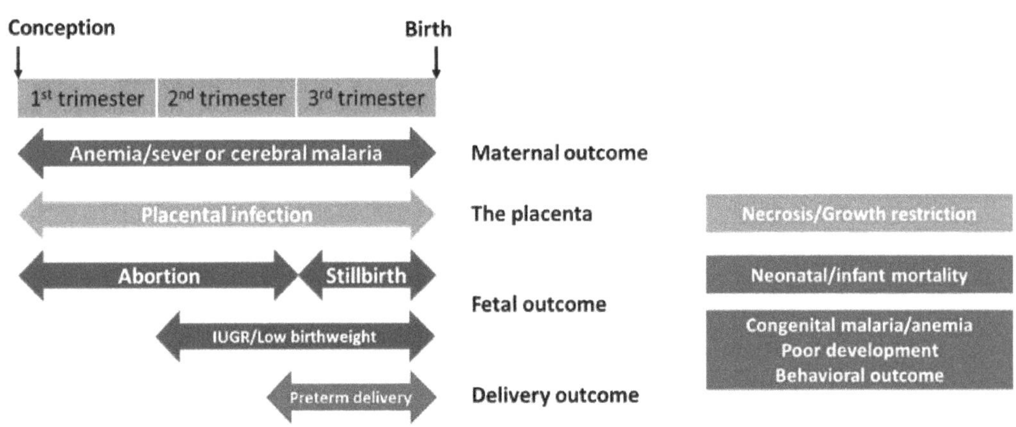

Figure 11.5: The consequences of malaria in pregnancy. The parasite affects the placenta hard, affecting the pregnancy, the fetus, and the delivery, during pregnancy with consequences after birth of the offspring [34].

During the second and third trimesters, uncomplicated *P. falciparum* malaria must be treated using ACTs, although safety assessment of artemether and lumefantrine is still ongoing, pharmacokinetics and effectivness as well as its effectiveness [10]. Safety studies in more than 4000 pregnancies, report no adverse effects on both mother and fetus. Certain antimalarial drugs, however, such as primaquine should not be used during pregnancy. The fetus is constantly growing. First slowly, but during second and third trimester it starts growing rapidly, making the fetoplacental compartment (11.4) under constant change. The volume of this compartment (V_{preg}) can be described by the Gompertz equation:

$$V_{preg} = ae^{\left(\frac{b}{c}\right)\left(1-e^{-cGA}\right)} \tag{11.10}$$

where GA indicates the gestational age in weeks and a, b and c are constants, that are equal to 0.01, 0.37 and 0.52, respectively [31]. After the intake of a drug, the changes in the drug concentration in the fetoplacental compartment can be described by [32] as follows:

$$\frac{d\left(V_{\text{preg}}C_{\text{preg}}\right)}{dt} = Q_{preg}\left(C_{ab} - \frac{C_{\text{preg}}}{\frac{K_{preg:P}}{B:P}}\right) \tag{11.11}$$

Here, the C_{preg} is the drug concentration in the fetoplacental compartment, Q_{preg} is the blood flow to the compartment, C_{ab} is the concentration in the incoming arterial blood, $K_{preg:P}$ is the fetoplacental compartment:plasma partition coefficient and B:P is the blood:plasma concentration ratio (0.7 for artemether and 0.6 for lumefantrine,[33]). To complicate things even more, all these parameters are dependent on the gestational time.

Malaria affects the placenta quite hard, resulting in spontaneous miscarriage, stillbirth, or neonatal mortality [15]. If the fetus survives the placental sickness, it will probably have lower birth weight. Due to this, all pregnant women are recommended to use antimalarial drugs such as sulfadoxine-pyrimethamine during pregnancy, reducing the placental parasitaemia by about 50%. Pregnant women in their first trimester should avoid using artemether/artesunate and lumefantrine, but to use quinine and clindamycin instead [15].

11.6 TREATMENT OF INFANTS AND YOUNG CHILDREN

After birth, the organs are continuing their maturation and necessary functions such as the liver and the kidneys. Elimination, for example, of drugs from newborns can be very slow. So, infants and children may metabolize and excrete drugs, such as antimalarial drugs, quite differently from adults. It takes time for the liver enzymes to mature. The maturation of the liver enzymes, expressed as the ratio of enzymes compared with humans can be described as follows [35], for each enzyme:

$$CYP2C9 = 0.17 + \frac{0.81.\text{Age}^{0.53}}{0.0157^{0.53} + \text{Age}^{0.573}} \tag{11.12}$$

$$CYP2C19 = 0.3 + \frac{0.68\text{Age}^{2.44}}{0.29^{2.44} + \text{Age}^{2.44}} \tag{11.13}$$

For children under the age of 2 years, the CYP1A2 enzyme follows following equation:

$$CYP1A2 = 0.24 + \frac{1.47\text{Age}^{1.73}}{0.36^{1.73} + \text{Age}^{1.73}} \tag{11.14}$$

where children above 2 years, they follow:

$$CYP1A2 = 0.83 + 0.79e^{-0.06(Age-1.8)} \tag{11.15}$$

For CYP3A4 and CYP3A5, the enzyme maturation changes their maturation rate around 2.3 years, so for children under the age of 2.3 years it is as follows:

$$CYP3A4 = CYP3A5 = 0.11 + \frac{0.95\text{Age}^{1.91}}{0.64^{1.91} + \text{Age}^{1.91}} \tag{11.16}$$

where children above 2.3 years, they follow:

$$CYP3A4 = CYP3A5 = 1.1 - 0.123e^{-0.05(Age-2.2)} \tag{11.17}$$

So, the total degree of enzyme maturation (MFA) in children (under the age of 25) can be expressed using following equation, where adults, 25 years or older, have $MFA = 1$:

$$\begin{aligned} MFA = (0.21CYP1A2) &+ (0.23CYP2C9) + (0.29CYP2C19) + \\ &+ (0.19CYP3A4) + (0.08CYP3A5) \end{aligned} \tag{11.18}$$

The body fat proportions in children, plasma proteins, organ sizes etc. are not as they will be when they grow up. Therefore, *children cannot be regarded as small adults* and caution must be taken when dosing are decided and when administrating drugs to this population. Different methods have been suggested to extrapolate dosage from adults (D_{adult}) to children (D_{child}) such as [36]:

Table 11.2: Different dosing rules.

Young's dosing rule:	$D_{child} = \frac{Age\ (y)}{Age\ (y)+12} D_{adult}$
Salomon (Fried) dosing rule:	$D_{child} = \frac{Age\ (mo)}{150} D_{adult}$
Webster dosing rule:	$D_{child} = \frac{Age\ (y)+1}{Age\ (y)+7} D_{adult}$
Clark dosing rule:	$D_{child} = \frac{Weight\ (lbs)}{150} D_{adult}$
Area dosing rule:	$D_{child} = \frac{BSA\ (m^2)}{1.73} D_{adult}$

A different method has also been proposed based following equation [37]:

$$D_{child} = 1.5 \left(\frac{W_{child}}{70}\right)^{\frac{3}{4}} D_{adult} \tag{11.19}$$

Table 11.3: Estimating that a 6 month old child is about 5kg, the dosing will be as follows as well as the maximal plasma concentration.

Method	**Artemether** $\mathbf{D_{child}}$ **(80 mg adult)**	$\mathbf{C_{max}}$ μ**g/mL**	**Lumefantrine** $\mathbf{D_{child}}$ **(480 mg adult)**	$\mathbf{C_{max}}$ μ**g/mL**
WHO guidelines	20 mg	4.44	120 mg	7.50
Yong's	3.2 mg	0.71	19.2 mg	1.20
Salomon (Fried)	3.2 mg	0,71	19.2 mg	1.20
Webster	16 mg	3.56	96 mg	6.00
Clark	6 mg	1.33	35 mg	2.19
Metabolic ratio	17 mg	3.56	99 mg	6.19
Adult dose	80 mg	0.37 *	480 mg	4.66

* Based on adult values of V_d, being 3.1 L/kg for artemether [20] and 1.47 L/kg for lumefantrine [39].

where W_{child} is the weight of the child in kilograms.

Using the pharmacokinetic values available, however, the dose (D) may be based on the target plasma concentration (C_p) and calculated using following equation:

$$C_p = \frac{\mathrm{FD}k_a}{V_d\,(k_a - k_e)}\left(e^{-k_e t} - e^{-k_a t}\right) \tag{11.20}$$

where F is the bioavailability and k_a is the absorption rate constant. Here, the target concentration could be 186 ng/mL for artemether [38] and 8 µg/mL for lumefantrine [38], which is the measured plasma concentration 2 and 6 hours after the administration of an adult dose to adults, respectively. Using the equations, the new dose may be calculated as shown in Table 11.3. Here, an important factor that must be taken into the account, is that the pharmacokinetics in children, such as volume of distribution (V_d) and the half-life, is quite different, compared to adults.

For artemether the V_d has been found to be around 8 L/kg and the half-life is about 1.6 hours for adults [38, 40], compared to V_d for the central compartment of 2.8 L/kg and 15.3 L/kg for the peripheral compartment, in children [41]. The half-life in children was found to be 3.9 hours [42]. The bioavailability for artemether tablets is found to be 43.2% [40]. For lumefantrine the V_d has been found to be around 1.5 L/kg and the half-life is about 95 hours [38] for adults, compared to V_d for the central compartment of 0.75 L/kg and 3.2 L/kg for the peripheral compartment, in children. Tchaparian et al. [43], however, found significant higher V_d for lumefantrine, or 53,2 L/kg. The half-life in children was found to be 17.9 hours [44]. The bioavailability for lumefantrine tablets is found to be 57% for crushed tablets, and 65% with dispersible tablets [23]. Based on the short half-life in children, compared to adults, they may need more frequent and longer dosing scheme, than with adults.

When uncomplicated *P. falciparum* malaria is treated in infants, young children and the malnourished ones, ACT should be the first line of treatment, since the safety of artemisinin derivatives in children is good. Certain drugs like sulphadoxine – pyrimethamine should not be given during the first weeks of life as it causes competitive displacement of bilirubin which can exacerbate hyperbilirubinemia in neonates. Primaquine should not be given in babies under 6 months and tetracyclines (doxycycline) should not be given during infancy. Other issues that need to be considered with pediatric dosage forms are the taste, volume, consistency in addition to gastrointestinal tolerability.

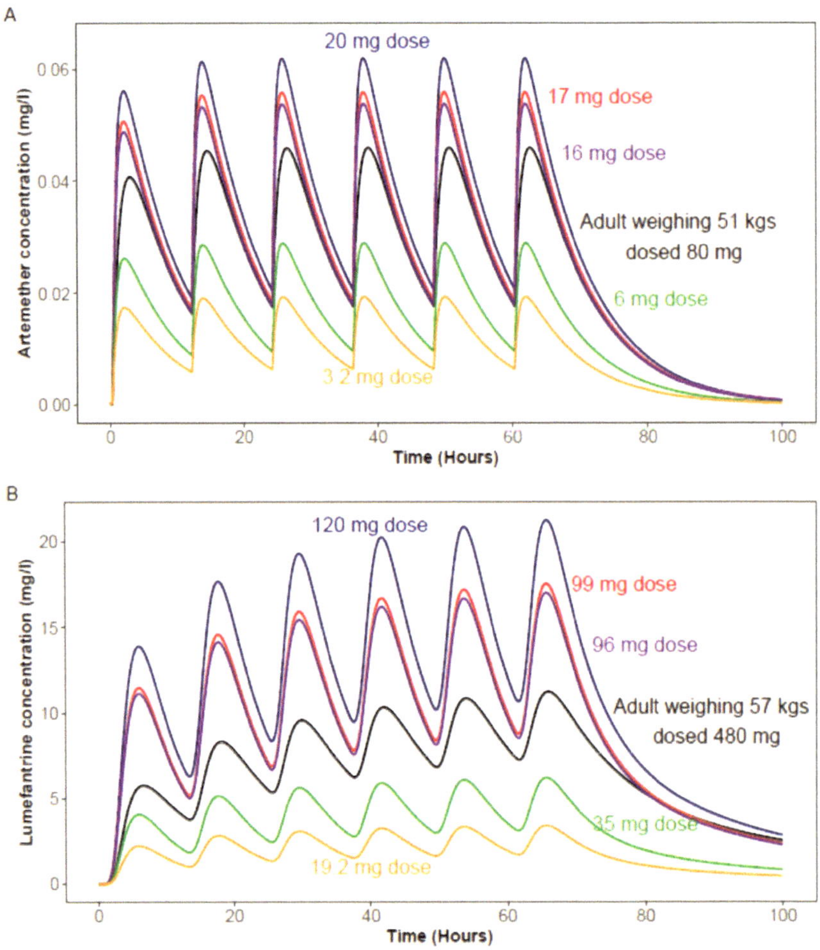

Figure 11.6: Showing the plasma concentration time curves for artemether (A) and lumefantrine (B) over time when administered as 80+480 mg, respectively, to an adult (70 kg) [black lines] or as 20+120 mg, respectively, to a child (5 kg) in different concentrations [colored lines]. Lumefantrine calculations are based on Francis et al. [45] and artemether on Gordi et al. [46].

11.7 CONCLUSION

mosquitoes of the genus *Anopheles* are responsible for transmitting malaria, that accounts for a large proportion of deaths in Africa. Worldwide, a child perishes every two minutes because of that vector, and sadly, Africa bears about 90% of all malaria mortalities especially among children under the age of 5 years. This is also the age group that suffer the greatest burden of the disease. The principal objective of treatment is to necessitate the quick and complete removal of the *Plasmodium* parasites from a patient's circulation to prevent an uncomplicated malaria from progressing to severe infection or mortality.

Finding the right dosing for children is dependent on several factors, including their age, weight, health status etc. Early treatment and careful consideration and estimation of dose should be done to ensure successful dose to complete removal of the parasite, because children are hit hard, and if untreated, they are at risk of getting severe malaria and even cerebral malaria. The first line of treatment is the use artemether and lumefantrine together. A combination product is becoming more and more vital because the parasite has been developing resistance towards many of the drugs available. Not getting the right drugs can have a long lasting neurological and/or behavioral impact on young children that get severe and cerebral malaria.

ACKNOWLEDGMENTS

This chapter is partly based on work performed within the framework of IMAAC (`https://imaac.eu/`) related to COST Action CA16227 (*Investigation & Mathematical Analysis of Avant-garde Disease Control via Mosquito Nano-Tech-Repellents*, `https://cost.eu/actions/CA16227/`), supported by COST Association (European Cooperation in Science and Technology).

GLOSSARY

The definitions of some commonly-used special terms: related to immunity, and that of some general epidemiological terms are given here:

Table 11.4: Glossary of definitions for commonly-used special terms in this chapter.

A	Distribution coefficient
ACT	Artemisinin based combination therapy
AUC	Area under the curve
a	Distribution rate constant
B	Elimination coefficient
B:P	Blood-plasma concentration ratio
BSA	Body surface area
β	Elimination rate constant
C_{ab}	Drug concentration in the incoming arterial blood
Cl	Clearance
C_{max}	Maximal plasma concentration
C_p	Plasma concentration
C_{preg}	Plasma concentration in the fetoplacental compartment
C_{preg}	Plasma concentration in the fetoplacental compartment
CYP	Cytochrome P enzyme, with different subclasses
D	Dose
D_{child}	Dosage to a child
D_{adult}	Dosage to an adult
DHA	Dihydroartemether
EC50	50% of maximum achievable effect
E_{max}	Maximum achievable effect
F	Bioavailability
F_t	Fraction of drug absorbed at time t
GA	Gestational age
K_a	Absorption rate constant
K_{10}	Elimination rate constant
K_{12}	Rate constant from central to peripheral compartment
K_{21}	Rate constant from peripheral to central compartment
$K_{preg:P}$	Fetoplacental compartment:plasma partition coefficient
m	meters (hight)
MFA	Total degree of enzyme maturation
mo	Months (age)
P.	Plasmodium

FURTHER READING

See the references attached to this chapter or contact the authors directly.

To whom correspondence should be addressed:
Prof. Sveinbjorn Gizurarson,
Faculty of Pharmaceutical Sciences, School of Health Sciences,
University of Iceland, Hofsvallagata 53, 107 Reykjavik, Iceland
E-mail: sveinbj@hi.is, Phone: +354 898 0318.

VII

Using Natural Oils Combatting Mosquitoes: An Overview

CHAPTER 12

Plant Based Repellents: Green Mosquito Control

Kiril Lisichkov*
Faculty of Technology and Metallurgy, Skopje,
University Ss. Cyril and Methodius, North Macedonia
** corresponding author, e-mail: klisickov@yahoo.com*

Katerina Atkovska
Faculty of Technology and Metallurgy, Skopje,
University Ss. Cyril and Methodius, North Macedonia

Erhan Mustafa
Faculty of Technology and Metallurgy, Skopje,
University Ss. Cyril and Methodius, North Macedonia

Stefan Kuvendziev
Faculty of Technology and Metallurgy, Skopje,
University Ss. Cyril and Methodius, North Macedonia

Mirko Marinkovski
Faculty of Technology and Metallurgy, Skopje,
University Ss. Cyril and Methodius, North Macedonia

CONTENTS

12.1 Introduction 214
12.2 Plant essential oils - composition and extraction 215
12.3 Efficacy of different essential oils as mosquito repellents 216
12.3.1 Lemon eucalyptus oil 216
12.3.2 Immortelle oil 216
12.3.3 Lavender oil 216
12.3.4 Citronella oil 217
12.3.5 Basil oil 217
12.3.6 Thyme oil 217
12.3.7 Neem oil 218
12.3.8 Rosemary oil 218
12.4 Improving the repellent efficiency of essential oils 218
12.5 Conclusion 219

DOI: 10.1201/9781003035992-12

12.1 INTRODUCTION

Mosquitoes are vectors for some of humanity's most deadly illnesses, and they are public enemy number one in the fight against global infectious disease. Mosquito-borne diseases cause millions of deaths worldwide every year. There are more than 3000 species of mosquitoes, but the members of three bear primary responsibility for the spread of human diseases. *Anopheles* mosquitoes are the only species known to carry malaria. They also transmit filariasis and encephalitis. *Culex* mosquitoes carry encephalitis, filariasis, and the West Nile virus. And *Aedes* mosquitoes, of which the voracious Asian tiger is a member, carry yellow fever, dengue, and encephalitis [1]. Global warming has moved the mosquitoes on the way to some temperate and higher altitudes, affecting people who are vulnerable to such diseases [2].

The most important way to prevent the transmission of mosquito diseases is to reduce or disable the contact of the vector transmitters with a human. This can be achieved by using different types of mosquito repellents. The most used and effective mosquito repellents are DEET-based chemical repellents. However, the use of DEET and other synthetic repellents like DMP and allethrin has raised several concerns in terms of environmental and human health risks [3]. With an increasing concern for public safety, a renewed interest in the use of natural products of plant origin is desired because natural products are effective, environmentally friendly, biodegradable, inexpensive, and readily available [4, 5, 6]. Many studies have reported evidence of repellant activities of plant extracts or essential oils against mosquito vectors around the world. Thus, plant essential oils with low toxicities for the environment and humans are considered as an alternative to conventional synthetic insecticides [7, 8]. Essential oil has been the active principle of most important herbal remedies since ancient times. Ancient Greek and Roman scholars wrote about using plants on skin and clothing, so it is no surprise that the new resurgence of essential oils in popular culture is entering the fight against the bite.

There are many plant essential oils extracted from different families that can be applied as green repellents against mosquito vectors, such as: citronella, peppermint, clove, eucalyptus, catnip, immortelle, basil, thyme, lavender, rosemary and others. These oils are considered safe by the Environmental Protection Agency (EPA) at low concentrations but provide a limited duration of protection against mosquitoes ($< 3\ h$). Most of these essential oils are highly volatile and that is the reason for the short duration of their repellent effectiveness. As a result, repellents containing only essential oils in the absence of an active ingredient such as DEET should not be recommended as repellents for use in disease-endemic areas, whereas those containing high levels of essential oils could cause skin irritation, especially exposed to sunlight [9]. Even though many studies have shown that almost all plant-based repellents offer limited protection and require frequent reapplication, the growing demand for natural alternative repellents indicates the need for development of natural repellents with improved efficiency, long-lasting protection and enhanced safety [5, 8, 10].

12.2 PLANT ESSENTIAL OILS - COMPOSITION AND EXTRACTION

Essential oils are volatile natural complex secondary metabolites characterized by a strong odor and have a generally lower density than that of water [11]. Many chemical compounds can be found in essential oils, but in general essential oils consist of chemical compounds which have hydrogen, carbon, and oxygen. The volatile components of essential oils can be classified into four main groups: terpenes, benzene derivatives, hydrocarbons and other various compounds. Terpenes and terpenoids are the main components found in essential oils and are present either as hemiterpenes, monoterpenes or sesquiterpenes and as their derivates. Most essential oils contain monoterpenes at around 90%, which allow a great variety of structures with diverse functions [12]. There are different hydrocarbons or their related compounds such as: alcohols (citronellol, linalool, geraniol, terpeniol, menthol, borneol), phenoles (eugenol, thymol, carvacrol), aldehydes (citral, citronellal, neral, cuminic aldehyde), ketones (camphor, menthone, jasmone, carvone, thujone) [13]. There are also some other groups of compounds that may occur in certain essential oils: acids (alantic acid, benzoic acid, phenyl acetic acid, and anisic acid), oxides (ascaridol, bisabolol oxide, bisabolone oxide, and cineol) [14]. Here are some examples for common constituents in some essential oils having mosquito repellent activity: 1,8-cineole, the major constituent of oils from rosemary (*Rosmarinus officinale*)and eucalyptus (*Eucalyptus globus*); eugenol from clove oil (*Syzygium aromaticum*); thymol from garden thyme (*Thymus vulgaris*); and menthol from various species of mint (*Mentha species*) [15].

There are a variety of methods employed in extracting essential oils from aromatic plants. The processes of extraction must result in a minimal chemical change of the compounds present in the oil, in order to maintain its natural aroma. The economy of the process and the yield and recovery of active components are important. Essential oils can be extracted from the plant materials by simple expression as is the case in most of the citrus oils including lemon and bergamot. The process of distillation, steam and water distillation is the main method for extracting the aromatic parts of plants. Hydrodiffusion and water infussion as well as use water or steam as solvents. Other methods use alcoholic tinctures, extraction of oleoresins, using organic solvents such as methanol, ethanol, isopropanol, ethyl acetate or acetone. However, the use of non-toxic solvents during the extraction process is an important issue because of regulatory restrictions. New techniques using supercritical or subcritical CO_2 have been developed with significant advantages compared to the use of organic solvents. CO_2 extraction is a relatively recent development over the last few decades [16]. It produces oils that are very pure and with a unique quality, such that they can differ greatly from steam distilled essential oils. Other advantages include the fact that CO_2 is inert which means that it does not react chemically with the oil being extracted, it is non-toxic, colorless and odorless, temperatures are kept very low, so thermally labile compounds do not suffer damage. Methods such as gas-and high-performance liquid chromatography, mass spectrometry and nuclear magnetic resonance have been used to determine the composition of oils, the quantities present in the extracts, as well as the nature of the oils components [17].

12.3 EFFICACY OF DIFFERENT ESSENTIAL OILS AS MOSQUITO REPELLENTS

12.3.1 Lemon eucalyptus oil

Used since the 1940s,lemon eucalyptus oil is one of the most well-known natural repellents. Oil of lemon eucalyptus extract or PMD (para-menthane-3,8 diol) is highly effective and long-acting mosquito repellent, similar to DEET, because it has a lower vapor pressure than volatile monoterpenes found in most plant oils [18]. The Centers for Disease Control and Prevention (CDC) have approved eucalyptus oil as the only plant - based repellent, for use in disease endemic areas because of its proven clinical efficiency to prevent malaria and having no risk to human health [19, 20]. Several papers have been published examining the repellent effectiveness of lemon eucalyptus essential oil on different types of mosquitoes. Two research works found that plant-based spray that contains oil of lemon eucalyptus, was the only DEET-free formula to deliver strong and long-lasting results on repellency of disease-carrying mosquitoes *Aedes albopictus* and *Aedes aegypti* [21, 22]. 20% PMD applied topically can provide 100% protection from *A. Stephensi* for 11 - 12 hours and 100% protection for 2 hours against *Ae. aegypti* [23, 24]. *Another study showed that 32%* lemon eucalyptus oil provided around 95% protection from mosquitoes for 3 hours [25].

12.3.2 Immortelle oil

One of the most common used plant for obtaining immortelle essential oil is *Helichrysum italicum*. Immortelle essential oil is distilled from the flowering tops of the plant. It is a fantastic oil that can promote normal healing of cuts and bruises, but it is also packs a punch against mosquitoes. An Italian study showed that immortelle oil from *H. italicum* caused a high mortality rate against the mosquito *A. albopictus*. The results from this study has shown that immortelle oil has significant amounts of oxygenated monoterpenes and the highest level of sesquiterpenes (Neril acetate, α-Pinene, Limonene, γ-Curcumene, Neril propionate and Nerol). By increasing the applied oil dosage from 200, 250 to 300 ppm, there is an increase in efficiency in terms of the mortality rate of *A. albopictus* from 41.7, through 81,7 to 100% mortality, respectively [26].

12.3.3 Lavender oil

Lavender essential oil, and the plant from which it derives, contains a compound known as linalool, which produces a strong odor that is pleasant to humans and detestable to mosquitoes. This is primarily because it overloads their sensitive olfactory organs, pretty much in the same manner as DEET [27]. A 2009 study found that lavender oil possessed a 93% repellant rate against mosquitoes indoors and only around a 53% repellant rate against mosquitoes outdoors [28]. Taken together, lavender oil is one of the most effective natural mosquito repellants, especially when used as part of a larger natural repellant regimen. Barbara Conti et al. studied the insecticidal activity of essential oils extracted from six Mediterranean plants, among which was *Lavandula angustifolia* against the larvae of the *Culicidae* mosquito *Aedes albopictus*. At a dosage of 300 ppm lavender essential oil showed 55% larval mortality rate [26].

12.3.4 Citronella oil

Essential oils and extracts belonging to plants in the citronella genus (Poaceae) are commonly used as ingredients of plant - based mosquito repellents. Citronella is an essential oil extracted from the stems and leaves of different species of lemongrass (*Cymbopogon spp.*). It is used on humans and their clothing – in the form of oil, liquid and patch. The active compounds in citronella oil for repelling mosquitoes are camphor, eucalyptol, eugenol, linalool, citronellal and citral [29]. Citronella oil is a natural, non-toxic alternative to chemical insect repellents such as DEET, therefore, is usually the preferred choice. Disadvantage is that citronella oil rapidly evaporate and the effectiveness to deter mosquito biting lasts very short [30]. A field study from Bolivia has shown that a 100% of citronella oil (*C. citratus*) applied topically provide 74% protection against *An. darlingi* for 2.5h and 95% protection against *Mansonia* for $2.5h$ [29]. One research team have tested the repellency protection of the citronella essential oil (*C. winterianus*) against the three mosquito species, *Ae. aegipty, C. quinquefasciatus* and *A. dirus* and the results show100% efficiency for 3h, 8h and 3.5h, respectively [31]. Trongtokit and his coworkers have shown that the topical application of 100% citronella oil (*C. nardus*) can provide complete protection against same three mosquito species for a particular time in a laboratory setting [30].

12.3.5 Basil oil

Basil is an annual plant of the *Ocimum* genus, which belongs to the Lamiaceae family and is used in traditional medicine in many parts of the world. In the laboratory trial, 20% basil oil solution, with mean percentage repellency of 66.7%, had 100% protective impact against *An. stephensi* for $3.5h$ [32]. Phasomkusolsil and colleagues used basil essential oil at 0.02, 0.10, and $0.21 mg/cm^2$ concentrations against *An. dirus*. The percentage repellency was dose–response and was reported to be 66%, 74% and 96%, respectively [33]. Adam and the associates have analyzed the repellent efficiency of topically applied essential oil extracted from *O. basilicum,* against malaria vector *Anopheles* mosquito. Three different concentrations of basil oil were tested, 2, 4 and 6% of the oil. The obtained results show relatively high repellency effect of 6% concentration of the oil, more than 250 min [34]. One work has found that basil oil of *O. americanum* provides 100% efficiency for 3 h, 3.5 h and 8 h against *Ae. aegipty, A. dirus* and *C. quinquefasciatus*, respectively [31].

12.3.6 Thyme oil

Thymus species have been reported to possess various beneficial effects, such as antiseptic, carminative, antimicrobial, and antioxidant properties. The 20% oil solution of thyme in the study conducted by Amer et al. with 100% protection against *An. stephensi* for 7.5 h, had a good effectiveness in preventing *Anopheles* mosquitoes [31]. Thyme essential oil of *T. vulgaris* had potent repellent activity against Culex pipiens pallens, with a protection rate of 91% at a concentration of 0.05% topical treatment. Thyme essential oil significantly extended the duration of protection [35].

12.3.7 Neem oil

The Neem tree (*Azadirachta indica*) is a tropical evergreen tree native to India and is also found in other southeast countries. A study evaluated repellent action of neem oil against different mosquito species. 2% neem oil mixed in coconut oil provided 96 - 100% protection from *Anophelines,* 85% from *Aedes*, 37.5% from *Armigeres* whereas it showed wide range of efficacy from 61% to 94% against *Culex* spp. Therefore, neem oil can be applied as a personal protection measure against mosquito bites [36]. The 20% Neem oil in a field trial conducted by Amer et al. with mean percentage repellency 71%, had a complete protection time for 3 h against *An. arabiensis* [32].

12.3.8 Rosemary oil

Rosemary is an evergreen aromatic shrub with a Mediterranean origin, which belongs to Lamiaceae (Labiatae) family. Rosemary essential oil is obtained by steam distillation of the flowering tops of the plant. It is widely used as culinary herb. However, rosemary oil has been shown to be an effective repellent. The 20% oil solution of rosemary had a good effectiveness in preventing *Anopheles* mosquitoes, enabling 100% protection against *An. stephensi* for 8 h [32]. Govindarajan et al. reported that rosemary at 1, 2.5 and $5mg/cm^2$ concentrations completely repels *An. subpictus* for 1, 1, and 1.5 h, respectively [37].

12.4 IMPROVING THE REPELLENT EFFICIENCY OF ESSENTIAL OILS

In order for the application of plant-based mosquito repellents to be a suitable alternative to chemicals, it is necessary to develop methods that will increase their effectiveness and extend their protection time. Many methods have been described for the improvement of repellent efficiency of essential oils. Synergistic interaction is the most used method which is obtained by combination of several essential oils from different plants. A mixture of active components present in various essential oils was found to efficiently enhance the repellent effect, comparable to the effect of the sum of the individual components [38, 39].

Microencapsulation technique is one of the latest technologies used in the development of plant- based repellent products. This technique encapsulates or entraps the plant's active ingredient within the shell or wall materials using a natural or synthetic polymer to form microcapsules. Microencapsulation results in an increase in repellency duration via controlled release of the essential oils [40].

An increase in repellent efficiency was also reported when fixative agents including vanillin, liquid paraffin and salicyluric acid were used. The most widely used fixative agent is vanillin and the duration of repellency is notably enhanced when vanillin is mixed with the essential oils. In addition, microencapsulation or nanoemulsification combined with vanillin treatment improve the effects and protection time of natural repellents [40, 41].

A variety of essential oils have significant repellent effects. However, the effects tend to dissipate quickly due to their high volatility. Essential oils generally act in the vapor phase being active only for a short period. For example, citronella oil is highly volatile, and thus, mosquito repellents with citronella oil as the major component need to be reapplied every 20 - 60 minutes. The drawback of the short protection time could be improved via formulation technology development, by retaining the active components on the skin for longer periods. Cream-based formulations and polymer mixture-based formulations led to an increase in the repellent effect [42].

Currently, nanotechnology is extensively used to prepare repellents with essential oils for better efficiency. Nanoparticle fabrication by using plant components as reducing and stabilizing agents has several advantages compared with conventional methods. The size, shape and efficiency of nanoparticles against mosquitoes vary depending on the plant sources. For example silver nanoparticles containing neem are mostly spherical, whereas silver nanoparticles fabricated using leaves from bush plum are cubical [43, 44]. In addition, the use of nanotechnology for essential oil delivery could reduce the costs, steps for development process an risks associated with pressure, temperature and energy.

12.5 CONCLUSION

Repellency is an important way of preventing vector-borne diseases by reducing man - mosquito contact. Because of the possible negative impact on human health and environment, the synthetic repellents are gradually being replaced by plant-based repellents. Many studies show that different plant essential oils can be effectively used as "green" repellents for mosquito control. Considering that essential oils are highly volatile, evaporate quickly and leave the user unprotected, the biggest challenge in applying essential oil-derived repellents is to increase their effectiveness and extending their longevity. For this purpose, various techniques and methods are being developed and applied.

ACKNOWLEDGMENTS

This chapter is partly based on work performed within the framework of IMAAC (`https://imaac.eu/`) related to COST Action CA16227 (*Investigation & Mathematical Analysis of Avant-garde Disease Control via Mosquito Nano-Tech-Repellents*, `https://cost.eu/actions/CA16227/`), supported by COST Association (European Cooperation in Science and Technology).

Microencapsulation of Essential Oils for Antimicrobial Function and Mosquito Repellency

Katie Lair*
Leicester School of Pharmacy,
Infectious Disease Research Group,
De Montfort University, The Gateway,
Leicester, United Kingdom
** corresponding author[1], e-mail: klaird@dmu.ac.uk*

Anita Soroh
School of Fashion and Textiles,
Textile Engineering and Materials (TEAM) Research Group,
De Montfort University, The Gateway,
Leicester, United Kingdom

Jinsong Shen**
School of Fashion and Textiles,
Textile Engineering and Materials (TEAM) Research Group,
De Montfort University, The Gateway,
Leicester, United Kingdom
*** corresponding author[2], e-mail: jshen@dmu.ac.uk*

CONTENTS

13.1 Introduction 222
13.2 Microencapsulation technology 223
13.2.1 Complex coacervation 223
13.2.2 Ionic-Gelation 225
13.2.3 Freeze-Drying 225
13.2.4 Spray-Drying 225
13.2.5 Emulsification 226
13.3 Characterization of microcapsules 226
13.3.1 Particle size and size distribution 226
13.3.2 Surface charge 226
13.3.3 Release of the core material 227

DOI: 10.1201/9781003035992-13

13.4 Antimicrobial activity and mosquito repellency of encapsulated essential oils 227
13.5 Conclusion 229

13.1 INTRODUCTION

Essential oils (EOs) are very promising in the biomedical industry due to their antiseptic, antibacterial, antifungal and antioxidant properties. Especially, natural plant-based ingredients like EOs have grown in popularity as they represent an eco-friendly and biodegradable alternative for use in antimicrobial textile finishing. However, EOs have shown to be difficult to achieve their full potential because of the chemical volatility and instability they possess. This makes EOs prone to deterioration and loss of compounds when exposed to environmental factors such as oxygen, heat, light and moisture. To overcome these challenges, microencapsulation has been used as a viable technique to preserve the essential biological and functional characteristics of the oils. The microencapsulation can prevent the loss of volatile oil compounds while also allow for the controlled and sustained release of the essential oils, enhancing bioavailability and efficacy against pathogens (Chouhan et al. 2017).

Biopolymers, specifically natural occurring polysaccharides like chitosan and alginates, are becoming popular carriers in encapsulation processes or nanoparticle forming processes. The deacetylated form of chitin, chitosan, has been used to protect compounds like EOs using methods like ionic gelation (Xu and Du 2003) and spontaneous emulsification (Wilson et al. 2010). Keawchaoon and Yoksan (2011) prepared Carvacrol-loaded chitosan nanoparticles using a two-step method combining emulsification and ionic gelation, and showed that the resulting particles effectively inhibited the growth of *E. coli, S. aureus* and *Bacillus cereus* with an MIC of 0.257 mg/mL and MBC of 8.225, 4.113 and 2.056 mg/ml respectively. Chitosan has also been used to successfully encapsulate oregano EO, showing a two-phase release profile of the initial burst release and followed by a slow drug release (Hosseini et al. 2013). Sayed et al. (2017) applied a nanoemulsion encapsulating neem EO on cotton fabric and reported 71.73% and 65.69% reduction of *S. aureus* and *E. coli* after 4 washes. In addition to their antimicrobial activity, a number of EOs also possess mosquito repellent properties. Azeem et al. (2019) reported greater than 50% repellency of Aedes aegypti mosquitoes by Conyza sumatrensis, Erigeron canadensis, Mentha spicata, Parthenium hysterophorus and Tagetes minuta EOs. M. spicata EO demonstrated complete (100%) repellency and was comparable in activity to the commercially available mosquito repellent N,N-diethyl-3-methylbenzamide (DEET). Specos et al. (2010) reported greater than 90% repellency for up to 21 days when cotton fabric was treated with microencapsulated citronella EO.

Alginates are natural polymers extracted from brown algae and have been widely used in the form of sodium alginate to encapsulate pharmaceutical actives and EO's such as clove, thyme and cinnamon (Shinde and Nagarsenker, 2011; Soliman et al., 2013). The formulation of sodium alginate particles is achieved through cross-linking, such as ionic cross-linking. A study on lemon balm-loaded sodium alginate beads cross-linked with calcium chloride found that there was no interaction with the extract and its antioxidant activity was not affected by the encapsulation (Najafi-Soulari et al. 2016).

Due to the rise in antibiotic resistance, the ecological concern created by current synthetic antimicrobials and the increased demand for eco-friendly antimicrobials and textile products, the development of "green" formulations based on natural antimicrobials such as EOs and natural formulation ingredients such as biopolymers should be explored for safe and functional textiles.

13.2 MICROENCAPSULATION TECHNOLOGY

A microcapsule is comprised of a core (usually the active component needing protection) and wall materials (also referred to as the coating or shell) which are commonly polymers, carbohydrates or proteins (Bakry et al. 2016; Haidong et al. 2012). The process of microencapsulation involves the coating of droplets or particles of a substance (e.g. drugs, hormones, proteins, fertilizers, cosmetics, oils) with a thin wall of natural or synthetic polymers that acts as a protective barrier, to create individual particles (Butstraen and Salaün 2014). There are various methods of microencapsulation including physical (e.g. spray-drying and freeze-drying), chemical (e.g. solvent evaporation and *in situ* polymerization) and physicochemical (e.g. ionic gelation, coacervation and emulsification) methods (Tomaro-Duchesneau et al. 2013). Methods of encapsulating the active material to be used are depending on the nature of the core material, the desired particle size, desired release of the core and the intended application of the final product (Ghayempour and Montazer 2016; Haidong et al. 2012).

13.2.1 Complex coacervation

Complex coacervation technique for microencapsulation is based on the coacervation of two or more types of polymers under specific conditions that are dependent on the charge and charge density of the wall polymers used, the processing temperature and the process itself, such as cooling and stirring (Piacentini et al. 2013). During complex coacervation a spontaneous reaction occurs between two polymers of opposite charge, leading to a phase separation in which an aqueous phase and a polymer phase are formed once the charges are neutralized as illustrated in Figure 13.1 (Piacentini et al. 2013).

Butstraen and Salaün (2014) prepared the microencapsulation of oils using chitosan and algination. In the microencapsulation process, the oil-in-water emulsion containing an anionic emulsifier was added to an aqueous chitosan solution and subsequently converted into microcapsules by the addition of a suitable electrolyte such as alginate. Microencapsulation requires the cross-linking of the wall polymers to increase the thermal and mechanical properties of the capsules (Butstraen and Salaün 2014; Zhang et al. 2012). Most of the cross-linking agents used to enhance microcapsules are toxic in nature and have to be washed out with a solvent to reach a biologically acceptable level, restricting

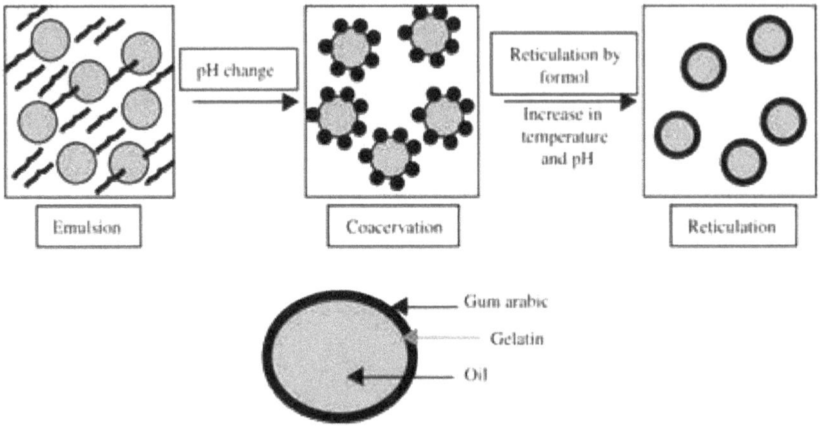

Figure 13.1: Complex coacervation process (Madene et al. 2006).

its use in many applications; such cross-linkers include aldehydes i.e. glutaraldehyde and formaldehyde (Butstraen and Salaün, 2014; Yang, et al. 2014; Zhang et al. 2012). Sodium tripolyphosphate (TPP) is non-toxic cross-linker that has been proposed as an alternative to aldehyde crosslinkers (Butstraen and Salaün 2014).

Complex coacervation is a promising technique for the production of micro/nanoparticles or microcapsules within industry. It is simple without the use of solvent, allowing high payloads, good controlled release, heat resistant properties and high efficiency (Lv et al. 2014; Nakagawa and Nagao 2012; Yang J. et al. 2015). In a microencapsulation process based on coacervation, the pH is a key parameter. Aziz et al (2014) evaluated the effects of core material (krill oil) to wall material (gelatin-gum Arabic) ratio, stirring speed and pH on the encapsulation efficiency. It was found that pH had the most significant effects on the encapsulation efficiency (EE). Stable microcapsules, with 92% EE were synthesized using optimal conditions of pH 3.8, stirring speed 3, and a ratio (of core material to wall material) of 1.75:1 (Aziz et al. 2014). Stirring speed is important because the microcapsules can be significantly affected by the homogenization rate during the process of emulsification. When a lower rate is used during preparation, the microcapsules release the core material more rapidly than those prepared with a higher rate during the process (Zhang et al. 2012).

Microcapsules produced by complex coacervation are also affected by the polymer properties including molecular mass, ionic charge density and concentration in the formulation (Nakagawa and Nagao 2012). Microencapsulation of *Melaleuca alternifolia* (tea tree) EO by complex coacervation led to an increase in the evaporation temperature of tea tree EO from 140 °C to 230 - 260 °C because of the core protection provided by the polymers gelatine (G) and sodium carboxymethyl-cellulose (C). The ratio of these polymers (G/C), affected the formation of the coacervate during synthesis and the EE of tea tree EO. The increase in G/C ratio lead to an increase in EE ($63.3 \pm 1.4\%$) up to $G/C = 10$, because of the amount of coacervate formed, and above this value, the amount of oil in the microcapsules decreased again (Pérez-Limiñana et al. 2014). The process, however, is not without its challenges; aggregation and release problems (burst) have been reported, which are not desirable for most of its applications (Yang X. et al. 2015).

13.2.2 Ionic-Gelation

Ionic-gelation is a method that has received a lot of attention specifically in the preparation of chitosan and sodium tripolyphosphate (TPP) microcapsules, which are used for the *in vivo* administration of drugs (Fàbregas et al. 2013). The process is non-toxic, convenient, controllable without the need of organic solvents. The method involves the complexation of physical crosslinking by electrostatic interaction between the negative and positive charges of tripolyphosphate and chitosan instead of chemical crosslinking (Dong et al. 2013; Fàbregas et al. 2013; Fan et al. 2012). This method has the advantage to avoid the use of chemical cross-linkers and emulsifiers which are usually harmful or toxic (Fan et al. 2012). The ionic gelation method is less expensive when comparing to the efficient coacervation method. Abang et al (2012) proposed the use of inverse gelation to produce spherical capsules with diameters around $3mm$, but Martins et al. (2015) optimized the process by adjusting the experimental conditions (wall material ratio and concentration, curing time, stirring rate) and achieved core-shell microcapsules with a smaller $500\mu m$ mean diameter.

13.2.3 Freeze-Drying

Freeze-drying, known as lyophilization, is a method used to dehydrate heat-sensitive substances such as oils. It has been used to encapsulate fish oil and olive oil (Calvo et al. 2012; Heinzelmann et al. 2000). Freeze-drying operates by lowering pressure and freezing the microencapsule material, followed by sublimation of ice into water vapour under reduced pressure (Krokida and Philippopoulos 2006). Advantages of freeze-drying include ease of operation, simplicity and protection of heat sensitive materials (Bakry et al. 2016). Velasco et al. (2003) found that freeze-drying reduced sensitivity of oils to oxidation but decreased the encapsulation efficiency. Freeze drying involves a long process using high amounts of energy, resulting in high cost. Additionally, the material (e.g. the oil) could be more exposed to the environment because of high porous structures of microcapsules produced from freeze-drying, though this feature is advantageous when a high drug release is required (Bakry et al. 2016; Sinha et al. 2007).

13.2.4 Spray-Drying

Spray drying is one of the oldest and most established process of encapsulation and has been used to prepare pharmaceutical products such as granules, suspensions and dry powders. Spray drying involves forming an emulsion by dispersing the core material in a polymer solution; the emulsion is then homogenized and atomized into a drying chamber. The method is commonly used to encapsulate core materials that are sensitive to heat, and functional lipophilic ingredients (Berendsen et al. 2015; Dima et al. 2016; Munoz-Ibanez et al. 2016). A disadvantage of spray drying is that the release properties can be affected due to the formation of amorphous systems, which are thermodynamically unstable and can change back to the crystalline state on storage. Spray drying can also affect particle size; dexamethasone acetate containing PLGA nanoparticles were formulated and spray dried, the spray drying processes significantly ($p < 0.05$) increased the nanoparticle sizes. The mean particle size increased from $200 \pm 60\ nm$ to $230 \pm 100\ nm$, however particle density and size distribution seemed to be unaffected (Gómez Gaete et al. 2008).

13.2.5 Emulsification

Emulsification is a simple and cheap method used to encapsulate bioactives (such as EOs and extracts) within aqueous solutions. Emulsions comprise two phases, usually oil and water, which are immiscible (hydrophilic and hydrophobic); the hydrophobic (oil) phase can be dispersed within an aqueous phase, forming an oil-in-water (O/W) emulsion or the opposite can be true forming a water-in-oil (W/O) emulsion (Bakry et al., 2016). These emulsions are then ready to be further processed using the microencapsulation methods described above. Polymer microcapsules have been created using this method with polymethyl-methacrylate (PMMA) and jasmine EO; spherical PMMA microcapsules, with smooth surfaces were achieved when the PMMA to jasmine EO weight ratio was 2:1 and 3:1. At a 1:1 ratio, the polymer capsules could not be achieved, as the capsules comprised holes, possibly due to insufficient amounts of PMMA required to coat the jasmine oil droplets. Encapsulation efficiency was determined to be 72%, as $4.78\ mg$ of jasmine oil was found, when analysing $20\ mg$ of dried capsule (Teeka et al. 2014).

13.3 CHARACTERIZATION OF MICROCAPSULES

13.3.1 Particle size and size distribution

Microcapsules often come in different sizes and size distributions depending on the methods used and their size are related to their mechanical properties e.g. smaller microcapsules will have lower rupture force compared to a larger microcapsule. A study by Sun and Zhang (2002) showed that the bursting force and deformation of melamine-formaldehyde, urea-formaldehyde and gelatine-formed microcapsules increased proportionally with their diameter. To determine the particle size of microcapsules, dynamic light scattering (DLS), laser diffraction and microscopy are used. There are limitations with the use of laser diffraction, as the refractive index of the shell material must be known for the measurement. Microscopy has an advantage over laser diffraction as it gives the true image of the microcapsule but it time consuming and is therefore, mostly used for individual size analysis rather than size distribution (Gray et al. 2016). DLS method provides the average particle size and the size distribution within the sample elucidating the homogeneity of particles being analyzed.

13.3.2 Surface charge

The zeta potential (the charge at the interface between a particle and the surrounding medium) needs to be controlled to prevent microcapsule aggregation. The zeta potential should be analyzed to identify what needs to be done to move the zeta potential away from the isoelectric point in order to prevent aggregation. Electrophoresis is one of the methods used to calculate the zeta potential by measuring the electrophoretic mobility of the microcapsules in a medium (Gray et al. 2016). A study on chitosan coated microemulsions (CH-MEs) found that the zeta potential of CH-MEs was increased after being coated with chitosan solution but decreased when surfactant concentrations increased. This was led to develop CH-MEs with optimal stability and acceptable physicochemical behaviour (Kesavan et al. 2013).

13.3.3 Release of the core material

The release of the core material from the microcapsule is measured by using gentle agitation to achieve a well dispersion and then the changes in the solute concentrations over time are measured either in intervals or continuously. The release kinetics and the diffusion coefficient can therefore be calculated (Gray et al. 2016). The release rate of an active ingredient from the microcapsule depends on different factors including: the wall material, the core material itself, the morphology and geometry of the particle, the degree of cross-linking, the conditions (e.g. pH, temperature, ionic strength) and the method of microencapsulation (da Silva et al. 2014; Dima et al. 2016). A study on chitosan-encapsulated menthol microcapsules observed that the amount of crosslinkers used (TPP) had an effect on the release time of menthol, and generally the higher the TPP concentration, the slower the release time. At 1% w/w TPP, 95% of menthol was release within 60 h, whilst at 15% w/w TPP used, only 38.3% was released at 60 h (Nuisin et al. 2013).

It is important that the release of the core material occurs at the appropriate time and place. A study by Nuisin et al (2013) shows that the release rate is mainly related to interactions between the core and wall material (da Silva et al., 2014). The pH of the microcapsule environment can also have an effect on the release rate of the core material. The drug containing alginate-pectin microcapsules showed higher drug release percentages in acidic pH 1.2 compared to an alkaline pH 8.2, with maximum drug release of 75.6% and 42% respectively (Jaya et al. 2009). The characteristics and the quantity of the core material can also affect release rate. Dürrigl et al. (2011) found that their calcium loaded microparticles, showed greater drug release with a higher drug load and a 2:1 drug: polymer ratio. Release studies are conducted using mathematical models that describe the different ways that molecules are transported across the capsule wall. Larger microcapsules are more suited to controlled release applications, because there is a reduced protection of the core material by the wall material and therefore the release rate of the core material is improved (Dong et al. 2011).

13.4 ANTIMICROBIAL ACTIVITY AND MOSQUITO REPELLENCY OF ENCAPSULATED ESSENTIAL OILS

Essential oils (EOs) are aromatic natural products typically extracted from plant matter by distillation (Georgiev et al. 2019). EOs have been a subject of interest as alternative antimicrobial agents, because they convey broad spectrum antimicrobial activity against bacteria, fungi and viruses (Tariq et al. 2019; Winska et al. 2019). For example, cinnamon bark inhibited *E. coli, S. aureus, Pseudomonas aeruginosa* and *Acinetobacter baumannii* with minimum inhibitory concentrations (MICs) ranging 0.015% - 0.125%, and all tests species except *P. aeruginosa* were inhibited by cinnamon leaf, clove, lemongrass, rosewood and thyme EOs with MICs ranging (0.125 - 1.0)% (Elcocks et al. 2020).

EOs could potentially be incorporated into textiles to create antimicrobial fabrics, however EO compounds are often volatile, and sensitive to light and oxygen. The successful application of EOs onto textiles requires a formulation that protects the EOs from volatilization and degradation and controls its release rate to prevent unacceptable deterioration of the final product (Ali et al. 2014; Aziz et al. 2015; Bakry et al. 2016). Encapsulation of EOs may preserve the functional and physicochemical properties of the oil and allow for greater durability of the final product (Aziz et al. 2015; Javid et al. 2014). Biopolymers including chitosan and alginates are an attractive option for encapsulation due to their favorable biodegradable, biocompatible and mucoadhesive properties (Pedro et al. 2009).

A litsea and lemon EO blend (1:2 ratio, previously shown to be antimicrobial) was encapsulated with chitosan and sodium alginate within an emulsion. The litsea and lemon EO encapsulated emulsion showed significant antimicrobial activity; *E. coli, S. aureus* and *S. epidermidis* were reduced by 7 $\log_{10}$ CFU ml^{-1} within 5 minutes of contact with 1% w/v emulsion (Figure 13.2). *T. rubrum* was less susceptible to the EO-encapsulated emulsion, with a complete inactivation (7 $\log_{10}$ CFU ml^{-1}) after 120 minutes of contact. Tian et al. (2016) reported that a 10% cinnamaldehyde nanoemulsion only reduced the bacterial load of *E. coli* by less than 1 $\log_{10}$ after 4 hours, and between 4 and 9 hours the bacterial load returned to nearly initial levels. A 0.25% lemon-myrtle oil emulsion achieved an 8 $\log_{10}$ reduction after 15 min of contact (Buranasuksombat et al. 2011).

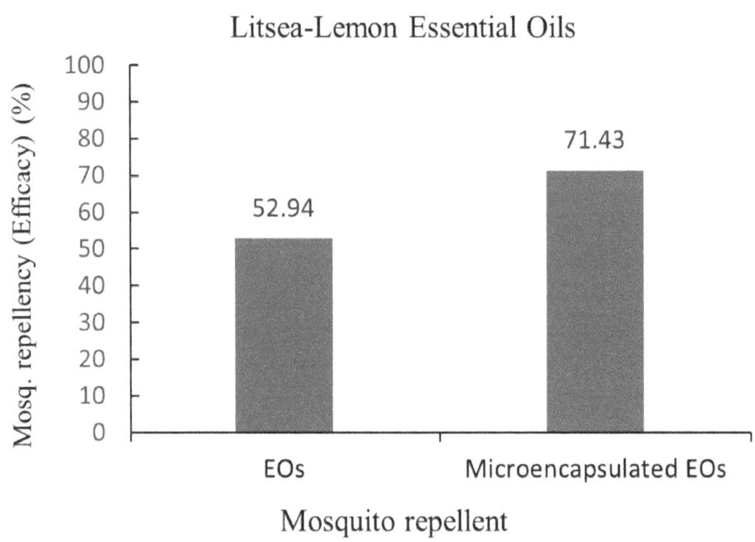

Figure 13.2: Mosquito repellent efficacy of the cotton fabrics treated with the microencapsulated litsea-lemon EO emulsion against *Aedes aegypti* by using Y-tube olfactometer.

The microencapsulated litsea and lemon EO blend emulsion was treated on cotton fabrics for testing the mosquito-repellent efficacy against Aedes aegypti mosquito species using Y-tube Olfactometer (Anuar and Yusof 2016). The cotton fabrics treated with microencapsulated EOs achieved 73.43% mosquito repellency, whereas the cotton fabrics treated EOs alone reached 52.94% repellency (Figure 13.2). This confirmed the importance of encapsulation of EOs. The EOs treated fabric has shown to have a potential application not only for wound dressing or sportswear to control bacterial and fungal contamination, but also for antimosquito repellency.

13.5 CONCLUSION

Natural plant-based essential oils (EOs) have grown in popularity as they represent an eco-friendly and biodegradable alternative for use in antimicrobial textile finishing. The main challenges faced with the application of natural EOs is their durability, shelf-life and antimicrobial efficiency due to volatility and oxidative degradation. Microencapsulation could be used as a viable technique to preserve the essential biological and functional characteristics of the volatile components of the essential oils and control their release during use. A litsea and lemon EO blend was encapsulated with chitosan and sodium alginate and applied on the cotton fabrics. The EOs treated fabric has shown to have a potential application not only for wound dressing or sportswear to control bacterial and fungal contamination but also for antimosquito repellency.

ACKNOWLEDGMENTS

This chapter is partly based on work performed within the framework of IMAAC (`https://imaac.eu/`) related to COST Action CA16227 (*Investigation & Mathematical Analysis of Avant-garde Disease Control via Mosquito Nano-Tech-Repellents*, `https://cost.eu/actions/CA16227/`), supported by COST Association (European Cooperation in Science and Technology).

VIII

Textiles and Paints as Mosquito Control Tools

CHAPTER 14

Mosquito Repellent against *Anopheles SPP.* and *Aedes Aegypti* on Cotton Fabric

Ana Marija Grancaric*

co - Chair of IMAAC (COST Action CA 16227) &
University of Zagreb, Faculty of Textile Technology (TTF),
Zagreb, Croatia
** corresponding author, e-mail: amgranca@ttf.hr*

Lea Botteri

University of Zagreb, Faculty of Textile Technology (TTF),
Zagreb, Croatia

Peyman Ghaffari

Chair of IMAAC (COST Action CA 16227) &
Center for Research and Development in Mathematics
and Applications (CIDMA), University of Aveiro,
Aveiro, Portugal

Jose Heriberto Oliveira do Nascimento

Universidade Federal do Rio Grande do Norte Centro de Tecnologia
Lagoa Nova Natal/RN, Brazil

Renata Antonaci Gama

Laboratory of Entomology, Department of Microbiology
and Parasitology, Universidade Federal do Rio Grande do Norte,
Natal, Rio Grande do Norte, Brazil

Rivaldo Leonn Bezerra Cabral

Universidade Federal do Rio Grande do Norte Centro
de Tecnologia Departamento de Engenharia Têxtil –
DET Nanociências e Têxteis Funcionais
Lagoa Nova Natal/RN, Brazil

Renato Cesar de Melo Freire

Laboratory of Entomology
Department of Microbiology and Parasitology
Universidade Federal do Rio Grande do Norte
Natal, Rio Grande do Norte, Brazil

DOI: 10.1201/9781003035992-14

CONTENTS

14.1 Introduction 234
14.2 Material and Methods 236
14.3 Results 237
14.4 Conclusion 239

14.1 INTRODUCTION

From the early 20th century discovery it is well known that mosquitoes are transmitting the vector-borne diseases such as malaria, dengue, chikungunya, West Nile virus, yellow fever, zika fivcr, etc. These diseases have spread from Asia and Latin America to other continents in last decades because of certain climatic conditions. These infections are transmitted mainly by *Anopheles spp*, *Culex pipiens,Aedes aegypti* and *Aedes albopictus* mosquitoes which spread rapidly world-wide. Vector control is the primary means of preventing vector-borne disease. There is a hope mosquito bites can be reduced by repellents applied on textiles and paint for walls, too. This chapter discuss about mosquito repellents applied on cotton fabric for protecting people against *Anopheles spp* and *Aedes aegypti*. For this purpose, scoured and bleached cotton fabric were treated with natural immortelle essential oil and ingredients, such as water glass and vibroactivated zeolites. Standard scouring of cotton use, mostly NaOH, with high textile cleaning effects from acquired and added impurities. Harsh boiling conditions from fiber leach fat, remove waxes, proteins, pectins and more. The fiber becomes hydrophilic, but loses weight, its feel worsens and the cellulose is partially damaged. From an ecological point of view, NaOH is unfavorable because it pollutes wastewater, and in the technological process, large amounts of water are used for rinsing textiles. For these reasons, the cotton fabric have been scoured according to a new technology, with pectinase, the production of which this fabric has been chemicaly bleached with hydrogen peroxide, using the standard procedure.

Immortelle oil is obtained from Helichrysum italicum plant. It is mediterranean shrubby plant that grows on sunny rocks along the coast and blooms with yellow flowers. It has been used for centuries in the traditional medicine of Mediterranean countries. Back in Homer's time, the Greeks valued immortelle as an excellent remedy for wounds. Today's science confirms that immortelle essential oil contains special properties that give it antioxidant, antibacterial, antifungal, regenerative and anti-inflammatory effects. It is rich in italodiones, intolerant diketones. Vibroactivated zeolite is natural minerals zeolite (crinoptilolite), treated with a special and protected technology of vibroactivated natural minerals which gives a completely new nanoparticle that has the ability to enter the cell of a living organism. The difference between tribomechanical and vibroactivated zeolite is in particle size, ion exchange capacity, electrostatic potential of the particle and most importantly in the activation of natural Silicon.[2].

Treated cotton achieved very good efficacy results without and with mentioned ingredients in treated bath. SEM images clearly showed different cotton surface when applied water glass and vibroactivated zeolites. Repellent efficacy methods used are WHO modified efficacy method (WHO/ CTD/ WHO PES/IC/96.1) and "human lending counts" ("glove") test method according to Coleman, Govere and Durrheim.

Vector-borne diseases are human illnesses caused by parasites, viruses and bacteria that are transmitted by vectors and 80% of the world's population is at risk of one or more vector-borne diseas. Every year there are more than 700,000 deaths from diseases such as malaria, dengue, schistosomiasis, human African trypanosomiasis, leishmaniasis, Chagas disease, Yellow fever, Chikungunya, Zika Japanese encephalitis and onchocerciasis [3, 4]. Since 2014, major outbreaks of dengue, malaria, chikungunya, yellow fever and zika have afflicted populations, claimed lives, and overwhelmed health systems in many countries. For instance in recent years, dengue fever has also reached in Europe (Croatia, France, Italy and Portugal) [5]. These infections are transmitted mainly by *Anopheles spp.* and *Aedes aegypti* mosquitoes which spread rapidly world-wide.

Species of the *Anopheles* mosquito can be found throughout the world in temperate, subtropical, and tropical areas. The *Anopheles* mosquito is the vector for malaria, which is caused by *Plasmodium spp.* parasites, with *P. falciparum* and *vivax* malaria being responsible for most of the mortality worldwide. While these parasites have been largely eradicated throughout much of the temperate zone (although risk remains due to the proliferation of the Anopheles spp. vector), malaria continues to be an enormous burden to tropical and subtropical regions of the globe, and particularly in sub-Saharan Africa [6].

Aedes aegypti is the best characterized species within the *Culicinae*, primarily due to its easy transition from the field to laboratory culture, and has provided much of the existing information on mosquito biology, physiology, genetics and vector competence. It maintains close association with human populations and it is the principal vector of the etiological agents of yellow fever and dengue fever , as well as for the recent Chikungunya fever epidemics in countries in the Indian Ocean area and Zika virus [7].

The "Global Vector Control Response (GVCR) 2017 – 2030" was approved by the World Health Assembly in 2017. It provides strategic guidance to countries and development partners for urgent strengthening of vector control as a fundamental approach to preventing disease and responding to outbreaks. Most vector-borne diseases can be prevented by vectorcontrol, if it is implemented well. Major reductions in the incidence of malaria, onchocerciasis and Chagas disease have been largely due to strong political and financial commitment. For other vector-borne diseases, vector control has not yet been used to its full potential or had maximal impact [8]. There is a hope mosquito bites can be reduced by repellents applied on textiles and paint for walls, too. This chapter represent mosquito repellents on textile for protecting people against invasive mosquitoes (*Anopheles spp.* and *Aedes aegypti*). The current research was involved in the development of mosquito repellent cotton fabrics with natural essential oils and further improvement of mosquitoes repellent efficacy on cotton fabrics. Cotton fabric treated with natural mosquito repellents (immortelle oil, water glass and vibroactivated zeolites) that achieved very good efficacy results [9]. WHO modified efficacy method, `WHO/CTD/WHOPES/IC/96.1` and "human lending counts" ("glove") test method according to Coleman, Govere and Durrheim [10, 11] were used for testing efficacy.

14.2 MATERIAL AND METHODS

Cotton fabric has been treated with Immortelle oil (I), natural vibroactivated zeolites (Z), water glass (WG) in the impregnation bath, combined Immortelle oil and vibroactivated zeolites (I_Z), Immortelle oil and water glass (I_WG) by using a Pad-Roll-Dry system. In the continuous impregnation process the fabric wet pick was 100%, followed by drying at 120 °C for 2 min. To every impregnation bath wetting agent Felosan RG-N (Bezema) has been added. For better durability organosilane (F) was added in some combination of baths. Samples that have organosilane in their bath were cured at 140 °C for 3 min.. The samples labels and treatment are listed in Table 14.1.

This chapter will discuss the *Anopheles spp.* and *Aedes aegypti* mosquito repellents efficacy, based on different products nature. For *Anopheles spp* mosquito the repellents efficacy is calculated by using the results of WHO modified test method (`CTD/WHOPES/IC/96.1`) which essentially is a chamber method, where mosquitoes are released on treated fabric. For textile fabrics with mosquito repellency properties, the mosquito will be repelled to the bait through the gap provided. In this way their effective repulsion i.e. their ability to migrate away is observed and calculated as Percentage Repellency (resp. efficacy).

Table 14.1: The samples labels and treatment.

Sample	**Treated with**
UN	Untreated
Z20	20 g/l vibroactivated zeolite
I _5	5 g/l Immortelle essencial oil
WG10	10 g/l water glass
I_5 _WG10	5 g/l Immortelle essencial oil, 10 g/l water glass
I _5 _Z20	5 g/l Immortelle essencial oil, 20 g/l vibroactivated zeolite
I_5_F10	5 g/l Immortelle essencial oil, 10 g/l organosilane
I_5 _WG10_F10	5 g/l Immortelle essencial oil, 10 g/l water glass, 10 g/l organosilane
I _5 _Z20_F10	5 g/l Immortelle essencial oil, 20 g/l vibroactivated zeolite, 10 g/l organosilane

For *Aedes aegypti* mosquito the repellent activity of each compound the assessment was based on the human landing counts [7, 8]. The study was conducted into a cage (33 × 33 × 33 cm) with a 32 × 32 mesh and with a 20 cm diameter circular opening fitted with cloth sleeve. Each cage contained 100 adult mosquitoes (sex ratio, 1:1), 5 to 10 days old, starved for 12 h at 25 ± 2 °C, and 70–80 % relative humidity. A plastic glove with an opening measuring of 5 × 5 cm was employed for all the bioassays. Different doses (from 0.05 to 1 $\mu l cm^{-2}$) for DEET were applied and found that the lowest dose, where

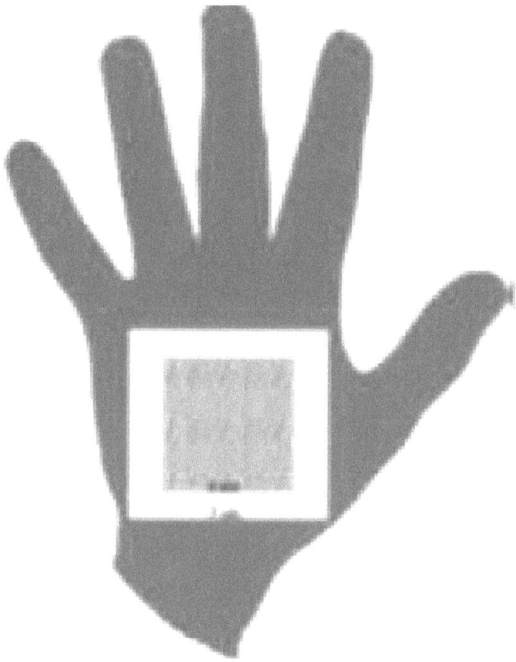

Figure 14.1: Human landing counts. A plastic glove with an opening (5 × 5 cm) on the upper side was used. The testing material was loaded to a filter paper or treated textile (7 × 7 cm) with an opening (5 × 5 cm) and placed in order to surround the glove opening [12].

zero landings were counted, was $\approx 0.2\,\mu l cm^{-2}$. All testing materials were applied on paper (Whatman chromatography paper) of 24 cm^2 total area and tested at two doses: 50 μl ("low", $\approx 0.2\,\mu l cm^{-2}$ of testing material) and 100 μl ("high", $\approx 0.4\,\mu l cm^{-2}$ of testing material) of 100 $\mu g \mu l^{-1}$ stock solution.

The paper was placed around the glove opening (Figure 14.1). Five minutes after treatment with the testing material (to ensure the solvent evaporation), the treated area (glove with filter paper) was inserted for 5 min through the sleeve into the cage. Control treatments without the components and with DEET were also included for the repellency tests as standards (control and positive control, respectively). Each treatment was repeated eight times and four human volunteers were used [11].

The physical structure and elemental composition of cotton fibers were analyzed by Hitachi SU3500 scanning electron microscopy equipped with energy dispersive spectrometer detector (SEM-EDS). The imaging was made with 3 kV accelerating voltage. The samples were coated with a 10 nm thick layer of gold before analysis [13].

14.3 RESULTS

Present work attempt to find suitable natural repellents for effective mosquito control measure and by this to contribute, in the near future, to human protection from the vector transmitted diseases.For this purpose, natural vibroactivated zeolite, Immortelle Oil and

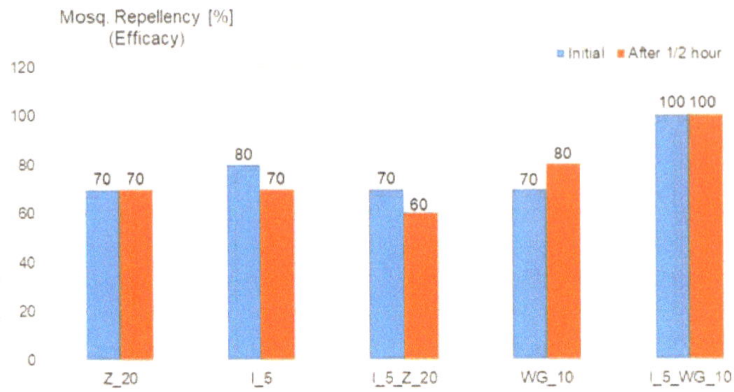

Figure 14.2: Repellents efficacy for *Anopheles spp.* mosquito repellents on cotton fabric.

water glass are currently applied on cotton fabric. The surface mass of cotton fabrics and Add-on of treated of all samples are given in Table 14.2.

During the repellency test procedure, mostly mosquitoes migrated to untreated fabric and achieved a high efficacy. From Immortelle oil treated cotton, mosquitoes migrated to untreated cotton already at the very beginning of the applied test (I_5 – Initial efficacy = 80% and 70% after ½ hour). The same phenomenon happened with another treated cotton (Figure 14.2). When cotton fabrics treated in combination with vibroactivated zeolites results were a little bit lower (I_5_Z_20 – Initial efficacy = 70% and 60% after ½ hour) but when fabrics treated in combination Immortelle oil with Water glass the repellent activity were incredible 100 %. Repellents efficacy for *Aedes aegypti* mosquito repellents on cotton fabric were given in Table 14.3 and Figure 14.3.

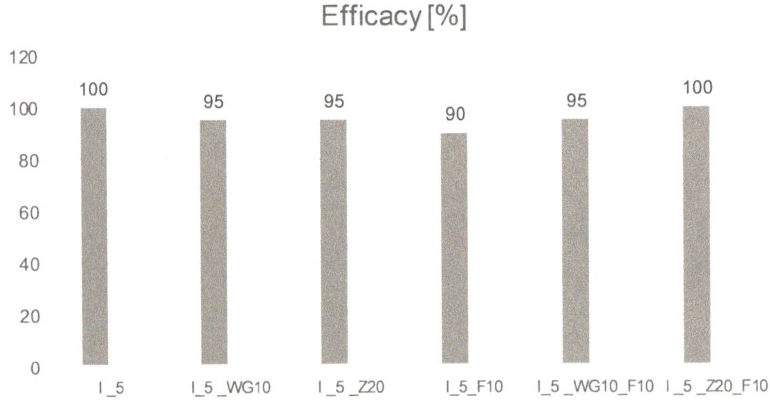

Figure 14.3: Repellents efficacy for *Aedes aegypti* mosquito repellents on cotton fabric

Table 14.2: Mass per m^2 and Add-on of treated samples.

Samples	**Mass per m^2**	**Add-on [%]**
UN	208,42	
Z20	214,13	2,74
I _5	211,11	1,29
WG10	211,54	1,36
I_5 _WG10	212,40	1,91
I _5 _Z20	213,67	2,52
I_5_F10	212,15	1,79
I_5 _WG10_F10	213,52	2,32
I _5 _Z20_F10	215,29	3,30

Cotton material treated with Immortelle oil and additions such as vibroactivated zeolites, water glass. For better durability Organosilane was added in some bath with Immortelle oil. Repellents efficacy was measure According to Coleman, Govere and Durrheim [6, 7]. Samples I_5 and I_Z20_F10 have the best efficacy – even 100%. No mosquitoes landed on these two samples. Another samples also have very good repellents efficacy for *Aedes aegypti* mosquito (I_5 _WG10, I _5 _Z20, I_5 _WG10_F10 = 95%, and I_5_F10 = 90%).

Figure 14.4 shows SEM images of the surfaces of the cotton fibers after treatment with different mosquito repellents. It can be seen that untreated cotton shows fibrilar surface structure. Cotton fibers surface looks smoother and uniform when impregnated with immortelle oil, vibroactivated zeolite or water glass. vibroactivated zeolite (Z_20) and water glass (I_WG_10) particles are clearly seen on the fiber surface. The zeolites particles are uniform in the range from 5 μm to 10 μm . It is found that water glass (sodium silicates) particles are smaller and located only in the spaces between fibers [13].

14.4 CONCLUSION

Mosquito repellents such as Immortelle oil, vibroactivated zeolite and water glass are successfully applied on cotton fabric and gave a high repellents efficacy for *Anopheles*

Table 14.3: Number of landings *Aedes aegypti* mosquito on treated cotton.

Sample	**n° of Landings**
Negative control	22
I _5	0
I_5 _WG10	1
I _5 _Z20	1
I_5_F10	2
I_5 _WG10_F10	1
I _5 _Z20_F10	0

spp. mosquitoes. During the repellency test procedure, from all treated cotton fabrics most of the mosquitoes migrated to the untreated fabric resulting in high efficacy even 100 %. Repellency test for *Aedes aegypti* mosquitoes also gave high efficacy which is 90 – 100 %.

ACKNOWLEDGMENTS

This chapter is partly based on work performed within the framework of IMAAC (`https://imaac.eu/`) related to COST Action CA16227 (*Investigation & Mathematical Analysis of Avant-garde Disease Control via Mosquito Nano-Tech-Repellents,*

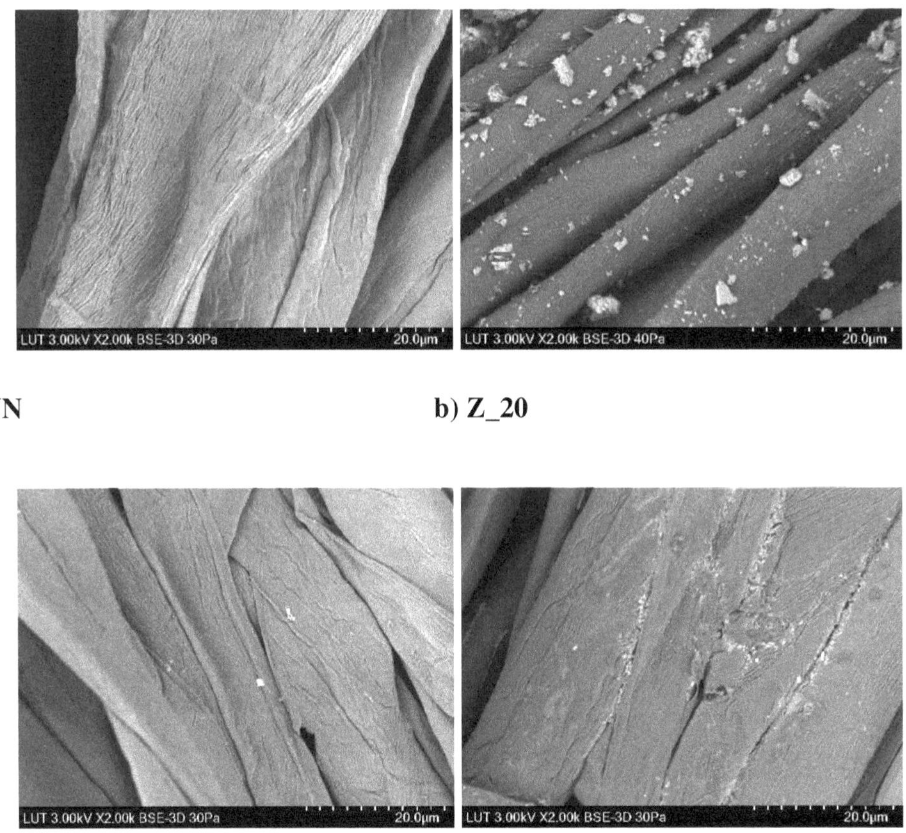

a) UN **b) Z_20**

c) I_5 **d) I_5WG_10**

Figure 14.4: SEM images of cotton fabrics: a) untreated, b) treated with vibroactivated zeolite, c) immortelle oil, and d) immortelle oil and water glass [13].

`https://cost.eu/actions/CA16227/`), supported by COST Association (European Cooperation in Science and Technology).

FURTHER READING

See the references attached to this chapter or contact the authors directly.

To whom correspondence should be addressed:
Prof. Ana Marija Grancaric,
Department of Textile Chemistry and Ecology,
Faculty of Textile Technology (TTF), University of Zagreb,
Prilaz baruna Filipovića 28a, HR-10000 Zagreb, Croatia;
E-mail: amgranca@ttf.hr.

CHAPTER 15

Silica-Based Organic-Inorganic Hybrid Treatments as Anti-Mosquito Textile Finishing

Veronica Migani

University of Bergamo, Department of Engineering and Applied Sciences, Dalmine, Bergamo, Italy

Ana Marija Grancaric*

co - Chair of IMAAC (COST Action CA 16227) &
University of Zagreb, Faculty of Textile Technology (TTF), Zagreb, Croatia
** corresponding author, e-mail: amgranca@ttf.hr*

Maria Rosaria Plutino

Institute for the Study of Nanostructured Materials, ISMN – CNR, O.U. Palermo, Department of ChiBioFarAm, University of Messina, Vill. S. Agata, Messina, Italy

Valentina Trovato

University of Bergamo, Department of Engineering and Applied Sciences, Dalmine, Bergamo, Italy

Giuseppe Rosace

University of Bergamo, Department of Engineering and Applied Sciences, Dalmine, Bergamo, Italy

CONTENTS

15.1 Introduction 244
15.2 Encapsulation techniques and sol-gel chemistry 245
15.3 Anti-mosquito finishing by sol-gel technique 247
15.4 Conclusions 249

DOI: 10.1201/9781003035992-15

15.1 INTRODUCTION

Chemical treatments are extensively used in textile finishing procedures to improve different properties of natural and synthetic fibers. A survey of the updated literature (Schindler W.D.; Hauser P.J. 2004) reveals that several chemicals are commonly used as finishes but, due to the intense pressure to ban harmful molecules, various attempts have been made to replace environmentally hazardous products and to use new procedures in the preparation of functional coatings for medical applications (Puoci et al. 2020), which allow combining the entrapment of bioactive compounds with their controlled release. Among the different methods proposed, the sol-gel process has demonstrated its exceptional potential with respect to the synthesis of new coatings with a high degree of homogeneity at the molecular level and exceptional physicochemical properties (Mahltig et al. 2005) and the application on clothes of derivatives from the plant world, which can be used both as insecticides, to kill insects, and as repellents to keep them away from the human body (Tseghai 2016), can provide an additional layer of protection to the skin, especially in tropical areas.

Protective textiles are among the innovative applications of smart technology and refer to those textiles that provide protection from something, such as antibacterial, UV protection, fire protection (flame retardant textiles), self-cleaning, hydrophobicity, or multifunctional materials, all of which are developed with the application of functional finishes to textile fabrics and can be prepared by sol-gel assisted immobilization of bioactive agents, biomolecules and biopolymers. High economic growth rates are expected in the world market of technical textiles (Haufe et al. 2008) because sol–gel nanocomposite hybrids have been shown to enable the chemical modification of natural fibres and produce a solid-state material from a chemically homogeneous precursor onto the textile substrate. By trapping the "randomness of the state of the solution" and thus ensuring the atomic mixing of the reagents, you should be able to produce complex inorganic materials such as ternary and quaternary oxides at lower processing temperatures and shorter synthesis times.

For the immobilization of biomolecules, the sol-gel technique provides mild processing conditions (physiological, pH and temperature) and single-step processing, employing conventional machinery used in industrial textile finishing, such as pad application or exhaust processes, to impart multifunctional properties to the finished fabrics, thus allowing variations in the composition and structure of the matrix, while keeping the immobilized biomolecules stable over time. Besides, it is possible to easily make large films during processing because the sol-gel method is a liquid phase process (Li et al. 2007), to control over morphology and particle size (Kakihana 1996) and to ensure excellent adhesion on cotton, attained through condensation between the –OH groups of the hydrolyzed silanes and those present on the surface of cellulose.

As already demonstrated (Ardanuy et al. 2014), the resulting silica-based layers can act as a matrix for embedding additives or active ingredients homogeneously into fabrics, leading to novel textile finishing, with controlled delivery properties (Haufe et al. 2008), thus presenting an alternative to toxic carriers. Accordingly, silica precursors should be in-

Table 15.1: Main micro/nanoencapsulation techniques

Methods	Micro/nanoencapsulation techniques
Chemical	Interfacial polymerization, In situ polymerization, polycondensation, polymer-polymer incompatibility, emulsion hardening, mini emulsion, liposome formation
Physico-chemical	Coacervation, polyelectrolyte multilayer, supercritical fluids, sol-gel, solvent evaporation
Phisico-mechanical	Spray-cooling/chilling, extrusion, air-suspension coating, fluidized-bed technology, microwave processing, ultrasonic atomizer, electrospray

volved in the immobilization of bio-based repellents (e.g. immortelle oil) that, in a previous study, showed good to excellent anti-mosquito repellent efficacy (Grancaric et al. 2020).

15.2 ENCAPSULATION TECHNIQUES AND SOL-GEL CHEMISTRY

Encapsulation techniques are generally divided into chemical and physical methods (which are also divided into physical-chemical and physical-mechanical processes) (Ghayempour and Montazer 2016) and are summarized in Table 15.1 some are applied with a gaseous and others with a liquid suspension medium.

Among the encapsulation methods listed in the table, the sol-gel process is considered the most feasible method to prepare chemically homogeneous coatings that are able to open promising applications in many areas such as optics, electronics, mechanics, energy, environment, biology, solar and fuel cells, catalysts, sensors and functional intelligent coatings such as antimicrobial coatings (Amiri and Rahimi 2016).

Sol-gel chemistry is based on hydrolysis and condensation of metal alkoxides or between hydrated metal species. Among many examples of alkoxide-based sol–gel chemistry, a large number of precursors involves early transition group metals (e.g. Ti, Zr) or early p-block elements (e.g. Al, Si) (Danks et al. 2016). Metal alkoxides can be prepared in different ways depending on the metal's nature, such as the reaction of metal chlorides with alcohols or the anodic dissolution of the metal into alcohol with an electroconductive additive. The suitability of alkoxides for sol-gel chemistry and the outcome of the reactions depend on several factors, such as the differences in electronegativity between oxygen and metal, which affect the ionic character of the M-O bond, as well as the ability of donation/withdrawal of electrons of the alkyl/aryl chain on the stability of the alkoxyl groups. These factors ultimately direct the gel structure by influencing the relative rates of hydrolysis and condensation as well as the degree of oligomerization or polymerization.

Finally, viscosity and volatility, as physical factors, can influence the suitability of alkoxides for sol-gel chemistry, along with process parameters such as the ratio of water to alkoxide and the presence or concentration of catalysts, since silica sol-gel chemistry is typically driven by acidic or basic catalysts that influence the structure of the resulting gel. Hydrolysis leads to the replacement of an alkoxyl group by a hydroxyl group with a

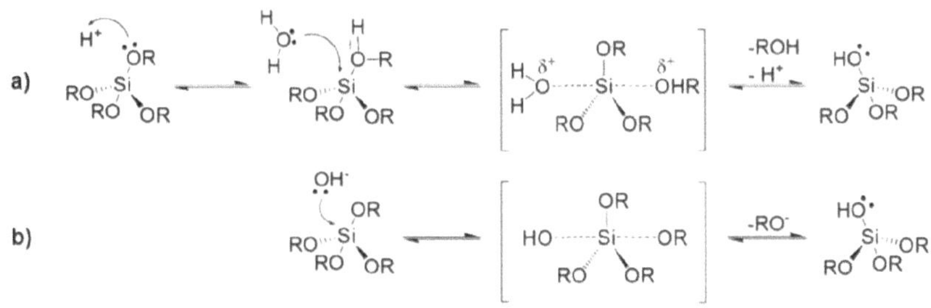

Figure 15.1: Schematic representation of acid (a) and base (b) catalyzed hydrolysis of silane precursors.

pentacoordinated transition state in both acid and basic catalyzed systems (Scheme 15.1.a and 15.1.b , respectively) (Danks et al. 2016, Gonzalez et al. 2019).

Depending on the conditions and the Si/H_2O ratio, more than one alkoxyl group can be hydrolyzed. The speed of each hydrolysis phase relies on the stability of the transition state, which in turn depends on the relative electron withdrawal or donation power of the -OH versus -OR groups. The result is that subsequent hydrolysis phases become progressively slower under acidic conditions and faster under alkaline conditions. The condensation depends on the degree of hydrolysis that has already occurred because a silanol group is required on at least one silicon center and is also catalyzed by acids or bases (Scheme 15.2.a and 15.2.b, respectively) with the formation of siloxane/methaloxanic bonds.

If the hydrolysis is complete before the first condensation phase occurs, the resulting product $(OH)_3Si\text{-}O\text{-}Si(OH)_3$ has 6 sites for the subsequent condensation phases in an alkaline environment. Multiple condensation phases give rise to small, highly branched agglomerates in the sol step, which eventually cross-link to form a colloidal gel. Under acidic conditions, where the first hydrolysis phase is typically the fastest, condensation begins before the hydrolysis is complete. Condensation often occurs on terminal silanols, resulting in chain-like structures in the sol and mesh gel. The consequences for the gel morphology are represented in Figure 15.1 (Danks et al. 2016).

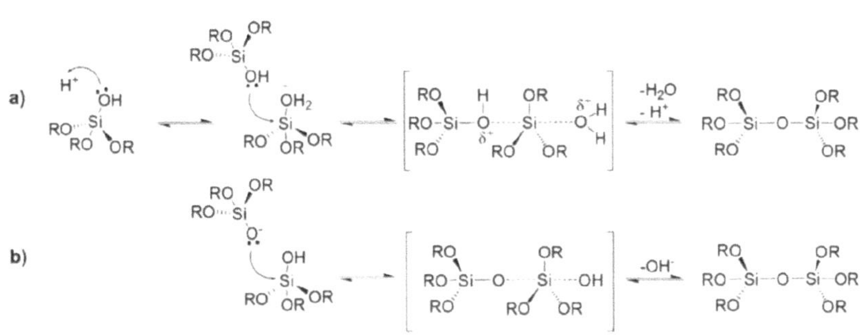

Figure 15.2: Schematic representation of acid (a) and base (b) catalyzed condensation reactions of hydrolyzed silane precursors.

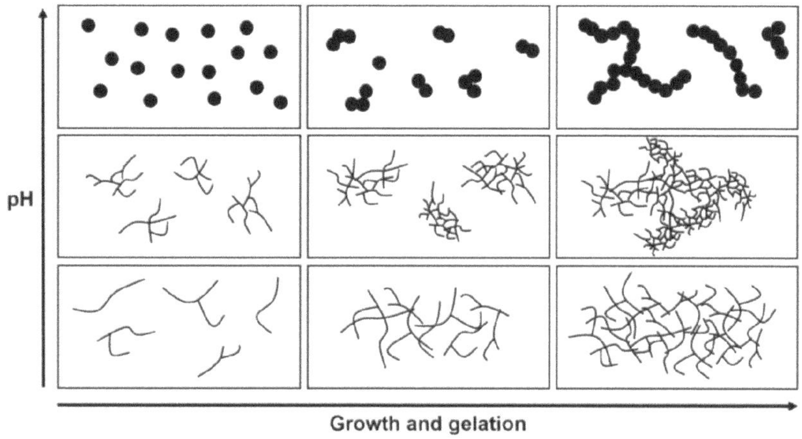

Figure 15.3: Influence of pH on the structure and growth of gel.

Hydrolysis and condensation rates, and therefore the structure of silica gels, can also be influenced by solvents due to their interaction with the silicon center. Indeed, many silicon alkoxides are insoluble in water and the alkoxide ratio/ water is often adjusted to limit hydrolysis. In addition, the molecular chemistry of silicon is much more diverse than simple tetra-alkoxides, and many compounds exist with the general structure $SiR(OR)_3$, $SiR_2(OR)_2$ or SiR_3OR. Finally, the presence of chelating agents can reduce hydrolysis and condensation rates.

Sol-gel coatings have high mechanical, chemical and thermal stability, controllable porosity and they do not show absorbance in the visible range. Thanks to these features, it is possible to develop innovative properties in the sol-gel matrices, mixing additives up to a level of about 30% of precursors (Böttcher et al. 1999). The so obtained solutions, after deposition, gelification and drying, form stable film onto coated materials. The release of encapsulated liquids from the silica film can be controlled by adjusting the silica/agent mass ratio, chemically modifying the silica matrix, adding soluble or swelling pore-forming substances and managing the preparation conditions. Generally, the use of encapsulated products offers greater convenience, better storage stability and controlled release of encapsulated organic substances. In the last years, investigations have been conducted on the immobilization and controlled release of different bioactive liquids through a modified silica coating to evaluate possible applications for functionalized fabrics (Haufe et al. 2008). The study was mainly focused on antimicrobial and anti-allergic effects due to natural oils and treatment of diseased respiratory tract by immobilized high volatility biological agents. A single-phase hybrid network combining organic and inorganic components, with molecular-scale interactions, then provides a new path to customize the desired thin-film coating properties for different applications (Amiri and Rahimi 2016).

15.3 ANTI-MOSQUITO FINISHING BY SOL-GEL TECHNIQUE

The development of innovative technologies can introduce new functionalities to textiles without modifying their appearance, thus introducing barrier properties for many application fields such as antibacterial and mosquito-repellent textiles. In particular, anti-mosquito finishing protects people from the bite of mosquitoes and, consequently, ensure safety from the infectious diseases they commonly spread (Amiri and Rahimi 2016, Raja, ASM; Kawlekar, Sujata; Saxena, Sujata; Arputharaj, A; Patil 2015). Recently, investigations have been conducted to improve the properties of textile fabrics by incorporating various finishes into the sol-gel coating to give them many important properties, such as wear resistance, flame retardancy, UV protection, controlled release of oil and flavour, antimicrobial properties, bio-catalytic properties and washing fastness of dyestuffs, showing no cytotoxicity (Plutino et al. 2017), thus the sol-gel technique resulting potentially attractive to develop anti-mosquito fabrics.

For example, this technique was used to immobilize permethrin molecules into cotton fabrics by a silicon oxide nanocoating applied by conventional padding followed by curing (Ardanuy et al. 2014). The effect of the process parameters, such as silica precursor content and permethrin/silica precursor ratio, on the insect-repellent activity, textile properties and stability during washing was studied. This new method provided the possibility of fine-tuning the amount of insecticide incorporated, maintaining the maximum dosage of permethrin in clothing less than 500 mg/m^2, according to the recommendation by the World Health Organization (WHO).

The paper confirmed that silica-based coating, under experimental conditions, did not influence mechanical properties of treated fabrics, maintaining the fabric softness and the wrinkle resistance close to the untreated textile. The final result showed high washing fastness of anti-mosquito coatings: after 50 laundering cycles, permethrin-containing sol–gel finishing provided a total mosquitoes mortality in one day of exposition, suggesting an alternative to well-established treatments for textiles.

Furthermore, the lavender oil distilled from Lavandula Angustifolia was used as a core material in combination with chitosan as a shell obtained by sol gel-emulsion method with starch as a template (Mulyani and Sunendar 2013). The obtained microcapsules, prepared at room temperature, showed a nanosizing structure in a rod shape that proposes the lavender-containing silica coating as a good candidate to develop anti-mosquito textiles. Unfortunately, no results were reported concerning the repellent properties of the so obtained textile samples. A more recent paper (Abdelhameed et al. 2017) investigated a titanium-bearing metal-organic framework (MOF) with the chemical formula $Ti_8O_8(OH)_4(BDC\text{-}NH_2)_6$, built up from octahedral titanium units connected via oxygen atoms to the organic linker 2-aminoterephthalic acid. For that investigation, MOF was immobilized onto the silica modified fabrics via covalent bonding. With this goal, the authors used 3-glycidyloxypropyltrimethoxysilane, as a sol-gel precursor, to finish plant-based fibres (100% cotton, linen) or regenerated cellulosic fibres (viscose). The composites were tested in the control of the adult stage of mosquitoes. At low MOF concentration, the mosquito mortality depends on the type of modified fabrics (cotton > linen > viscose), and on NH_2-MIL-125 concentration on the samples, high MOF content leading to higher killing efficacy. Modified textiles show good washing resistance, surviving more than five washing cycles. In short, the in situ formation of NH_2-MIL-125 on the surface of cellulose-based fabrics affords composite materials with excellent anti-mosquito properties that do not require the presence of any insecticide.

Other authors investigated a straightforward synthesis of silver nanoparticles using Moringa Oleifra water extract (El-Sayed et al. 2020). The obtained silver nanoparticles in the presence of Moringa were mixed with hydrolyzed 3-Glycidyloxypropyltrimethoxysilane silane, as a sol-gel precursor, in combination with a modified dimethylol dihydroxyethylene urea low formaldehyde reactant resin. The anti-mosquito activity of the treated fabric was assessed on cotton, polyester/cotton blend, viscose and linen textile samples. The test was carried out according to the reported procedure. A cage, inside which the treated fabric was fixed in one side, was filled with 100 adult mosquitoes, 3 days old, checking for the time the mosquitoes stayed away from the fabric. As a reference, the same experiment was conducted using an untreated textile sample. Results show that mosquito mortality depends on the type of treated sample and duration of exposure. The in-situ treatment of fabric surface by AgNPs@Moringa suspension offers the formation of composite materials with excellent anti-mosquito properties that do not require the presence of any harmful insecticide material.

15.4 CONCLUSIONS

The economic impact that mosquitoes cause is really high, so much so that the development of efficient repellents is of huge importance, especially if they are of natural origin and harmless to human health. The use of different essential oils extracted from plants and immobilized on tissues can prove to be one of the winning weapons in this battle due to their recognized repellent properties as well as antimicrobial and antioxidant characteristics. The high volatility and uncontrollable delivery of these oils can be solved through the sol-gel technique, which can control their release. In this way, essential oils can be encapsulated within sol-gel based coatings, providing composite materials with excellent anti-mosquito properties that do not exhibit significant toxic characteristics for the environment and human beings.

ACKNOWLEDGMENTS

This chapter is partly based on work performed within the framework of IMAAC (`https://imaac.eu/`) related to COST Action CA16227 (*Investigation & Mathematical Analysis of Avant-garde Disease Control via Mosquito Nano-Tech-Repellents*, `https://cost.eu/actions/CA16227/`), supported by COST Association (European Cooperation in Science and Technology).

Cotton and Polyester Fabrics Plasma Coated with Hydrogenated Amorphous Carbon Films

Melanie Fritz
Department of Physics, University Koblenz-Landau, Koblenz, Germany

Ana Marija Grancaric*
co - Chair of IMAAC (COST Action CA 16227) &
University of Zagreb, Faculty of Textile Technology (TTF), Zagreb, Croatia
** corresponding author, e-mail: amgranca@ttf.hr*

Lea Botteri
University of Zagreb, Faculty of Textile Technology (TTF), Zagreb, Croatia

Christian B. Fischer
Department of Physics, University Koblenz-Landau, Koblenz, Germany &
Materials Science, Energy and Nano-Engineering Department, Mohammed VI Polytechnic University, Ben Guerir, Morocco

CONTENTS

16.1 Introduction 252
16.2 Coating process and analytics 253
16.3 Results 254
16.4 Conclusion 256

DOI: 10.1201/9781003035992-16

16.1 INTRODUCTION

In the second half of the 20th century, cold plasmas were found suitable for surface modification of temperature-sensitive textile materials [1]. Recently, there has been a trend in textile engineering toward green finishing processes such as plasma technology [2,3]. Cold plasma can be classified into atmospheric pressure and low-pressure plasma like plasma enhanced chemical vapor deposition (PECVD) [4,5]. PECVD requires a closed system with good vacuum condition including appropriate equipment and operation, which is considered as drawback for commercial applications [1]. Furthermore, the sample size to be treated is limited to the chamber size and it must be operated off-line in batch mode. But it provides good control of the gas atmosphere and process parameters being a reproducible technique that results in high-end products with good stability and uniformity in the surface modification of textiles [6]. Plasma treatment of fabrics shows a great potential as an environmentally friendly and economical dry finishing technique, as conventional textile finishing processes require large amounts of chemical agents, water, and energy. Pretreatments of textiles are carried out to clean fibers from natural or manufacture-related impurities like oil, grease and volatiles [7]. This is essential to make the fiber receptive to water, dyes [8], and finishing chemicals [9].

The plasma supported deposition of hydrogenated amorphous carbon (a-C:H) films is proven to be very beneficial for modifying and improving material properties. Well-known are mechanical stability, hardness, low friction, chemical inertness, high corrosion resistance, biocompatibility and changed barrier properties that can also be generated on polymeric materials [2, 10 - 23]. Also textile properties such as wettability [7, 9], hydrophobicity [24 - 26], super hydrophilicity [7, 27], flame-retardant properties and fire-resistance [28], antimicrobial effects [29, 30], crease resistance, UV protection, or aesthetic properties are modified to be adapted for special applications e.g. in self-cleaning good progress was achieved with plasma-treated cotton [27]. Furthermore, Kitahara et al. investigated imparting wash-resistant properties to fabrics in combination with a-C:H films to make them more chemically resistant and mechanically stable [29].

For the plasma treatment it is irrelevant if the textiles are natural or synthetic fibers, yarns, woven, nonwovens or knitted fabrics, they can all be modified according to their intended functionality. The plasma substrate interactions are caused by the bombardment of reactive plasma species (ions, electrons, radicals, neutrals and ultraviolet photons) resulting in different surface reactions in the outermost layer (~10 nm) [3, 10]: (a) Cleaning the surface from contaminations, (b) activation by generating chemically reactive sites increasing surface energy and enhancing the affinity for other substances, (c) surface etching by plasma reactive species followed by desorption, and (d) coating or plasma polymerization using gases for thin film deposition [31,32]. Depending on the reactive gas or gas mixtures used, different functional groups can be formed like amino (-NH_2), hydroxyl (-OH), carbonyl (-C=O), carboxylic (-COOH) etc. The groups formed often have a tendency to revert to their original state, meaning plasma activation is thermodynamically non-stable and should be performed just before further treatment [33, 34]. Synthetic fibers often have a hydrophobic nature due to the absence of polar functional groups limiting their application. Whether a liquid is repelled or absorbed depends on the chemical composition and the morphology of the surface [35]. Previous studies determined that oxygen plasma pretreatment is more effective than argon and hydrogen for the super-hydrophilic/ultra-hydrophobic properties for a-C:H film layers [27]. The textile structure and construction depend on the type of weave patter, g/m^2 of fabric, type of the fiber content, fiber fineness, and also the yarn parameters like the twist factors [36]. Textile materials consequently have a complex surface composed of the inter-fiber/filament space, inter-yarn space and the pore size distribution. Therefore, plasma treatment of textile fabrics is more challenging than for solid polymeric materials [37, 38].

The present study investigates a-C:H films (30 and 60 nm thick) on cotton, polyethylene terephthalate (PET), and cotton-PET mixture (COT/PET, 50:50) fabrics that serve as intermediate layer for subsequent impregnation with immortelle oil and water glass. Before the textile substrates are coated via PECVD using acetylene (C_2H_2) an oxygen (O_2) plasma was previously applied for cleaning and activation. Overall the three textile types as pure, oxygen treated and coated with two a-C:H coatings are individually refined or combined with immortelle oil (IO) and water glass (WG) in preparation for enhanced repellency properties to suppress mosquito attacks that cause vector-borne diseases.

16.2 COATING PROCESS AND ANALYTICS

The used PECVD vacuum system is sized 600 x 600 x 750 mm and suitable for coating sensitive samples as the temperature does not exceed 40°C [16 - 18]. The fabric samples cotton, PET and COT/PET were cut into pieces of 210 x 279 mm. Each fabric sample is fixed along short edge top and bottom between two full-length aluminum poster clamps. To avoid swinging, the bottom clip is extra weighted. The as prepared fabric samples are mounted with the top clip in the chamber freely hanging on rotating rods, which in turn are mounted on a rotating plate. This planetary-like system is operated with 2 rpm to ensure uniform coating. The deposition process is described in detail in [16]. In brief: Exposition to plasma is conducted at 10^{-3} Pa with firstly O_2 (10 min, 1 Pa, 200 W) and subsequently with C_2H_2 (15 and 30 min, 0.65 Pa, 107 W, deposition rate 2 nm/min). This has proven to be very efficient for textile fabric treatments, because the mean free path in the gas phase is higher, so that gas-textile collisions are favored over gas-gas collisions [36]. The a-C:H coated fabrics are treated afterwards using a pad-dry-cure procedure (Benz pad-dry system, Germany), impregnated with a finishing bath containing 10 g/L WG and/or 5 g/L IO, squeezed, dried at 110°C for 2 min, and finally cured 4 min at 150°C [39].

The morphology of the a-C:H coated textiles were investigated by scanning electron microscopy (SEM, Philips SEM515), especially to check the quality of plasma treatments on the fibers. The air permeability was evaluated with a SDL ATLAS M021S in standard atmosphere. According to ISO 9237:1995 the rate of air flow which passes perpendicularly through a test surface area of 5 cm^2 under an air pressure drop of 100 Pa was measured [40]. The test was repeated at different locations on the sample at least five times and averaged. The tensile properties of the fabrics were performed according to ISO 13934-1:2013 for the determination of maximum force using a strip method strength tester/tensiometer

(TensoLab3 2512A Mesdan S.P.A., Brescia, Italy) [41]. Here only the warp of the fabric was tested. The test was conducted with a constant speed of 100 mm/min, the load cell ID/FS was 5/500 kg and pretension 5 N. In this way the maximum force and elongation at maximum force respectively the force and elongation at rupture can be measured.

16.3 RESULTS

SEM images presented in Figure 16.1, demonstrate clearly the preservation of the fiber structures of all three materials used after both plasma treatments. Depicted are the pure fabrics (first row), O_2 plasma treated (second row) and the two a-C:H coated ones (last two rows). In comparison to the pure fabrics the O_2 plasma treated ones appear more contrasted indicating a good cleaning process [16 - 23]. The images show clearly that the a-C:H coatings on each fabric sample are intact, except for the cotton fibers with 60 nm a-C:H (Figure 16.1 d), where the coating does not appear to be complete. Small delaminations are noticeable, which could be caused by the rougher overall structure of the fiber. It is also apparent that the thin films only coat the fiber surfaces and do not cover the entire fabric. A very smooth and uniform coating is especially achieved with PET fibers (Figure 16.1 k, l), in line with earlier studies for PET polymer [21]. This is also observable for the PET fiber content in the COT/PET mix (Figure 16.1).

The results for the air permeability tests, an important performance factor of textiles which can be used to provide an indication of the breathability of weather-resistant and rainproof fabrics, are shown in Figure 16.2 (two upper rows). The finishing with IO in combination with WG and the plasma treatments cause a change in the length of airflow paths through a fabric. Due to different fabric weaves (Cotton: Oxford, PET: single, COT/PET: 2/2 twill), findings are considered separately for each material used. The results for air per-

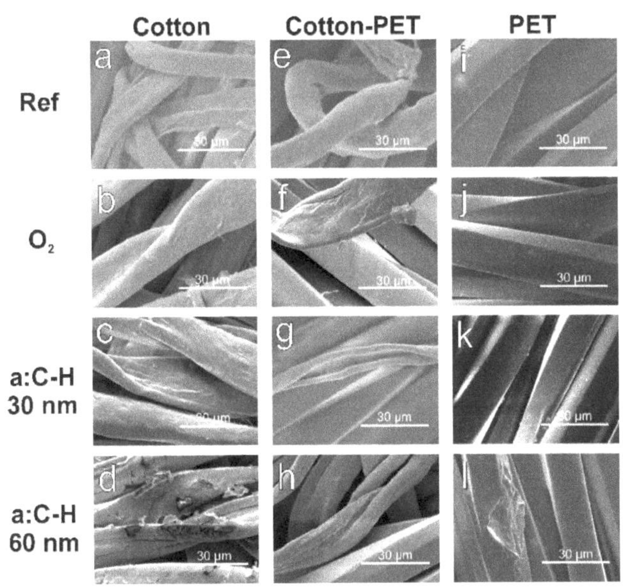

Figure 16.1: SEM images of the pure (first row), O_2 plasma treated (second row) and a-C:H coated fabrics (last two rows).

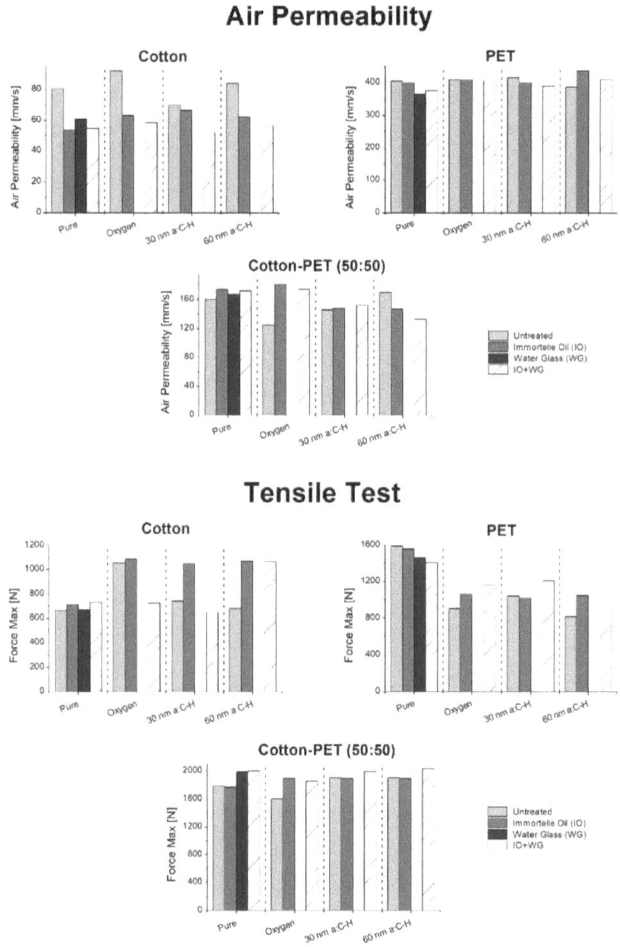

Figure 16.2: Air permeability (top) and tensile testing (below) for pure and plasma treated fabrics with IO and WG finishing.

meability R clearly indicate that the air flow passing vertically through all tested specimens does not affect breathing quality too much. For cotton, the highest value is determined for the O_2 treated fabric at around 90 mm/s. Followed by the 60 nm a-C:H layer, the untreated sample and finally the 30 nm a-C:H coating. Adding IO lowers R by 20 - 25 mm/s for all but the 30 nm thin coated fibers. The supplemental WG add-on to IO further lowers the plasma treated cotton from 5 to 15 mm/s.

For PET the 60 nm a-C:H film reduces R about 20 mm/s probably due to the smoothing of the fiber surface. Adding IO leads to a further slight reduction in R for all but the thicker a-C:H films. The decrease is amplified to another ~5 mm/s by the combination of WG. The lowest R is achieved with only WG finishing. For 30 nm a-C:H and IO add-on a fairly high air permeability is recognized on PET, leading to the assumption that the surface micro-roughness has changed.

For COT/PET fabric, the sample treated with O_2 only and the 30 nm a-C:H is 20 - 30 mm/s lower than the reference. The thicker coating shows a higher R of about 15 mm/s, which is probably due to the fact that the cotton content is more susceptible to damage, as shown previously. Here, all refinements increase R, except the fabric with 60 nm a-C:H, where it is 20 mm/s less for IO add-on and even 15 mm/s more for the IO+WG combination. For the IO finished samples, there is a slightly increased R of about 10 mm/s, which is significantly higher for the oxygen plasma-treated samples with around 60 mm/s. It could be that the oxygen treatment activates or etches the surface more strongly, and subsequent finishing results in a smoother surface that increases R.

Tensile tests (Figure 16.2, two lower rows) are used to check whether there are stability changes caused by the applied surface treatments. Cotton fabrics tear most easily, the maximum force (F_{max}) is reached at about 700 N. The O_2 treatment strengthens the tensile resistance by about 500 N. For the combined IO+WG finishing it reverts to the initial value. The 30 nm a-C:H deposition on cotton increases in stability only with an additional IO treatment and even lowers with the IO+WG combination. While for the 60 nm, partially incomplete a-C:H layer on cotton both add-ons are an improvement, there is none for the carbon layer alone.

In the case of PET, there is no improvement due to plasma treatment and finishing detectable. In addition, the fabrics can only withstand an F_{max} of about 1000 N instead of 1600 N previously. A significant deterioration in stability compared with the initial condition, despite the more homogeneous coating.

The COT/PET withstands higher tensile strength due to its fabric structure, which is only slightly changed by the plasma treatment. The O_2 plasma reduces F_{max} by about 200 N first and in turn increases it by about 100 N for the subsequent a-C:H coating. Finishing with both add-ons improves it around 100 N for 30 nm and 200 N for 60 nm a-C:H, compared to the pure one. A closer inspection of the stretched fabric samples revealed that the cotton fibers have become more stretchable as a result of the oxygen treatment. In contrast, the PET fibers seem to have become more brittle and thus more unstable. For the COT/PET mix there is nothing observable, suggesting the two properties cancel each other out due to the balanced fiber proportions.

16.4 CONCLUSION

The results demonstrate firstly, the plasma treatment does not change the breathability nor does it reduce the tensile strength by stress generation, except for the PET fabric. Second, for cotton fabrics, the current a-C:H thicknesses are not suitable yet to ensure layer uniformity. The data indicates that the fabric structure is not significantly affected by current plasma treatments. Thus, the current plasma processes are appropriate for surface activation and the resulting surface modifications (O_2 treatment and a-C:H coating) serve as suitable platform with improved attraction for finishing agents, that can be used against vector-borne diseases, for example. In further investigations, the possible effects of durability, such as wash resistance and mechanical abrasion, but also the efficiency and adhesion to finishing agents should be considered in more detail.

ACKNOWLEDGMENTS

This chapter is partly based on work performed within the framework of IMAAC (`https://imaac.eu/`) related to COST Action CA16227 (*Investigation & Mathematical Analysis of Avant-garde Disease Control via Mosquito Nano-Tech-Repellents*, `https://cost.eu/actions/CA16227/`), supported by COST Association (European Cooperation in Science and Technology). The authors acknowledge Prof. Dr. Barbara Hahn and Lee Liu from the Department of Material Analysis, University of Applied Sciences, RheinAhrCampus, Germany for SEM equipment and imaging. We thank Dr. Heinz Busch, NTTF Coatings GmbH, Rheinbreitbach, Germany for providing plasma treatment equipment and Dr. Ružica Brunšek of the Faculty of Textile Technology, University of Zagreb, Croatia for the permeability tests.

IX

Testing Methods for Treated Textiles with Mosquito-Repellents: An Overview

CHAPTER 17

Testing Methods for Mosquito-Repellent Treated Textiles

Hitoshi Kawada
Department of Vector Ecology & Environment, Florida, USA Institute of Tropical Medicine, Nagasaki University, Nagasaki, Japan

Rui-De Xue*
Anastasia Mosquito Control District, EOC Drive, St. Augustine, Florida, USA
** corresponding author, e-mail: rxue@amcdfl.org*

CONTENTS

17.1 Introduction 261
17.2 Active ingredient 262
17.3 Treated method 262
17.4 Laboratory testing 262
17.5 Field Testing 269
17.6 Influencing factors 270
17.7 Challenges and conclusions: Towards an international standard 271

17.1 INTRODUCTION

The global threat of mosquito-borne infectious diseases continues to spread every year, in-part due to the worldwide horizontal and vertical expansion of vector mosquito species caused by increasing human movement, as well as global warming (Kawada et al. 2020). Accordingly, consumers' needs of anti-mosquito textiles with enhanced functionality for protecting against mosquito biting or limiting human exposure to mosquitoes is needed. The use of insecticide or repellent-treated bed nets, head nets, jackets, uniforms, and curtains are also increasing. Over the years, long-lasting insecticidal treated bed nets (LLIN) and uniforms have played a major role in the control of mosquito-borne diseases (Carnevale & Gay 2019). The World Health Organization (WHO) has established guidelines for laboratory and field testing of LLIN's (WHO 2005) which is similar to the repellent treated

DOI: 10.1201/9781003035992-17

textiles/clothing. However, there seems to be no international standard method for evaluating such mosquito repellent treated textile products, although there are some country-specific publicized methods. Standardization of commercial textile products by an official test method is, therefore, indispensable for authentic and objective evaluation of these products. In this chapter, repellents, treated methods, several bioassay methods in the laboratory and field for anti-mosquito textiles are briefly reviewed and advisable standard methods are proposed.

17.2 ACTIVE INGREDIENT

Repellents may be used to treat a variety of fabrics, materials, and textiles, including the materials for making bed nets, uniform, table clothing, loose jackets, curtains, and other clothing items. The most successful insecticide & repellent treated textiles are LLIN and the uniforms treated by permethrin, DEET, and picaridin. Since 1942, the Florida based Agricultural Research Services, Center for Medical, Agricultural, and Veterinary Entomology (U.S. Department of Agriculture 1967), tested notable repellents and insecticides on clothing/textiles such as Benzyl benzoate, 2-Butyl-2-ethyl-1,3-propanediol, Cedar oil and derivatives, DEET, Dibutyl phthalate, Dimethyl phthalate, Naphthalene, p-Dichlorobenzene, picaridin, and permethrin (Rutledge et al. 2015). Permethrin, a broad spectrum and synthetic pyrethroid insecticide was registered by the U.S. Environmental Protection Agency (EPA) in 1990 as a repellent on clothing by the military (Frances 2015). The repellents used, formulation, method of application, type of materials, and amount of repellent absorbed per unit area of textile should be reported.

17.3 TREATED METHOD

Insect repellent applications to textiles/fabric include: hand application by applying a liquid repellent into a gloved hand and rubbing the repellent material on clothing; impregnated by using solution to impregnated clothing; barrier application by applying the liquid material only to the openings of clothing by daubing;, with a sprayer or by drawing the mouth of the bottle along the clothing to apply a thin layer; application to clothing by the spray method; or dust for solid repellent application (McCain and Leach 2006). Factory pretreatment of uniforms and clothing in the United States (U.S.) is limited to permethrin, however, consumers may treat clothing to repel mosquitoes on their own using over-the-counter DEET, picaridin, and permethrin.

17.4 LABORATORY TESTING

1. It seems that almost all test methods for the conventional mosquito repellents directly applied to human skin such as DEET, picaridin, IR3535, natural essential oils, etc., are applicable to the test of textiles treated with those materials. Although pyrethroid insecticides are not recommended for direct treatment to human skin because of dermal toxicity (Brown and Hebert, 1997), they are used as contact repellents by treating textiles such as clothing/uniforms, hammock, curtain, and bed nets. Evaluation of

Table 17.1: Classification of the effect of anti-mosquito textiles and points of evaluation.

Category	Classification	Effect against mosquitoes	Evaluation
E-1	Blood feeding repellency Physical blocking	Blocking of mosquito biting or blood-sucking	Number of biting mosquitoes or number of bites
E-2	Contact repellency Spatial repellency	Inhibition of orientation or landing to host	Number of repelled or attracted mosquitoes
E-3	Excito-repellency	Inhibition of probing	Number of repelled or staying mosquitoes
E-4	Knockdown	Inhibition of flight or movement	Number of knocked-down mosquitoes
E-5	Killing	Death	Number of dead mosquitoes

excito-repellency, knockdown, and killing effects caused by pyrethroids, therefore, have to be involved in the test methods for textiles (Table 17.1). The most used test methods for repellent-treated textiles are cage, cone, and excito chamber tests (Anuar and Yusof, 2016). As Anuar and Yusof (2016) reported, test methods using mosquito attractants (Table 17.2) might imitate the more realistic situation of mosquito biting. Table 17.3 shows officially published test methods for anti-mosquito textiles.

Table 17.2: Classification of attractant.

Category	Attractive source	Remarks
A-1	Human	Exposed arms or legs.
A-2	Animal	Hair-shaved mice, rabbits, guinea pigs etc.
A-3	Artificial	Dark color, body temperature, carbon dioxide, blood or blood components.
A-4	Food	Sugar solution
A-5	None	

Table 17.3: Evaluation methods of anti-mosquito textiles.

		Classification / Attractive Source									
		E-1	E-2	E-3	E-4	E-5	A-1	A-2	A-3	A-4	A-5
Guideline or Standard	Test Method	Blood feeding re-pellency Physical blocking	Contact re-pellency Spatial re-pellency	Excito-re-pellency	Knock-down	Killing	Human	Animal	Artificial	Food	None
Guidelines for laboratory and field-testing of long-lasting insecticidal nets (WHO) [17.1]	Cone Test				√	√					√
	Tunnel Test					√		√			
	Field Test					√	√				
Guidelines for testing mosquito adulticides for indoor residual spraying and treatment of mosquito nets (WHO) [17.2]	Cone Test				√	√					√
	Tube Test				√	√					√
	Wire-ball Test				√	√					√
	Field Test					√	√				
Guidance on the Biocidal Products Regulation (European Chemicals Agency) [17.3]	Cage Test	√	√				√	√			√
	Experimental Hut Test	√	√				√				√

Table 17.3: *Continued.*

		Classification / Attractive Source									
		E-1	E-2	E-3	E-4	E-5	A-1	A-2	A-3	A-4	A-5
Guideline or Standard	Test Method	Blood feeding re-pellency Physical blocking	Contact re-pellency Spatial re-pellency	Excito-re-pellency	Knock-down	Killing	Human	Animal	Artificial	Food	None
GB National Standard (People's Republic of China) [17.4]	Cage Test	√	√				√				
	Arti-ficial blood-feeding Test	√	√						√ (Blood)		
Japanese Industrial Standard L1950-1 [17.5]	Arti-ficial blood-feeding Test	√	√						√ (Blood, Carbone-dioxide)		

[17.1] https://apps.who.int/iris/bitstream/handle/10665/80270/9789241505277_eng.pdf;jsessionid=8E7E6D112F1D26912BBE15C545060237?sequence=1.

[17.2] http://apps.who.int/iris/bitstream/10665/69296/1/WHO_CDS_NTD_WHOPES_GCDPP_2006.3_eng.pdf.

[17.3] https://www.echa.europa.eu/documents/10162/23036412/bpr_guidance_assessment_evaluation_part_vol_ii_part_bc_en.pdf/950efefa-f2bf-0b4a-a3fd-41c86daae468.

[17.4] In Chinese: http://www.texfunction.com/view746.html.

[17.5] https://webdesk.jsa.or.jp/books/W11M0090/index/?bunsyo_id=JIS+L+1950-1\%3A2018.

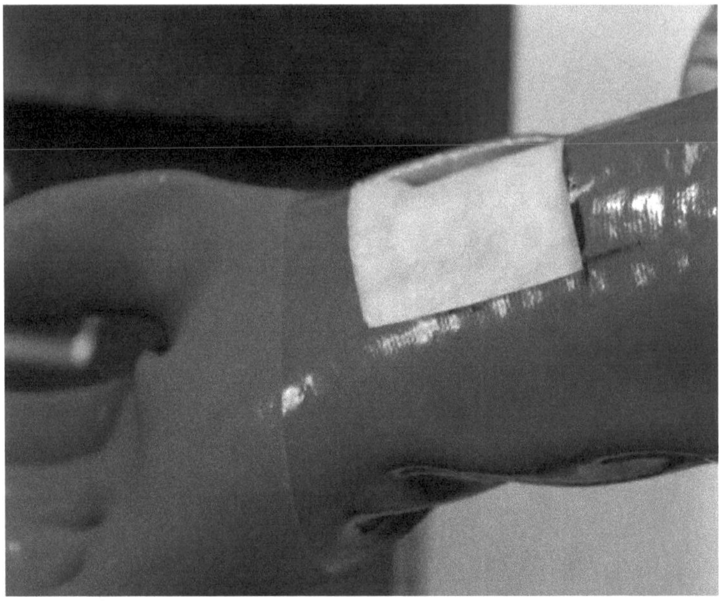

Figure 17.1: The rubber glove with a cut window (6 cm x 5 cm) on the human volunteer's forearm and the open area was covered with treated textile, then exposed to a testing cage holding 200 female mosquitoes.

2. The cage test: The cage test might be most common and simple test method for evaluation of repellents and repellent-treated materials, although it needs ethical approval by volunteers and requires the assurance of pathogen free mosquitoes. It also needs enough replications to reduce data discrepancies caused by individual variations among volunteers (i.e., participant sex, age, etc.). A screened cage (40 cm^3) containing 200, 7 - 8 day old starved female mosquitoes are used for each replicate of the evaluation. Participants will wear a long-sleeved rubber glove on one hand/arm that has a window cut out (6cm L x 5cm W) on the front sleeve of the glove. Next, a piece (7cm L x 6cm W) of treated textile is used to cover the window on the glove sleeve. The participant then exposes the treated arm into the screened cage with mosquitoes for 5 minutes. This exposure is repeated at 1 hr intervals until mosquitoes land/probe on the treated textiles on the window (Figure 17.1). Alternatively, wearing a short sleeved glove to protect the hand, a large piece of repellent treated textile can be used to wrap and cover all part of the forearm and exposed the treated forearm (Figure 17.2) to the testing cage for 5 minutes. Again, repeated at 1 hr intervals until the landing, probing and biting presents.

3. The cone and excito-repellency chamber test: These test methods are ethically more ideal because they do not use human volunteers or animals subjects as mosquito attractants. In cone test for *Anopheline* mosquitoes, five susceptible, non-blood-fed, 2–5-day-old female mosquitoes are exposed to each piece of netting (25 cm x 25 cm) for 3 min under standard WHO cones. Knock-down is recorded 60 min after exposure and mortality after 24 h. This procedure should be repeated until a total of 50 mosquitoes have been exposed to each piece. Excito-repellency chamber is

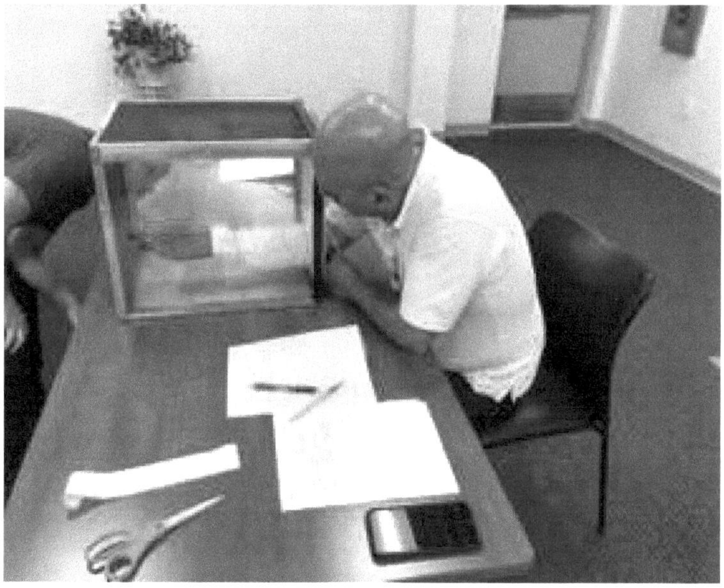

Figure 17.2: A human volunteer's whole forearm was covered and wrapped by repellent treated textiles or untreated textiles, and then exposed to the testing cage with 200 female mosquitoes.

composed of the outer chamber constructed with four metal sides (33.5 x 33.5 cm) and the screened inner chamber functioning as the test paper holder with four side-box slightly smaller than the outer chamber. The repellent-impregnated papers can be placed on the Plexiglas panel located either side of the wall of the inner chamber to allow or prevent mosquitoes from making physical contact with the test paper surface. The inner chamber with attached papers is carefully inserted into the outer chamber and the front door is then attached to the chamber together with the front escape funnel. A receiving box (6 x 6 x 6 cm) constructed of stiff paper carton material with screen netting on top for observation of escaped mosquitoes is attached to the exterior exit portal of the chamber. Both of these tests provide a simple and easy experiment for contact and excito repellency (Chareonviriyaphap et al. 2002; Kawada et al. 2014; Obermayr 2015). However, on the other hand, they are less adopted as mosquito repellent test for clothing.

4. Olfactometer and choice system test: In the laboratory, a pieces of repellent treated textiles or clothing/fabrics is used to cover an attractant object or a human volunteer's hand, then the covered attractant unit or human hand is placed or inserted to one of the ports of the olfactometer and an untreated attractant object or a human volunteer hand is placed or inserted into another port of the olfactometer for 5 minutes. The number of mosquitoes to enter each port are observed and counted. If the number of mosquitoes in the repellent treated textile is significantly less than the number of mosquitoes in the untreated control port, this means that the repellent treated textile works. The mosquitoes could be replaced every 4 hrs and the same testing be conducted many times to figure out the persistence.

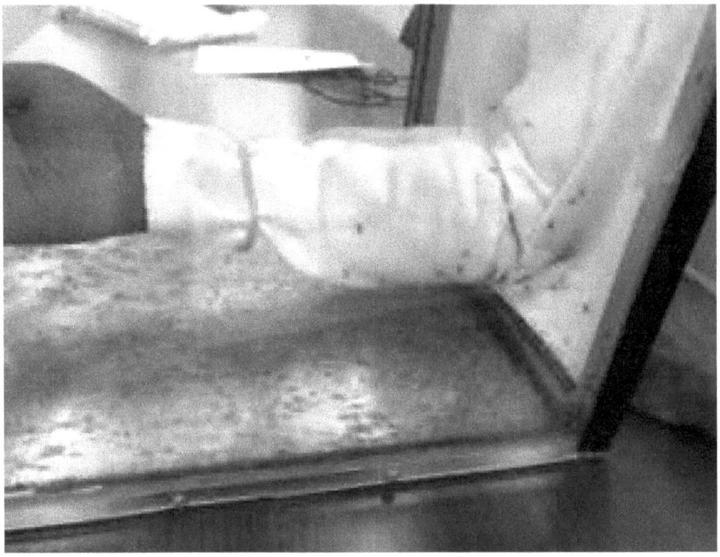

Figure 17.3: Outline sketch of the attractive blood feeding apparatus for anti-mosquito performance test (JIS L1950-1).

5. WHO bioassay: The World Health Organization (WHO) guidelines prescribe mainly on the test methods for insecticide-treated bed nets (ITNs). Laboratory studies such as the WHO cone bioassays and tunnel tests (phase I), small-scale field trials (phase II), and large-scale field trials (phase III) are involved in the above guidelines. The Guidance on the Biocidal Products Regulation (European Chemicals Agency, ECHA) basically follows the above WHO guidelines for insecticidal products. As for repellent-treated clothing, the similar test methods as those for repellents are stipulated by ECHA to be used (cage test and experimental hut test). The GB national standard in China (GB/T 30126-2013) might provide the only officially published test methods for anti-mosquito clothing. In the above standard, the modified cage test using human arms as mosquito attractant and the simulated blood feeding test using heated defibrinated animal blood (swine or chicken) and membrane (Parafilm®) are prescribed in the GB standard.

6. Attractive blood-feeding apparatus: Recently, the new anti-mosquito performance test method using attractive blood-feeding apparatus has been established as Japanese Industrial Standard (JIS L1950-1). The apparatus used in this method consist of a mosquito cage, the artificial blood feeding device (Hemotek®, http://hemotek.co.uk/starter-packs/), the carbon dioxide gas supply unit, and ventilation fans (Figure 17.3 and 17.4). Unfed female mosquitoes (*Aedes albopictus* Skuse) are released into a cage, one side of which is exposed to test textile specimens. Mosquitoes can feed the heated animal blood in Alsever's solution which is readily supplied by reagent manufacturers through the test textile specimens on the membrane (animal intestine) (Figure 17.5). Number of mosquitoes landed on the textile specimens is counted for 10 min. and successful blood feeding is observed after the test. The reproducibility and reduced discrepancies of the test were

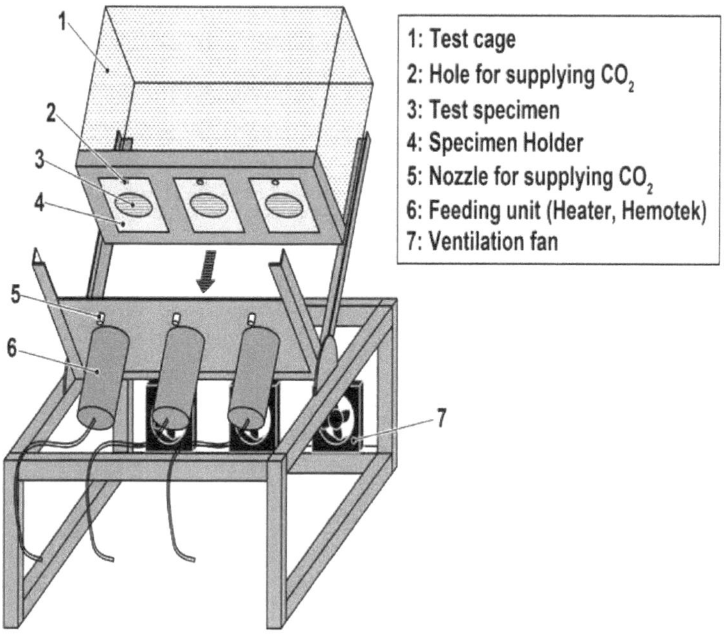

Figure 17.4: Cross-section view of the attractive blood feeding apparatus (JIS L1950-1).

demonstrated by the comparison experiments with the tests using human volunteers (Kuramoto and Kawada 2018; Kuramoto et al. 2019). This test method is now in the process of establishment for ISO (TC38/WG29).

17.5 FIELD TESTING

The final step for evaluation of repellent treated textiles against mosquitoes is conducting the field testing with a group of 6 - 13 human volunteers. The distance between each volunteer should be $\geq$ 10 meters. The population density of the target species of mosquitoes, activity peak period, and biting pressure in the testing location should be checked before conducting the field testing. The repellent treated textiles or uniforms will be worn by the human volunteers. Based on the testing textile products and purpose, the specific body part (i.e., arm or leg) of the participants will be selected to cover or wrap for the exposure. Unused body parts will be protected by thick clothing or plastic cover. Usually, repellent treated head netting, uniform, jackets, or t-shirt have been tested against mosquito bites in the field. Sometimes a large piece of treated textile have been used to cover/wrap the low part of legs or forearms and another one for untreated textile cover or wrap the other leg or forearm as control. The volunteers will sit or stand in the field to expose themselves to mosquitoes for 5 minutes. This exposure is repeated at 1 hr interval until mosquitoes land and probe on the treated materials. The number of mosquitoes landing/probing on the treated and untreated body parts (arms or legs) are collected and counted. In the meantime, the air temperature, humidity, wind speed, and other environmental condition will be detected and recorded. The report about the repellent treated

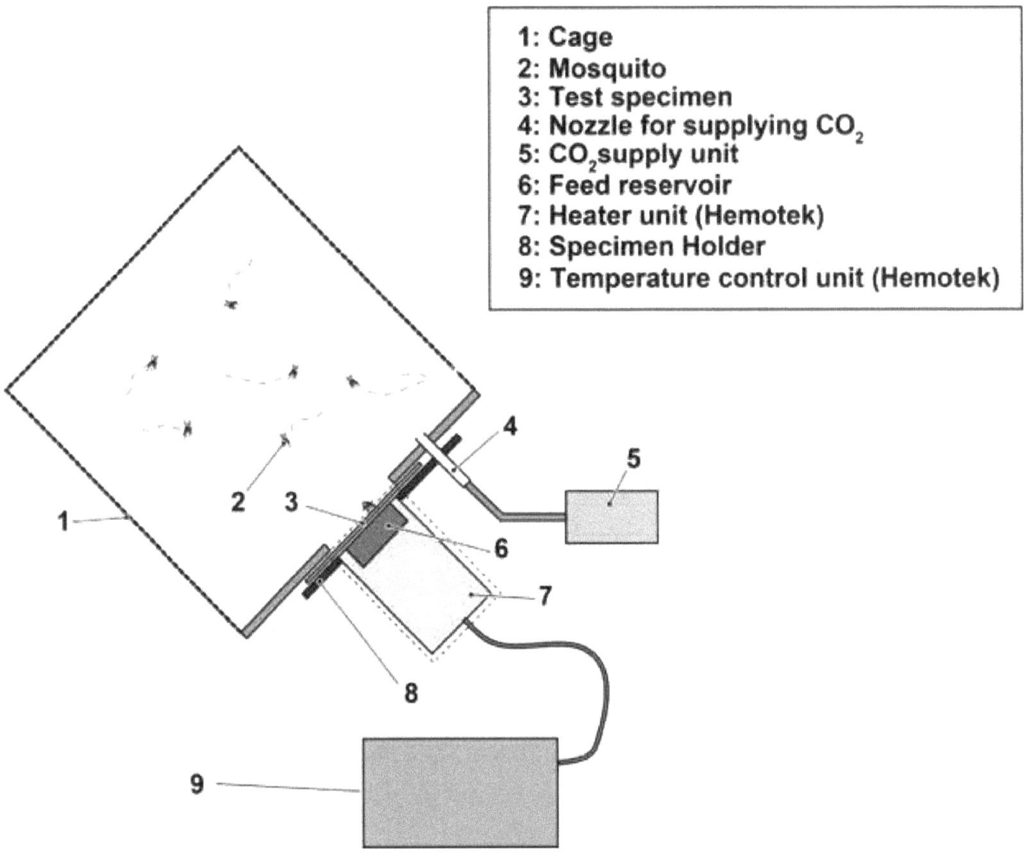

Figure 17.5: Enlarged drawing of a blood feeding part of the attractive blood feeding apparatus (JIS L1950-1).

textiles/clothing should include the materials used, repellent, formulation and amount used, method of treatment, and method of exposure (Govere and Durrheim 2006).

17.6 INFLUENCING FACTORS

There are many influencing factors that impact the testing results about repellents (Barnard et al. 2006) and repellent-treated textiles/clothing against mosquitoes. Major factors could be catalogued as the following:

- **Abiotic factors**: Major abiotic factors include the testing materials and the environmental conditions, such as different textile materials including cotton, polyesters, washing of materials, air temperatures, humidity, wind speed, lights, seasons, geographic location, vegetation, time of the day, testing methods, and the size of the testing cage.
- **Biotic factors**: There are two major parts about the biotic factors, such as human or animal as attractants and mosquito selves. Testing subjects' attraction, body part, age, and weight as attractants may influence the testing results. Target mosquito

species, population density and used number of mosquitoes, daily activity pattern, ages, parity, partial blood engorgement, and sugar availability are the major factors on the testing results (Barnard and Xue 2006).

17.7 CHALLENGES AND CONCLUSIONS: TOWARDS AN INTERNATIONAL STANDARD

There are no international standards or protocols and methods established for mosquito repellent treated textile testing and evaluation. The most common and recognized method is the WHO method, American Society for Testing and Materials Method, and U.S. EPA guideline. Recently, innovative vector control consortium (IVCC) and WHO evaluated and recognized several testing centers as Good laboratory practice (GLP) laboratories worldwide. The International Standard Organization (ISO) evaluated and established standard testing method for the insect repellent-treated textiles against mosquitoes. We hope that this chapter will help to define International standards, protocols, and methods for mosquito repellent treated textiles in the future.

ACKNOWLEDGMENTS

This chapter is partly based on work performed within the framework of IMAAC (`https://imaac.eu/`) related to COST Action CA16227 (*Investigation & Mathematical Analysis of Avant-garde Disease Control via Mosquito Nano-Tech-Repellents*, `https://cost.eu/actions/CA16227/`), supported by COST Association (European Cooperation in Science and Technology).

X

Case Studies: Putting the Knowledge into Action

CHAPTER 18

A Case Study: How the Rephaiah Project Combats Malaria in Young Children

Sveinbjorn Gizurarson*

Faculty of Pharmaceutical Sciences, School of Health Sciences, University of Iceland, Reykjavik, Iceland &
Department of Pharmacy, Kamuzu University of Health Sciences, Blantyre, Malawi &
Hananja plc, Reykjavik, Iceland
** corresponding author, e-mail: sveinbj@hi.is*

Precious Ngwalero Katundu

Department of Pharmacy, Kamuzu University of Health Sciences, Blantyre, Malawi &
Division of Clinical Pharmacology, University of Cape Town, Cape Town, South Africa

Emmanuel Mwathunga

Ministry of Natural Resources,Energy and Mining, Lilongwe, Malawi

Gudlaug Maria Sveinbjornsdottir

Faculty of Psychology, School of Health Sciences, University of Iceland, Reykjavik, Iceland

Urdur Njardvik

Faculty of Psychology, School of Health Sciences, University of Iceland, Reykjavik, Iceland

Titha Dzowela

UNC Project, Fleming Fund Country Grant Malawi, Lilongwe, Malawi

Wilfred Dodoli

Malaria Programme, World Health Organization (WHO), Lilongwe, Malawi

Kristin Linda Ragnarsdottir

Hananja plc, Reykjavik, Iceland

DOI: 10.1201/9781003035992-18

CONTENTS

18.1 Introduction 276
18.2 Mosquito transmitted malaria in Malawi 278
18.3 Geographical structure and demography of the country 278
18.4 WHO operation and mosquito control in Malawi 281
18.5 Successes and failures in mosquito control in Malawi 282
18.5.1 Successes 282
18.5.2 Failures 283
18.6 Consequences of cerebral malaria in young children 283
18.7 Supporting the project 284
18.8 Conclusion 285

18.1 INTRODUCTION

Malaria is responsible for a significant number of infections and deaths. According to the World Health Organization (WHO) [1], there were estimated 228 million cases of malaria in 2018, where 93% of them occurred in Africa. The incidence rate is about 229 cases per 1000 population, so the disease is still endemic in that part of the world. In the African region, the parasite *Plasmodium falciparum* is the most prevalent, accounting for 99.7% of estimated malaria cases, whereas *P. vivax* is accounting for 47% of the malaria cases in India [1]. These parasites are transmitted by mosquitoes. If not treated, malaria can quickly become life-threatening, affecting children under the age of five very hard with severe or even cerebral malaria. In 2018 it is estimated that 405,000 deaths occurred globally, due to malaria, of which 272,000 (67%) were children under the age of 5 years [1]. According to WHO, 94% of these deaths happened in Africa. That is about 750 deaths every day, or one child every two minutes in Africa alone.

It is important to keep in mind United Nations' (UN) central transformative promise of the 2030 Agenda for the UN Sustainability Development Goals (UN SDGs), which is summed up in one simple statement: *"leave no one behind"*. It is our responsibility, as citizens of the world, to take part in prioritizing different fast-tracking actions for the poorest and the most vulnerable and marginalized people. This includes seeing to their wellbeing and health (UN SDGs # 3).

If we take a closer look at the access to appropriate drugs to treat children with malaria, there is a lack of infant formulations and dosage forms for children. The drugs available are adult tablets that need to be divided, when dosing children, which can easily lead to inaccurate dosing [2]. Many families living in small villages, do not have access to hospitals, where they can bring their child if it has life-threatening severe malaria or cerebral malaria. The child may have emesis, poor consciousness, seizures or even be in a coma. Oral medication or a fraction of a tablet is, therefore, not an acceptable form of treatment in these conditions. If the parents live close to a hospital their child may be treated with injectable artemether or artesunate, subject to availability. For most parents, they need to carry their child a long distance, by foot, in order to receive treatment. Although injections are helpful, they are only found in hospitals and they only contain one drug, instead of two as recommended by WHO. Sadly, in many parts of the world, the *Plasmodium* strain has developed resistance to several drugs, which is why WHO has advocated two concurrent drugs, to minimize the risk of widespread resistance.

The Rephaiah project is based on the need for pediatric dosage forms to treat young children under the age of 5 years. There is a dire need for a simple dosage form, that can be used, even in the most rural areas. There is a need for a product that contains both drugs and can be stored in a hot climate, e.g. in health clinics in rural areas. The Rephaiah project is focusing on providing health and hope to these children, by establishing a not-for-profit pharmaceutical manufacturing entity in Malawi. The focus is on pediatric dosage forms for infants and children under the age of 5 years. The company will manufacture pediatric dosage forms to treat malaria as well as selected neglected tropical diseases such as schistosomiasis (bilharzia/snail fever) a parasitic infection transmitted with freshwater snails, living in lakes, rivers and even rice fields, and onchocerciasis (river blindness) a parasitic infection transmitted with small sand flies.

By establishing the entity in Malawi, the company will hopefully meet several needs and at the same time work toward different UN DSGs:

1. By manufacturing the drug in a country like Malawi, there is a possibility to provide a drug for affordable prices, even for parents that live on $\leqq$ \$ 1 per day. In the USA, the lowest price for the artemether and lumefantrine combination drug, to treat malaria, cost \$ 129,37 (January 2021). The majority of the population in Malawi cannot afford such a product, when the average monthly salary is around \$ 35.
2. Malawi is well located so the drug(s) may eventually be distributed from there to other Sub-Saharan countries.
3. Manufacturing these drugs where they are needed, will work towards achieving many of the UN SDGs e.g., lowering carbon footprints, and helping the country to be self-sustainable.
4. The only pharmacy education in Malawi is at Kamuzu University of Health Sciences. The BS program in pharmacy started in 2006 and the planning of a MS program is well on its way and will hopefully start in the near future.
5. Establishing a drug development entity and drug manufacturing company, where the production is made from raw materials, will strengthen the infrastructure of the country and make Malawians capable of formulate other drugs, e.g., in a case for emergency.

18.2 MOSQUITO TRANSMITTED MALARIA IN MALAWI

Malawi accounts for 2% of malaria cases worldwide having about 4 million cases every year. It is among the top 20 countries when looking at high malaria burden [1,3]. This is the most common cause of outpatient visits, hospitalization, and death in Malawi [4]. The disease is recurrent in most parts of the country, and increases during the rainy season, that normally begins in November and lasts through April [4]. The lowest risk areas are in the northern part of the country (in high altitude), where the highest malaria transmitted areas are in the southern part of the country, where the climate is warmer, wet and humid [4]. *Plasmodium falciparum* is the most common parasite species causing malaria in Malawi. It accounts for 98% of the infections, and all severe disease cases and deaths, where children under the age of 5 years and pregnant women are at highest risk [4, 5].

In addition to ill-health, malaria has a severe socioeconomic effect on households, communities, and the national levels, particularly those with low social economic status, mostly in the rural areas. For adults this includes loss of work and high levels of expenditure on malaria treatment, and for children they will lack education because of absence from school due to illness [5].

Since 2005, the Malawi government has been combatting the disease, and implementing malaria control programs. Focusing on >85% of its population, these strategies are directed at preventing the mosquitoes from biting people, by applying and providing insecticide-treated nets and insecticide that can be used indoors [6]. The government is also focusing on the case management, including the diagnosis and antimalarial medications [7].

In 2007, the Ministry of Health through the National Malaria Control Program, changed its national malaria treatment policy from using a known antimalarial drug. Instead of using sulfadoxine-pyrimethamine (SP) as the first-line treatment, they are now focusing on a more expensive, but also more effective artemisinin-based therapy. Currently, a combination of two drugs are used, artemether and lumefantrine [5,8]. The change was required, when the malaria parasite was found to be resistance to SP [5]. Other drugs that are also used for the treatment of malaria include artesunate-amodiaquine and quinine [5].

18.3 GEOGRAPHICAL STRUCTURE AND DEMOGRAPHY OF THE COUNTRY

Located in south of the equator, Malawi is a landlocked Sub-Saharan country surrounded by Tanzania in the north and northeast, Mozambique in the east, south, and southwest, and Zambia in the west and northwest. The country is 901 km in length and 161 km in width and occupies a total area of approximately 118,484 km^2. 94,276 km^2 of the total area is land, with the remaining area covered by water, mostly composed of Lake Malawi, the 3rd largest freshwater lake in Africa and the 9th largest world-wide. The lake is about 475 km long, delineating Malawi's eastern boundary with Mozambique. Lakes Chiuta, Chilwa and Malombe are the other smaller lakes found in the country.

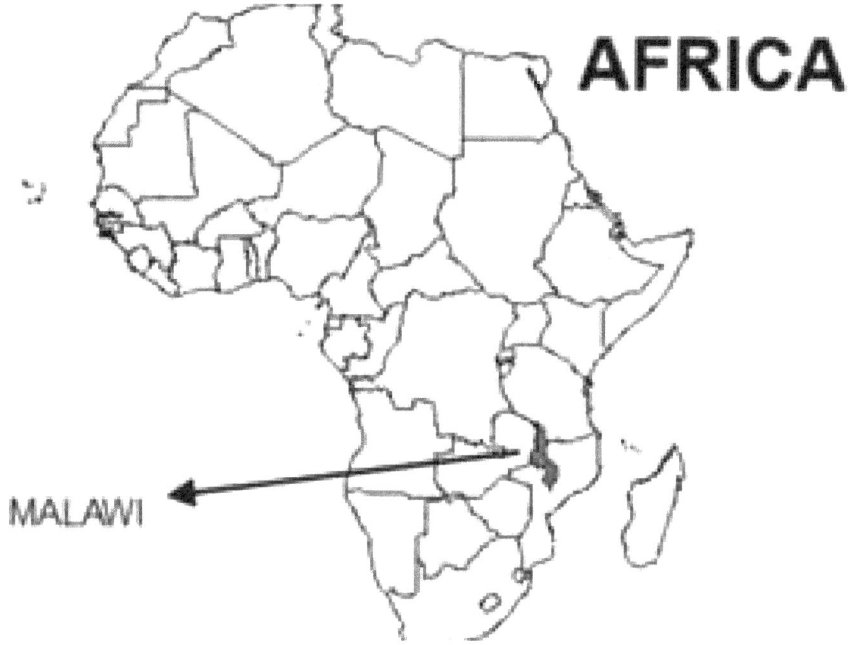

Figure 18.1: Location of Malawi in Africa.

The most striking feature on the geographical map of Malawi is the Great African Rift Valley. It runs through the entire length of the country, passing through Lake Malawi in the Northern and Central Regions to the Shire Valley in the southern part of the country. Shire is the largest river in the country and also its lowest point. It is the only outlet for Lake Malawi and drains into Zambezi river in Mozambique. In the western and southern areas of Lake Malawi there are fertile lowlands and mountain ranges, having peaks ranging from 1,700 to 3,000 meters. The southern areas of the country are largely low-lying except for Zomba plateau, which is approximately 2,100 meters high and Mulanje Massif, which is 3,002 meters high and also the highest mountain is south-central Africa.

Malawi has a tropical continental climate with some maritime influences. Altitude and proximity to the lake influences rainfall patterns and temperature variability. From May to August, the country experiences a cool dry season. A warm dry season is experienced from September to November. The rainy season begins in October or sometimes in November and proceeds through April, and this is the period that the country receives about 90% of the precipitation for the year. Annual rainfall ranges from 700 to 2,400 mm, with 1180 being the average. Maximum and minimum temperatures are 28 °C and 10°C, respectively, while rift valley plains have around 32 °C and 14 °C, respectively. The highest temperatures occur just before the rainy season, or in October-November. The lowest temperatures, however, are experienced in June or July.

In general, the different topographical and environmental features of the country also offer different weather conditions. Mountainous regions offer cooler temperatures, while lowlands offer warmer temperatures and rainfall. Climatic conditions in Malawi remain one of the contributing factors leading to the prevalence of tropical diseases like malaria and schistosomiasis [9]. Flood and drought cycles are also common in the country occurring almost on yearly basis, with the low-lying areas being the most affected.

The country is divided into three regions: the northern region, which is mostly mountainous, the upland central plateau region and the low-lying southern region. There are a total of 28 districts in the country. The Northern Region consists of six districts, The Central Region has nine districts while the Southern Region has thirteen districts. The three regions have also three different capitals. Mzuzu is the capital for the Northern Region, Lilongwe is the capital for the Central Region and also the capital city for the country, while Blantyre is the capital for the Southern Region and also the commercial city for the country. Administratively, the districts in Malawi are further subdivided into traditional authorities (TAs), headed by chiefs and each TA is comprised of villages, which are the smallest administrative units, and these are overseen by village headmen.

According to the sixth Population and Housing Census (PHC) that was carried out in 2018, Malawi registered a total of approximately 17.5 million people. Males make up 49% of this population while females make up 51%. This population size is almost 4 times that which was registered in Malawi's first census of 1966. There has also been a 35% increase in population size from the previous census, which was carried out in 2008, representing a growth rate of 2.9% annually. If such a growth rate remains constant, the country is expected to double its current population by 2042 [10].

Malawi's population density is regarded as one of the highest in Sub-Saharan Africa. The 2018 PHC indicated that Malawi's population density rose to 186 persons per km^2 compared with 138 in the 2008 census. Of the three regions of the country, the southern region remains the region registering the highest population density, or 244 persons per km^2. This is followed by the central region at 211 per km^2 and then the northern region at 84. Fertility rate is also regarded as one of the highest in the Sub-Saharan African region, which partly explains the country's high population density. The latest Demographic Health Survey of 2015/16, however, registered some significant declines in the fertility rate [11].

The country's population is regarded as youthful, with about 46% of the population under the age of 15. This results in a heavy burden on the working-age population, that need to provide basic needs and services like education and health to this young population [12]. Furthermore, it poses challenges for poverty reduction [13]. Malawi is also predominantly rural with 84% of the population living in rural areas and 16% in urban areas. While females make up the biggest percentage in the rural areas, it is almost equal, males and females in the urban areas.

According to the World Bank, Malawi falls in the category of the world's least developed countries, with a significant portion of its population living below the poverty line [13]. The country's economy is greatly dependent on agriculture (>80%). The country's high population density, however, has subsequently resulted into reduced landholdings.

Smaller farms coupled with soil erosion have degraded agricultural land consequently affecting agricultural production. This has, therefore, had serious consequences especially on marginalized groups in the country like the poor, women and children, making them highly vulnerable to food insecurity.

18.4 WHO OPERATION AND MOSQUITO CONTROL IN MALAWI

mosquitoes of the genus *Anopheles* transmit malaria, that accounts for a large proportion of deaths in Malawi. *Anopheles gambiae* and *Anopheles funestus* species groups are the principal malaria vectors in Malawi. The Ministry of Health with support from partners developed the first ever Malaria Vector Control Strategy, to guide and implement recommendations towards an effective malaria vector control intervention, that is also sustainable and cost-effective for malaria control and reducing morbidity and mortality caused by malaria. This strategy was developed within the context of Integrated Vector Management and universal access to key malaria vector control interventions in line with the national Malaria Strategic Plan (MSP) and Global Technical Strategy (GTS). The plan focused on major malaria prevention methods such as distribution of Long Lasting Insecticide-Treated Nets (LLITNs) and Indoor Residual House Spraying (IRS), other vector control measures such as Larval Source and environmental management, entomological monitoring and surveillance, and capacity building.

Control of malaria transmission conventionally relies heavily on two insecticide-based interventions: LLIN (Long Lasting Insecticide Nets) and IRS. Use of LLINs is the primary vector control intervention in the country. In the current Malaria Strategic Plan, the NMCP (National Malaria Control Program) has prioritized universal coverage of LLINs to reduce morbidity and mortality due to malaria by 50% by 2022. In order to achieve the set target, Malawi continues pursuing distribution of nets through the routine antenatal care and periodic nationwide distribution models. In 2008, first free mass distribution of LLIN was launched, targeting children and pregnant women. Since then national wide distribution of ITNs have been done at least every three years the last one to be done was in 2018. Apart from the mass distribution, routinely ITNs are being distributed through antenatal clinics targeting pregnant women and children under one years of age. Households in Malawi that own at least one LLIN greatly improved from 2% in 2007 to 82% by 2017. The 2017, 42% of households had at least one ITN for every two people. The LLIN use rate was 55% among the household population, 68% in children under five and 63% in pregnant women.

The first IRS pilot project was launched in Nkhotakota district in 2007 with support from President Malaria Initiative (PMI). In line with the national malaria strategic plan, IRS implementation was expected to be scaled up to 11 high burden districts. The program was extended to five then seven other districts for only one year. Due to the emergence of pyrethroid insecticide resistance, a switch to the organophosphate pirimiphos-methyl was necessary. By 2014, the spraying program was halted due to high cost of procuring organophosphate insecticides and lack of viable alternatives. In order to manage resistance in IRS implementing districts, annual rotation of insecticides has been adopted in line with Insecticide Resistance Management plan for the years 2019-2022. Although the resistance monitoring data shows that the major vectors are still susceptible to pirimiphos-methyl capsule suspension formulation, it will be rotated annually together with clothianidin or clothianidin and deltamethrin combination to minimize the pressure on the local vectors. One of the challenges facing vector control program in Malawi is development of resistance to most of insecticides recommended for indoor residual house spraying and in Long Lasting Insecticide-Treated Nets. In order to manage increased pyrethroid resistance in Malawi, the synergist piperonyl-butoxide (PBO) has been introduced.

18.5 SUCCESSES AND FAILURES IN MOSQUITO CONTROL IN MALAWI

Intervention mechanisms to malaria in Malawi have focused on reducing human exposure to infectious malaria vectors. These have generally included insecticides on mosquito nets, internal residual spraying, and other means. All these methods are aimed at mosquito control. Mosquito control is the management of the population of mosquitoes to reduce their damage to human health, economies, and comfortable living [14]. It is a vital public health initiative throughout the world, and especially Malawi where there is high prevalence of malaria, for which mosquitoes are the cause. Depending on the situation, source reduction or the killing of adults may be used to manage mosquito populations. This paper looks at the successes and failures of the initiative in Malawi.

Mosquito control as a public health measure was introduced in Malawi as an innovative measure to complement the existing strategies of combating malaria including health surveillance and mosquito nets. The currently known large scale project in mosquito control is led by Malawi-Liverpool Wellcome Trust Centre, who through UNICEF, introduced a drone project in 2017 to control mosquito populations. The first attempt at internal residual spraying were made in the late 1950s as a way of tackling mosquitoes right from the source and controlling their populations after post infection measures proved too costly. This was largely due to the successes from Zimbabwe (then Southern Rhodesia) [15].

18.5.1 Successes

The aforementioned methods have led to some successes in controlling mosquito populations in their target districts. The greatest impact on mosquito populations was in the ML-Wellcome Trust project in Kasungu, where mosquitoes were controlled at larvae stage. The idea was to use drones and spray insecticides and pesticides in concentration areas. The emphasis was on habitat management and controlling the immature stages, right from the eggs to the larvae, before mosquitoes turned into full blown adults. The involvement of the community was very essential in this intervention where the communities were also alerted on the need to remove any habitats including standing water bodies.

Another main success story in the mosquito control programs has been the larvae source management and the control of adult mosquito populations. These interventions mostly involved community mobilizations and then have them trained in habitat removals. It also involved spraying pesticides in other habitats to curtail the development of mosquitoes right from the source. In Southern Malawi, this project has had its fair share of successes as mosquito populations have decreased this way [16].

18.5.2 Failures

The main failure of the mosquito control programs has been the accelerated rate at which the vectors develop resistance to pesticides and insecticides. This is especially true with the female *Anopheles* mosquito which is the main malaria transmission vector. According to Hunt et. al. [17], widespread resistance to sprays was reported in many districts where data was collected. Further studies across 2011 and 2012 have also confirmed a widespread resistance rate, meaning that new means must be employed.

Another key failure which is attributed to social factors is the failure to remove mosquito habitats. This is an important aspect of mosquito control around the world, but it seems to be lacking in Malawi. Water in pools, ponds, fountains rain barrels and potholes and other standing water sources have not been adequately eliminated, this could be a result of lack of proper education for the communities, or the communities' lack of general interest in preventive measures [18].

Finally, one key feature which has been failing in the preventive aspect of mosquito control is the use of structural barriers. Mosquitoes largely bite indoors, and this requires proper structural barriers to deny them entry. However, most communities in Malawi still do not have window and door screens to prevent entry and covering on building gaps on walls and windows.

18.6 CONSEQUENCES OF CEREBRAL MALARIA IN YOUNG CHILDREN

Cerebral malaria is one of the most severe complication of malaria in children, consisting of seizures and coma with an estimated 20% mortality rate [19, 20]. It was previously believed that children would make full neurological recovery but there is increasing evidence of serious long-term effects of cerebral malaria and it is now considered a leading cause of neuro-disability in Sub-Saharan Africa [19, 20]. The long-term effects include epilepsy, blindness, hearing impairment, loss of speech, gross motor deficits, attention deficits and disruptive behavior problems [20, 31].

Some neurological effects appear to be transitory while others seem to be more persistent and may lead to life-long disabilities. Idro et al. [20], found that visual impairment seemed to improve after several months, while behavior problems seemed to be much more persistent. Many children have been found to display symptoms similar to Attention Deficit Hyperactivity Disorder (ADHD) and autism spectrum disorders with long-term impairments in academic performance and increased stress levels in the children's families [20]. Symptoms of ADHD appear to be especially common as research has shown that approximately 25% of children who survive cerebral malaria show deficits in attention and working memory two years after their recovery [24, 25, 27, 28]. In fact, after controlling for age, gender, nutrition, home environment, and child's education level, John et al. [28]

found that children who had survived cerebral malaria had a 3.67-fold increased risk of a deficit in attention and working memory and that although working memory seemed to improve somewhat over time, the attention deficit problems appeared to be persistent. Similarly, behavior problems also appear to be quite severe sequelae of cerebral malaria, with an increased risk of disruptive behavior disorders in children two years post cerebral malaria, both compared to children with a history of severe malarial anemia and children with no history of malaria [22, 27].

Onset of these behavioral and neurological difficulties is often delayed, with a mean onset of 111 days post malaria infection. Onset of ADHD symptoms appear to occur about 83 to 228 days after the recovery, with a mean of 150 days [22]. These results indicate that cerebral malaria puts children at an increased risk of developing behavioral and neurological difficulties in the months following infection, calling for increased follow-up care and cognitive testing up to a year after recovery and subsequently, appropriate interventions for the children and their families. Unfortunately, access to standardized mental health assessment and empirically validated mental health treatments is limited for children in sub-Saharan Africa and the children who do show deficits often do not receive any psychiatric or psychosocial help [22, 24].

In summary, cerebral malaria seems to place children at increased risk for the development of persistent neurodevelopmental and behavioral problems which lead to impairments in academic and social functioning. The course of these difficulties appears to develop over time, indicating a need for prolonged follow-up assessment and care for at least two years following cerebral malaria. More research in this area is called for and the development of testing protocols and appropriate intervention strategies for children who have survived cerebral malaria are sorely needed.

18.7 SUPPORTING THE PROJECT

Establishing a specialized not-for-profit pharmaceutical entity (developing and manufacturing age-appropriate formulations for 0 – 5 year old children) is a major undertaking. There is little or no experience in Malawi in manufacturing drugs from raw materials. Therefore, locally trained pharmacists have limited experience and due to lack of equipment, they will need to get specialized training. The Rephaiah Projects goal is to get this entity running and financially sustainable, while focusing on drug formulations for diseases that impact the lives of young children and their families. Our needs:

1. **Funding:** (a) for the construction of the building; (b) to purchase equipment to harvest water from the air, for a well, solar cells, generator etc.; (c) to purchase operational equipment such as ventilation, a water purification system etc.; (d) to purchase manufacturing equipment; (e) to purchase analytical equipment for quality control; (f) to purchase raw material and packaging materials; (g) to purchase office equipment etc.; (h) diverse starting expenses. As a not-for-profit entity, we deeply appreciate support in this area.

2. **Practical/technical training:** Our goal is that the entity will be fully operated by Malawians. Consequently, we need to train our future personnel in operating all the

equipment, be that operational-, manufacturing- or analytical equipment. This could e.g. be done by inviting an employee of Rephaiah to visit your company or your university, or by providing on-site training in Malawi.

3. **Quality assurance:** As the Rephaiah entity will follow international standards in all aspects of the organization, ongoing training concerning the following points will be necessary: (a) Good Manufacturing Standards (GMP); (b) Good Laboratory Practice (GLP); (c)Good Documentation Practice (GDP); (d) Good Transportation Practice (GTP) this also includes distribution; (e) Good Clinical Practice (GCP); (f) Good Financial Practice (GFP) and transparency; (g) Good Business Practice (GBP); (h) Good Safety Practice (GSP). Also, different ISO standards concerning e.g. sustainability, environmental, organizational and industrial requirements will need to be met. We welcome tools, advice, training, and other help in this area.

4. **Advice and consultation:** As Rephaiah works towards the UN Sustainability Development Goals, the company will be looking at: (a) different aspects of sustainability; (b) green chemistry such as 3R (Reduce, Reuse, Recycle) were purifying water, solvents and other chemicals and minimize waste is a high priority; (c) being environmentally friendly, by using biodegradable packaging materials and reducing the use of plastic; (d) carbon footprints, especially with respect to energy consuming operations such as the ventilation system and transportation; (e) management, including subjects such as teamwork, psychologically healthy workplaces etc.; (f) pediatric pharmacy, such as pharmacokinetics in infants and children, malnourished children, children with different health conditions etc.; (g) illiteracy, because of the need to provide information that is understandable and can be followed by illiterate, as well as literate people (e.g. prescription guidelines). All advice in these areas is welcome.

5. **Volunteers:** if you want to be hands on getting the Rephaiah Project in Malawi up and running, please let us know and together we will figure out the best way to do so. We are thankful for your help whether it is in Malawi or in your home country.

The Rephaiah Project's contact information: If you are interested in supporting this project, we would love to hear from you at [`info@rephaiah.com`].

18.8 CONCLUSION

Malaria is a serious disease that can be life-threatening, especially for children in the age group of 0 - 5 years. It affects a large percentage of the population of Malawi each year, particularly during the months of November to April. The very dense Malawian population is quite widespread over the country and in rural areas access to medical services can be difficult. Infants and young children that get infected with malaria, are as a group hit hard because they are not only at more risk of getting severe malaria and even cerebral malaria, but also malarial medicine does not come in dosage forms suitable for this age group. Not getting the right drugs can have a long lasting neurological and/or behavioral impact on young children that get severe and cerebral malaria.

Table 18.1: Glossary of definitions for commonly-used special terms in this chapter.

3R	Reduce, Reuse, Recycle
ADHD	Attention Deficit Hyperactivity Disorder
GBP	Good Business Practice
GCP	Good Clinical Practice
GDP	Good Documentation Practice
GFP	Good Financial Practice
GLP	Good Laboratory Practice
GMP	Good Manufacturing Standards
GSP	Good Safety Practice
GTP	Good Transportation Practice or Global Technical Strategy
IRS	Indoor Residual House Spraying
ITN	Insecticide Treated Nets
ISO	International Organization for Standardization
LLIN	Long Lasting Insecticide Nets
LLITN	Long Lasting Insecticide Treated Nets
ML	Malawi-Liverpool
MSP	Malaria Strategic Plan
NMCP	National Malaria Control Program
PBO	Piperonyl-butoxide
PHC	Population and Housing Census
PMI	President Malaria Initiative
SDG	Sustainable Development Goals
SP	Sulfadoxine-pyrimethamine
TA	Traditional authorities (each TA is headed by chiefs)
UN	United Nations
UNICEF	United Nations International Children's Emergency Fund
WHO	World Health Organization

The Rephaiah, not-for-profit, project aims to produce malaria medicine for children aged 0-5 years to be sold at a very reasonable price. This is possible because the drug will be produced in Malawi, by Malawians, not only influencing the access to, and the price of the medicine, but also boosting manufacturing and pharmaceutical knowledge and experience in the country. In the long run the Rephaiah Project is working on better health for young children, that will in due course, together with LLIN and other measures taken against the spread of malaria, enable children to do well in school, resulting in better job opportunities and improved quality of life.

ACKNOWLEDGEMENTS

This chapter is partly based on work performed within the framework of IMAAC (`https://imaac.eu/`) related to COST Action CA16227 (*Investigation & Mathematical Analysis of Avant-garde Disease Control via Mosquito Nano-Tech-Repellents*, `https://cost.eu/actions/CA16227/`), supported by COST Association (European Cooperation in Science and Technology).

GLOSSARY

The definitions of some commonly-used special terms: related to immunity, and that of some general epidemiological terms are given here.

FURTHER READING

See the references attached to this chapter or contact the authors directly.

To whom correspondence should be addressed:
Prof. Sveinbjorn Gizurarson,
Faculty of Pharmaceutical Sciences,
School of Health Sciences, University of Iceland,
Hofsvallagata 53, 107 Reykjavik, Iceland.
E-mail: sveinbj@hi.is, Phone: +354 898 0318.

CHAPTER 19

Strengthening the control of mosquito vectors in Cabo Verde; New Approaches to Improve Intervention Strategies

Lara Ferrero Gomez*
Unidade de Ciências da Natureza, da Vida e do Ambiente,
Universidade Jean Piaget de Cabo Verde, Praia, Cabo Verde
** corresponding author, e-mail: lara.ferrero.gomez@gmail.com*

Derciliano Lopes da Cruz
Departamento de Entomologia, Instituto Aggeu Magalhães,
Fundação Oswaldo Cruz-PE, Recife, Pernambuco, Brazil

Morgana do Nascimento Xavier
Secretaria Estadual de Saúde de Pernambuco, Recife, Brazil

Deinilson Conselheiro Mendes
Unidade de Ciências da Natureza, da Vida e do Ambiente,
Universidade Jean Piaget de Cabo Verde, Praia, Cabo Verde

Rosangela Maria Rodrigues Barbosa
Departamento de Entomologia, Instituto Aggeu Magalhães,
Fundação Oswaldo Cruz-PE, Recife, Pernambuco, Brazil

Helio Daniel Ribeiro Rocha
Unidade de Ciências da Natureza, da Vida e do Ambiente,
Universidade Jean Piaget de Cabo Verde, Praia, Cabo Verde

DOI: 10.1201/9781003035992-19

CONTENTS

19.1 Introduction 290
19.2 Study area 291
19.3 PILOT STUDY I 292
19.3.1 Assessment of the use of substances with attractive power in ovitraps 292
19.3.2 Material and Methods 292
19.3.3 Results 294
19.3.4 Discussion 295
19.3.5 Conclusion 295
19.4 PILOT STUDY II 295
19.4.1 Sticky BR-OVT evaluation 295
19.4.2 Material and Methods 297
19.4.3 Results 298
19.4.4 Discussion 299
19.4.5 Conclusion 299
19.5 PILOT STUDY III 299
19.5.1 Evaluation of the effectiveness of insecticide paints 299
19.5.2 Material and method 299
19.5.3 Results and discussion 300
19.5.4 Conclusion 301

19.1 INTRODUCTION

Cabo Verde is an insular country located in the Atlantic Ocean and plagued by vector-borne diseases since its origins, with malaria outbreaks registered since the 16th century, with epidemics of yellow fever and lymphatic filariasis in the past and currently with large outbreaks of emerging viruses such as dengue and Zika [1,5]. To respond to this priority health problem, the country has an integrated national program to combat vector-borne diseases, based on the use of insecticides (temephos for the control of breeding sites and deltamethrin for indoor and outdoor spraying). These control activities include the use of larvivorous fish, physical control of solid waste cleaning, and communication campaigns during outbreaks and periods of greater risk of epidemics [6]. Despite the efforts made, the epidemics of malaria and arboviruses (dengue and Zika) continue to be a reality [7].

Partly due to failures in the design and development of the control program itself, but also due to the weather and the geopolitical position that Cabo Verde plays, in the middle of the Atlantic between three continents, affected by the main traffic routes of trade and people. To help the health authorities implement more assertive vector control strategies, the Tropical Diseases Research Group at the Jean Piaget University of Cabo Verde – GIDTPiaget conducts research on control methodologies and interventions aimed at vectors mosquitoes in the country (*Aedes aegypti*, *Anopheles arabiensis* and *Culex pipiens sl*).

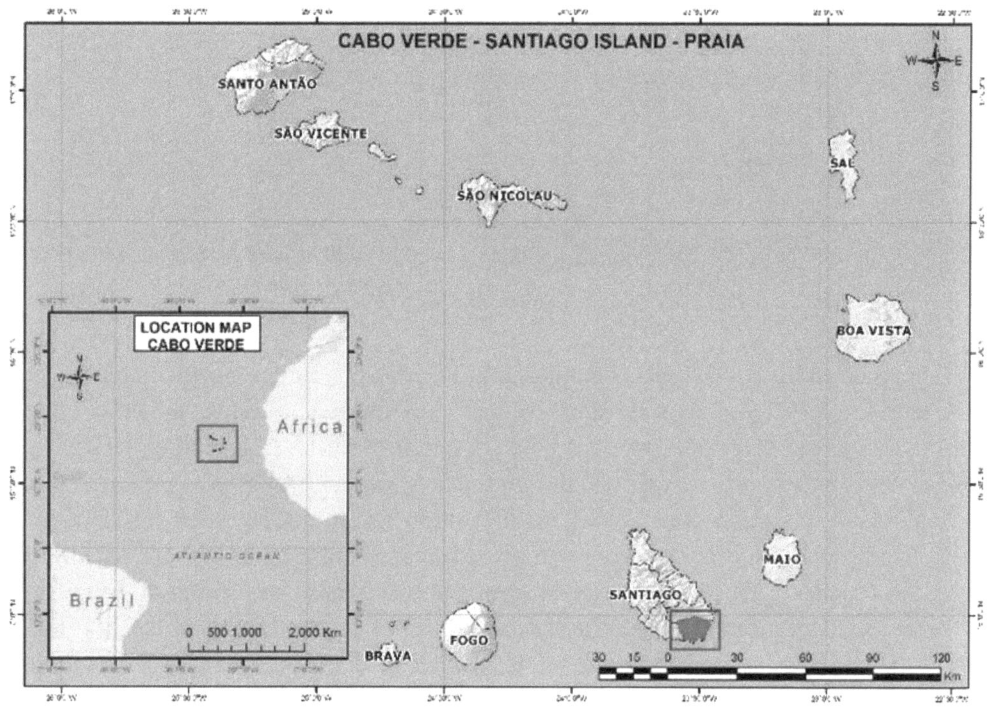

Figure 19.1: Cabo Verde, Santiago Island, City of Praia.

Next, we present three pilot studies integrated into two priority lines of research: improvement of tools for monitoring the main and potential arbovirus vectors in the country and search for new control strategies aimed at the implementation of a surveillance system stratified by risk of arbovirus outbreaks.

19.2 STUDY AREA

Three pilot studies were carry out on Santiago Island, the largest of ten islands in the volcanic archipelago of Cabo Verde and the most populated, with more than half the nation's population, 290,000 inhabitants out of 500,000 residents [8]. Located here is the nation's capital of the country, with 131,000 inhabitants and the focus for all vector-borne diseases (19.1)

The country, located in the subtropical region 560 km west of the Senegal coast, has an arid and semi-arid climate, with an average annual temperature of 25° C and little rainfall, average annual precipitation below 250 mm, concentrating in the rainy season (July to October) [9].

The island of Santiago is located in the southern island group or "Sotavento", of which Maio, Santiago, Fogo and Brava are part. The rest are included in the Barlovento group, located to the north and comprising the islands of Santo Antão, San Vicente, Santa Lucía, Sao Nicolau, Sal and Boa Vista. With rugged terrain, Santiago has a rural population located in the interior of the island and an urban population, concentrated in the capital, which is growing rapidly, giving rise to the appearance of overcrowded neighbourhoods without planning or urban infrastructure and with poor housing conditions [10].

19.3 PILOT STUDY I

19.3.1 Assessment of the use of substances with attractive power in ovitraps as a method of monitoring *Aedes aegypti*, the vector of Zare ika and dengue in Cabo Verde

The main strategies for vector monitoring and control based on methods for egg collection, larval research and adult mosquito collection. However, methods aimed at collecting mosquito eggs are more appropriate to the peculiarities of *Ae. aegypti* than larval research [11]. Oviposition traps (ovitrap) are the most sensitive and economical instrument for detecting *Aedes* species, especially when infestation levels not revealed by larval indices [12]. To improve the efficiency of ovitraps, attractant substances such as organic matter infusions are used [13, 14]. Different studies report the *Bacillus turigiensis* var. *israeliensis* (Bti)-treated ovitrap technique in vector control as a promising strategy for detecting *Aedes* species [15, 16]. In addition to being a biolarvicide, there is evidence that Bti acts as a stimulant of *Aedes* species oviposition, improving the efficiency of ovitraps [9, 15, 17]. In addition, household substances, like table salt, have been tested in ovitraps to control *Ae. aegypti* [14].

The aim of this study was to evaluate the attractiveness of substances tested in ovitraps (salt, Bti and Bti + acacia infusion), as a complementary tool for monitoring *Ae. aegypti*, the Zika and Dengue vector, in the city of Praia.

19.3.2 Material and Methods

Attractive and repellent substances for *Ae. aegypti*:

- Bacillus thurigiensis var. israeliensis, serotype 14, 0.2% (granules) VectoBac G, Kenogard, Valent Biosciences Corporation. Lot 217-317-N8.
- Table salt diluted to 1.2%
- 10% acacia infusion (100 ml infusion for 1 litre of water). To prepare the infusion, 15 grams of acacia leaves wee used (Prosopis sp) for each litre of water. The prepared solution rested for 7 days, before use, to allow for the fermentation of the organic material.

Simulated field study to evaluate the effectiveness of substances tested in ovitraps (Bti, Bti+infusion, Table salt) used to monitor *Aedes aegypti*:
For this test, oviposition traps (OVTs) were used to monitor *Ae. aegypti* in Praia [18], treated with Bti, Bti + infusion and table salt. They were setup semi-randomly in eight georeferenced locations in the Palmarejo district, distributed in a homogeneous way (19.2). Four OVTs, were installed in each location containing: OVT Control (800 ml tap water),

OVT + Bti (0.62g), OVT + Acacia infusion (10%) + Bti and OVT + Salt (1,2%). These were placed outdoors, in the shade, with a distance of 2 to 3 meters between them [19, 20]. The four points in each location were named A, B, C and D. The OVTs were monitored weekly for three months (August-October 2014). Their contents were reviewed, and the four OVTs were rotated to pre-established points (A,B,C,D) within each location to eliminate bias. Every two weeks the content of the traps were changed to ensure the effectiveness and attractiveness of the acacia infusion. Eggs were counted using a stereoscopic microscope (Lupa binocular Motic microscopes).

Weather data:

The National Institute of Meteorology and Geophysics (INMG-delegation from the City of Praia) provided the weekly weather data (temperature, relative humidity and rainfall) of the period in which the OVTs remained in the field, in Cabo Verde.

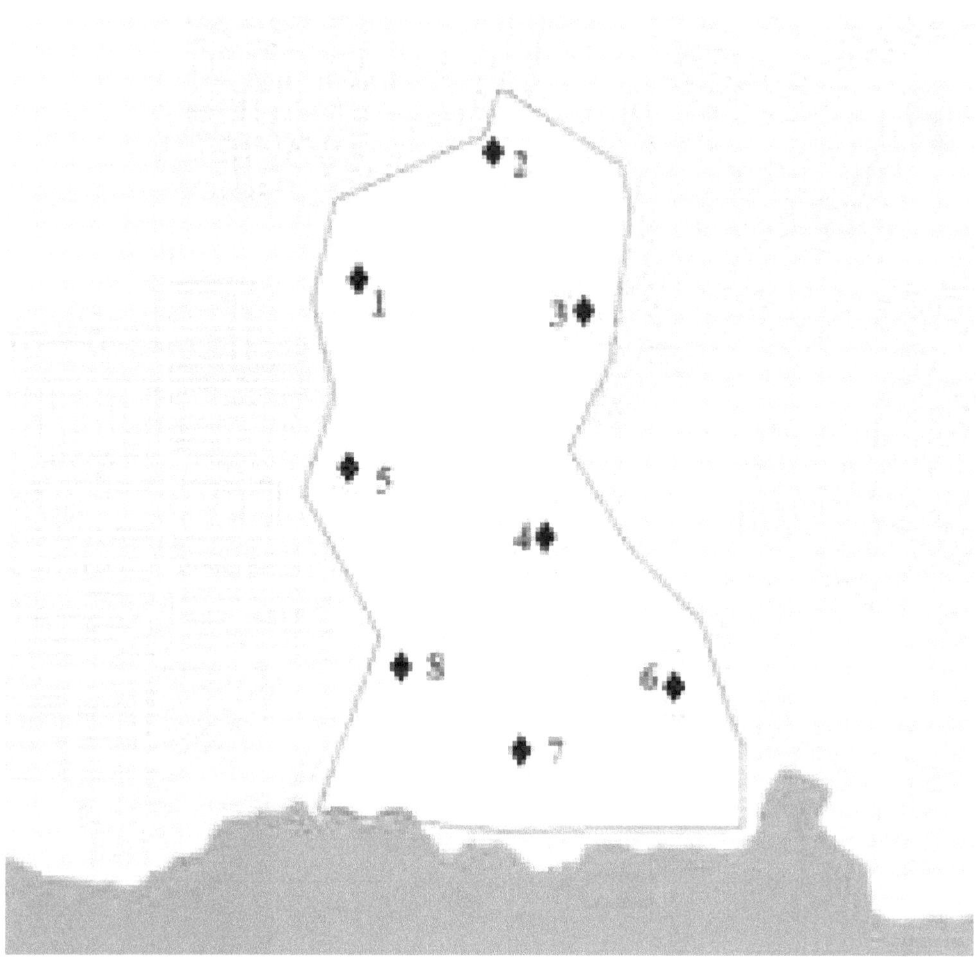

Figure 19.2: Delimitation of the study area (Palmarejo) and the locations of placed OVT.

Table 19.1: Total number of eggs of *Ae. aegypti*, number of positive OVTs, POI and DEI in the study period.

Month	N° OVT analyzed	N° OVT positive	N° eggs	IPO (%)	DEI
August	123	109	14079	88,62	129,17
September	127	111	13937	87,40	125,56
October	127	120	17621	94,53	145,69
Total	377	340	45643	90	134

Data analysis and calculation of rates of infestation and abundance of *Ae. aegypti*: Data obtained from the simulated field study Microsoft Excel software was used for data processing obtained from the simulated field study was processing using Microsoft Excel. SPSS version 21 was used for descriptive and comparative statistical analysis of the data. A Kruskal-Wallis test was used to compare the attractiveness of the different substances tested in the experiment, and to determine the degree of significance of the differences observed in the egg collections carried out in each point. A chi-square test was conducted to verify the existence of an association between the substances tested in the OVTs and the presence of larvae. Two different indices to estimate the vector population density and its distribution were applied: The positive ovitrap index (POI), which is the proportion of ovitraps positive for the presence of *Aedes* eggs, and the density eggs index (DEI), the average number of eggs per positive ovitrap.

19.3.3 Results

During the three months of monitoring the OVTs, 45643 eggs of *Ae. aegypti* were collected. The POI was 90% and the DEI was 134. Analysing the distribution and abundance of the vector, October was the month with the highest indicators (19.1). From the individual analysis of each of the eight locations, the presence of *Ae. aegypti* eggs was observed in all collections carried out, with differences in the amount of eggs collected in different locations, not following a distribution pattern over the period of this experiment (19.2).

Table 19.2: Total number of *Ae. aegypti* eggs, number of positive OVTs, POI and DEI, by locations.

Locations	N° OVT analyzed	N° OVT positive	N° eggs	IPO (%)	DEI
1	47	46	6512	97,87	141,57
2	46	42	7912	91,30	188,38
3	48	46	6288	95,83	136,70
4	45	33	2418	73,33	73,27
5	48	46	5766	95,83	125,35
6	47	41	4087	87,23	99,68
7	48	41	4691	85,42	114,41
8	48	45	7969	93,75	177,09
Total	377	340	45643	90	134

A comparative analysis (Kruskal-Wallis test) of the turnover of OVTs, at the four points in each location, shows that only location 6 ($P = 0,012$) showed a statistically significant difference ($P < 0.05$) in the number of eggs found at each point. After applying the Tukey test at location 6, it observed a significant difference for eggs collected between points A and B ($P < 0.05$). As a whole, the result of the comparative analysis demonstrated a distribution of OVTs, by locations, without influence of the position of OVTs in the oviposition of gravid females of *Ae. aegypti*.

Analyzing the POI obtained according to the type of substance tested in the OVTs, the differences were not appreciable except for the OVTs with salt in relation to the control (Figure 19.3 A). For the DEI the differences were notable. The OVTs with Bti + infusion collected a greater amount of *Ae. aegypti* eggs (20233) with a DEI of 229.92. The OVTs with table salt collected the lowest number of eggs (1508), having recorded a DEI of 16.39 (19.3 B).

Comparison of the different OVTs tested with the Control OVT (Kruskal-Wallis test) in relation to the number of eggs collected during the study period demonstrates that there is a statistically significant difference ($P < 0.05$) between them and the Control OVT ($P = < 0.001$). Regarding temperature and monthly relative humidity, there were no major variations during the study period, with mean values of 26.9 °C and 82% respectively. Average monthly rainfall was 37.7 mm, occurring almost entirely in September (108.8 mm). There is no significant relationship between climate data and infestation rates (POI and DEI).

19.3.4 Discussion

In this study, it was observed that the adaptation of the ovitrap from the model developed by [21] is promising for monitoring *Ae. aegypti* in the city of Praia, since the use of acacia infusion + Bti in the OVT collected twice as many eggs when compared to the use of tap water alone. The use of acacia infusion in OVTs is an innovation, used for the first time (in oviposition traps) in this study. The use of table salt in OVT worked as a repellent for female *Ae. aegypti* mosquitoes in Cabo Verde.

19.3.5 Conclusion

Of the substances tested in ovitraps, Bti and Bti+infusion work as attractants of *Ae. aegypti* from the city of Praia, whilst table salt having been verified as having an effect of repellency. The use of biological larvicide Bti, in ovitraps, allowed the permanence of OVTs in the field, safely, for at least 15 days. Monitoring with ovitraps in the Palmarejo neighborhood showed that it had a high infestation of *Ae. aegypti*, during the study period.

19.4 PILOT STUDY II

19.4.1 Sticky BR-OVT evaluation as a tool for monitoring mosquito vectors in Cabo Verde

Cabo Verde has a record of eleven species of Culicidae in the country, two of which are recognized vectors, *Ae. aegypti* and *Anopheles arabiensis* [22, 23]. This fact does not mean that in the future other potential vector species, such as *Culex pipiens* and *Culex*

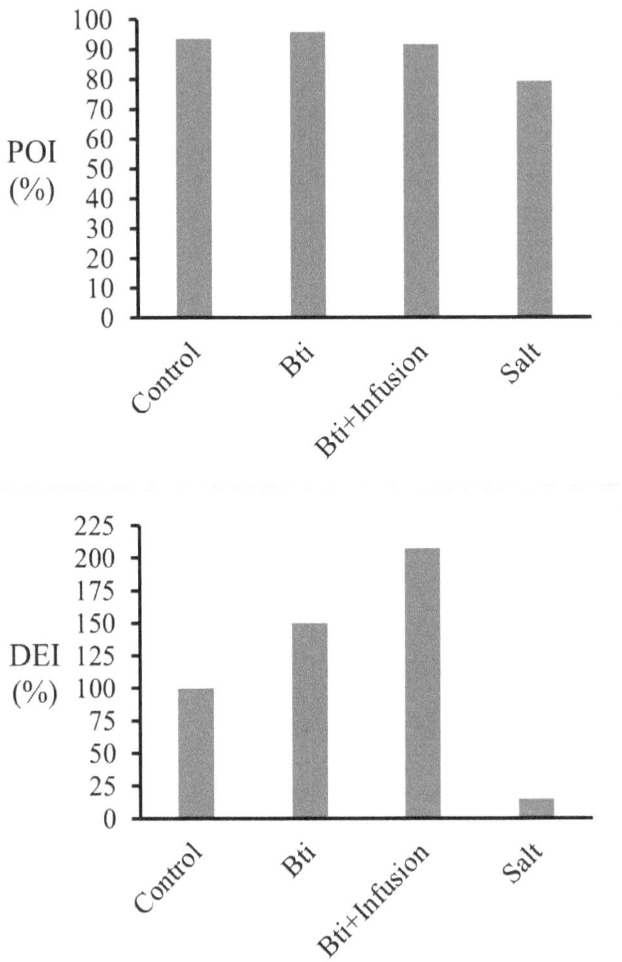

Figure 19.3: Ovitrap Positivity Index (IPO) and Density Eggs Index (DEI) of the substances tested in OVTs used to monitor *Ae. aegypti* in the Palmarejo district. The DEI of the tested substances is presented in relation to the number of eggs in the control, taking the value of 100%.

quinquefasciatus, will not be able to transmit other diseases in the country, such as West Nile. Currently, the vector control program does not monitor the vectors in space and time, limiting itself to intervention measures, with intra-household spraying (PID) (deltamethrin) for adults, and with temephos and diesel for the treatment of breeding sites. Larvivorous fish are also used as biological control agents in irrigation water tanks [6]. Experiments have been conducted in the country of monitoring populations of *Ae. aegypti* with ovitraps [18], but it is necessary to develop and adapt tools that serve, at the same time, to monitor and control of potential vectors in the country.

Methods that use biolarvicides (Bacillus thuringiensis israelensis (Bti)) with the sticky BR-OVT trap, for *Culex*, have proven to be efficient, safe and operationally simple [25, 26].

This composition (sticky BR-OVT and Bti) forms a continuous monitoring system, allowing the trap to remain in the field for months, and works as a good strategy to attract and eliminate mosquitoes [27]. Because of a project carried out in the Metropolitan Region of Recife (RMR), Pernambuco, Brazil, the sticky BR-OVT proved to be able to remove significant amounts of *Cx. quinquefasciatus* rafts from the environment [26, 27].

The aim of this study was to evaluate the efficiency of adhesive sticky sticky BR-OVT as a tool for monitoring the populations of *Culex pipiens* s.l. and *Ae. aegypti* in the main urban centers of the island of Santiago - Cabo Verde.

19.4.2 Material and Methods

Study area: The pilot study was carried out between July and August 2014 in two cities on the island of Santiago, Cabo Verde: Praia (14° 55 ' N 23° 30' W) and Assomada (15° 05' 45 " N 23° 40' 00" W). The country's capital, is located at sea level and has large urban agglomerations. Considered like a capital of the island's interior, the city of Assomada is predominantly rural, is located at 44 km from the capital and situated on a plateau at 391 m above sea level.

Study tool: Mosquitoes were collected using the sticky BR-OVT trap, developed by [27] and adapted to collect adult mosquitoes by [28]. This tool, made up of a black polyethylene box (13 x 35 x 24 *cm*), with a central opening (16 x 9 *cm*) on the upper face and containing, inside, a black container with a capacity of 4 L. Around this, there is an adhesive edge on the top face and a substrate (fabric) attached to the edge inside the container. Sticky BR-OVT is installed indoors (Figure). **Experimental approach:** For the development of this project, 40 indoors traps were installed, of which 25 in Praia and 15 in Assomada. In each trap, added an attractive solution of 500 *ml* of acacia infusion with 3 L of water

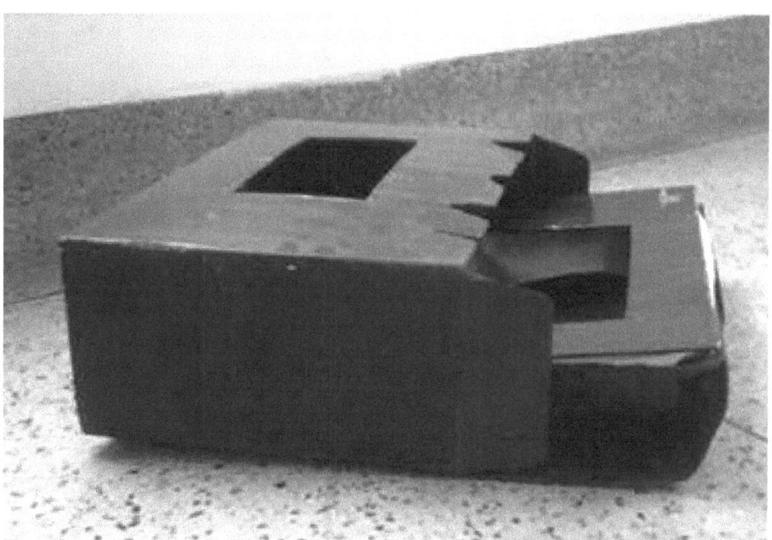

Figure 19.4: Sticky BR-OVT adhesive trap.

was added. Each sticky BR-OVT adhesive was treated with 2 g of the biolarvicide VectoBac G, based on *Bacillus thurigiensis* var. *israelensi*. Every 30 days the adhesive edges and the oviposition substrate for *Ae. aegypti* were replaced. The rafts of *Culex pipiens* sl. Were retrieved once a week and counted. All mosquitoes captured on adhesive edges and ovipositor substrates were taken to the laboratory of the Tropical Disease Research Group at the Jean Piaget University in Cabo Verde, for identification and quantification.

19.4.3 Results

During the study period in Praia and Assomada, 382 adult mosquitoes were collected, belonging to the species Cx. pipiens s.l. and *Ae. aegypti*. Of these, about 90% were captured in Praia. During the same study period, 207 rafts (*Culex* eggs) were also collected, the majority (88%) in the city of Praia. In Praia, from the total number of mosquitoes captured, 72% classified as *Cx. pipiens* s.l. and the rest as *Ae. aegypti*. Mosquito densities obtained in the two months showed little variation when compared. However, for egg collection, these traps presented results opposite to those described in Brazil: the positivity for *Aedes* eggs was higher than for *Culex* eggs (rafts), with positivity of 96% and 40% for the respective species. In Assomada, the collection of adult mosquitoes in adhesive sticky BR-OVT was lower than in Praia and about 50% of these traps were positive for adult mosquitoes, in both months. As in Praia, mosquito densities showed little monthly variation. However, of the total number of mosquitoes collected, there was a greater presence of *Ae. aegypti* (60%) captured over *Cx. pipiens* s.l. (40%). As for the presence of eggs, the positivity of adhesive sticky BR-OVT was 75% for *Aedes*, and 25% for *Culex* (19.5).

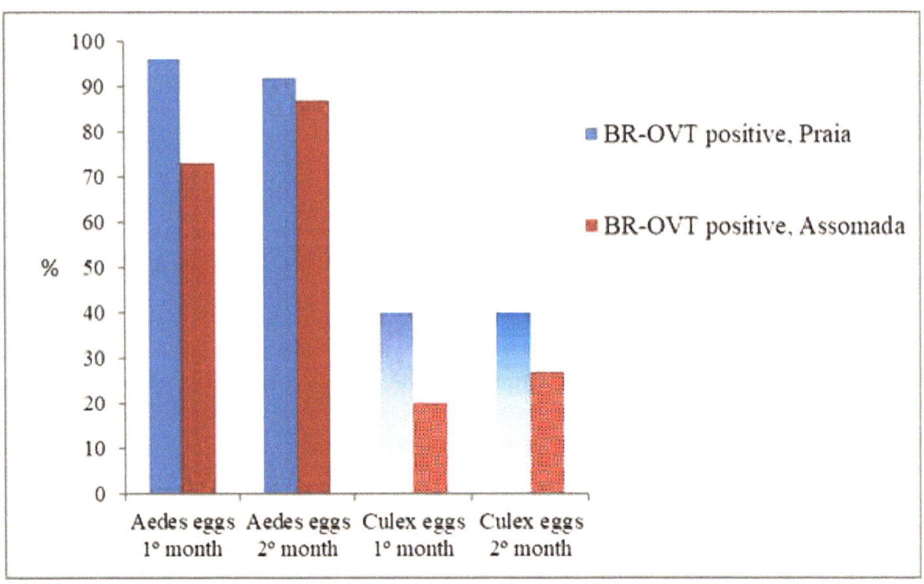

Figure 19.5: Percentage of positivity of the sticky BR-OVT trap for *Aedes* and *Culex* eggs, per month, in the cities of Praia and Assomada during July and August 2014.

19.4.4 Discussion

The results showed that sticky BR-OVT adhesive can be a good tool for monitoring the two species in Praia, Cabo Verde. Although it was developed to capture *Cx. quinquefasciatus*, this trap also captures *Ae. aegypti* at different stages of its cycle, both in Praia and Assomada. The presence of *Cx. pipiens* s.l. is associated with infusion activity, with a drop in the number of rafts collected over the months of observation. In contrast, *Ae. aegypti* colonizes sticky BR-OVT as the infusion loses its activity, given the known preference of this species for breeding sites with a low concentration of organic matter. Another factor that contributes to the collection of *Ae. aegypti* is its population size. According to [22], who carried out an entomological survey of the culicidological fauna of the leeward islands of Cabo Verde, this is the prevalent species at the expense of others.

19.4.5 Conclusion

Adhesive sticky BR-OVT is a potentially employable trap for monitoring *Cx. pipiens s.l.* and *Ae. aegypti* on the island of Santiago, Cabo Verde, as it is sensitive to the presence of different stages of the life cycle of both mosquitoes.

19.5 PILOT STUDY III

19.5.1 Evaluation of the effectiveness of insecticide paints for use in the control of *Ae. aegypti*, vector of dengue and zika in Cabo Verde.

The control strategies for invasive *aedine* species implemented in recent years have not been effective due to the tools used and the continuous need for repeated interventions that can hardly be sustainable. It is necessary to concentrate efforts on the focal control of the places detected with the greatest presence of the vectors and with residual tools that carry a constant and lasting pressure on the mosquitoes over time [29, 31]. Homes with poor hygiene and sanitation conditions constitute the ideal habitat for the proliferation of mosquitoes. Additionally, the high density of homes and people in these marginal peripheral urban areas enhance the rapid transmission of arboviruses [32, 33]. The mosquitoes' activity peaks in terms of their blood feeding coincide with moments of majority presence of the residents in their homes (evening), being necessary control activities in the houses and specifically to protect people from bites. Therefore, the use of insecticidal paints for the indoor control of arbovirus-transmitting mosquitoes is an important strategy to reinforce vector surveillance and control programs [34, 35].

The aim of this study was to evaluate the susceptibility of *Aedes aegypti* from Praia, the country's capital and main focus of vector-borne diseases (VBD), to insecticide paint candidates for introduction as a form of household vector control.

19.5.2 Material and method

Biological material: Three-five days old females of *Ae. aegypti*, unfed, from collected eggs of different locations of the city of Praia, Cabo Verde. Four collections of *Ae. aegypti* eggs were carried out, since October 2020, to conduct the bioassays at one, three, six and twelve months after painting the surfaces with insecticidal paints.

Substrate: Glazed ceramic (non-porous surface) and cement block (porous surface). Insecticidal Paints: Polymeric microencapsulated suspension of insecticides. Two paints carrying organophosphate compounds (5A IGR and ARES) and one carrying pyrethroids (VESTA), from Inesfly Corporation.

Method: WHO cone bioassay, corresponding to that defined by World Health Organization in WHO methodological guide for adulticides against mosquitoes used in indoor spraying [36].

19.5.3 Results and discussion

Females from populations of *Ae. aegypti* from cidade da Praia, Cabo Verde, show variations in the mortality and delayed mortality rates according to: the type of paint tested, the type of substrate painted and the period of time since they were painted. Figure 19.6 shows, in percentage, the delayed (24 h) mortality for *Ae. aegypti* in bioassays performed at one, three, six and twelve months after the surfaces were painted, for the three tested paints.

The low mortality observed, after 24 hours, in the bioassays carried out for the 5A IGR and ARES paints show the resistance to organophosphate insecticides of the populations of *Ae. aegypti* from the city of Praia, Cabo Verde.

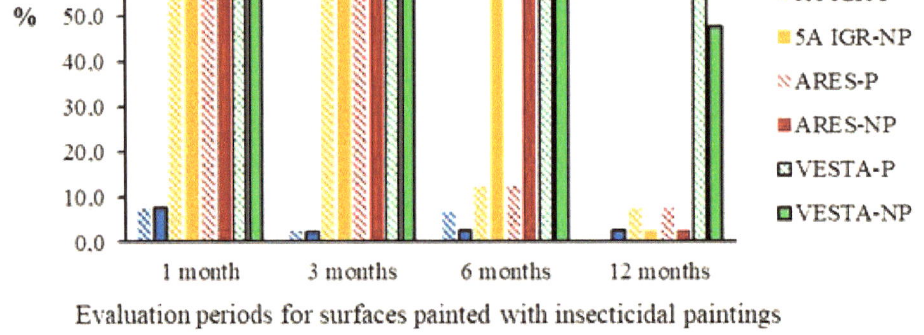

Figure 19.6: Mortality, at 24 h, of *Ae. aegypti* on porous and non-porous surfaces painted with insecticidal paints (P (Porous surface), NP (Non-porous surface).

19.5.4 Conclusion

Pyrethroid-based insecticidal paint can be an effective strategy for the intra-household control of *Ae. aegypti* from the city of Praia, Cabo Verde, however it is recommended to be used on porous surfaces and to prove, in a pilot field study, its effectiveness and residuality directly on painted surfaces in buildings.

ACKNOWLEDGMENTS

The authors thank to: the students of the Grupo de Investigação em Doenças Tropicais (GIDTpiaget) by their participation in field work, the University Jean Piaget (UniPiaget) by the logistical support, Dra. Marga Miquel for her collaboration in conducting pilot studies 1 and 2, Coordenação de Aperfeiçoamento de Pessoal de Nível Superior (CAPES) for financial support (Pró-Mobilidade CAPES/AULP Program) to carry out the pilot study 2, Dr. Iemke Postma for the correction of English, INESFLY for supporting insecticidal paints and SITA SA for entrusting us the evaluation of insecticidal paints. This chapter is partly based on work performed within the framework of IMAAC (`https://imaac.eu/`) related to COST Action CA16227 (*Investigation & Mathematical Analysis of Avant-garde Disease Control via Mosquito Nano-Tech-Repellents*, `https://cost.eu/actions/CA16227/`), supported by COST Association (European Cooperation in Science and Technology).

Bibliography

Part (I): Control of Mosquitoes and Their World: An Overview

Chapter 2: Practical Control Methods and New Techniques for Mosquito Control

1 Airs, P.M. and L.C. Bartholomay (2018),
Chapter 6. Molecular and nano-scale alternatives to traditional insecticides for in situ control of mosquito vectors. Advances in the Biorational Control of Medical and Veterinary Pests. ACS Symposium Series, Vol. 1289 75-99.

2 Alphey, L. (2013),
Genetic control of mosquitoes. Annu. Rev. Entomol. 59, 205-224.

3 Barnard, D.R. and R.D. Xue. (2004),
Laboratory evaluation of mosquito repellents against *Aedes albopictus*, *Culex nigripalpus*, and *Ochlerotatus triseriatus* (Diptera: Culicidae). J. Med. Entomol. 41, 726-730.

4 Barrera, R., M. Amador, V. Acevedo, B. Caban, G. Felix, and A. J. Mackay (2014),
Use of the CDC autocidal gravid ovitrap to control and prevent outbreaks of *Aedes aegypti* (Diptera: Culicidae). J. Med. Entomol. 51, 145-154.

5 Benelli, G. and J.C. Beier (2017),
Current vector control challenges in the fight against malaria. Acta Trop. 174, 91-96.

6 Bernardini, F., R.E. Haghighat-Khah, R. Galizi, A.M. Hammond, T. Nolan, and A. Crisanti (2018),
Molecular tools and genetic markers for the generation of transgenic sexing in Anopheles mosquitoes. Parasit Vector 11(Suppl. 2), 660, doi:10.1186/s13071-018-3207-8.

7 Bezirtzoglou, C, K. Dekas, and E. Charvalos (2011),
Climate changes, environment and infection: facts, scenarios, and growing awareness from the public health community within Europe. Anaerobe 17,337-340. doi:10.1016/j.anaerobe.2011.05.016.

8 Bibbs, C.S., C. Anderson, and R.D. Xue (2016),
Autodisemmination of insect growth regulator, methoprene, with two formulations against *Aedes albopictus*. J. Am. Mosq. Control Assoc. 32,247-250.

9 Bibbs, C.S. and P.E. Kaufman (2017),
Volatile pyrethroids as a potential mosquito abtement tool: a review of pyrethroid-containing spatial repellents. J. I. Pest Manage. 8, 21.

10 Bonds, J. (2012),
Ultra-low-volume space sprays in mosquito control: a review. Med. Vet. Entomol. 26, 121-130.

11 Brelsfoard, C.L., J.W. Mains, S. Mulligan, A. Cornel, J. Holeman, S. Kluh, A. Leal, L.J. Hribar, H. Morales, T. Posey, and S.L. Dobson (2019),
Aedes aegypti males as vehicles for insecticide delivery, Insects. 10, 230, Doi:10.3390/insects10080230.

12 Buckner, E.A, K.F. Williams, A.L. Marsicano, M.D. Latham, and C.R. Lesser (2017),
Evaluating the vector control potential of the In2Care mosquito trap against *Aedes aegypti* and *Aedes albopictus* under semi-field conditions in Manatee County, Florida. J. Am. Mosq. Control Assoc. 33, 193-199.

13 Caragata, E.P., S. Dong, Y. Dong, M.L. Simoes, C.V. Tikhe, and G. Dimopoulos (2020),
Prospects and pitfalls: Next generation tools to control mosquito-transmitted disease, Annu. Rev. Microbiol. 74, 455-475.

14 CDC (Center for Disease Control and Prevention) (2020),
A National Public Health Framework for the Prevention and Control of Vector-Borne Diseases in Humans, https://www.cdc.gov/ncezid/dvbd/pdf/Brochure_National_Framework_VBDs-P.pdf.

15 Fiorenzano, J.M., P. G. Koehler, and R.D. Xue (2017),
Attractive toxic sugar bait (ATSB) for control of mosquitoes and its impact on non-target organisms: a review. International Journal of Environmental Research and Public Health 14, 398.

16 Fulcher, A., J.M. Scott, W.A. Qualls, G.C. Muller, and R.D. Xue (2014),
Attractive toxic sugar baits mixed with pyriproxyfen sprayed on plants against adult and larval *Aedes albopictus* (Diptera: Culicidae), J. Med. Entomol. 51, 896-899.

17 Furnival-Adam, J.E.C., S. Camara, M. Rowland, A.A. Koffi, L.P. Ahoua Alou, W.A. Oumbouke, and R.N'Guessam (2020),
Indoor use of attractive toxic sugar bait in combination with long-lasting insecticidal net against pyrethroid-resistant *Anopheles gambiae*: an experimental hut trial in Mbe, central Cote d'Ivoire. Malaria J. 19, 11.

18 Gu, Z.Y., J. He, X.D. Teng, C.J. Lan, R.X. Shen, Y.T. Wang, N. Zhang, Y.D. Dong, T.Y. Zhao, and C.X. Li (2019),
Efficacy of orally toxic sugar baits against contact insecticide resistant *Culex quinquefasciatus*, Acta Tropica, https://doi.org/10.1016/jactatropica.2019.105256.

19 IAEA and WHO (2020),
Guidance framework for testing the sterile insect techniques as a vector control tool against *Aedes*-borne diseases, P. 1-184.

20 Kittayapong, P., S. Ninphanomchai, W. Limohpasmanee, C. Chansang, U. Chansang, and P. Mongkalangoon (2019),
Combined sterile insect technique and incompatible insect technique: The first proof-of-concept to suppress *Aedes aegypti* vector populations in semi-rural settings in Thailand, PLoS, https://doi.org/10.1371/journal.pntd.0007771.

21 Kline, D.L. (2006),
Traps and trapping techniques for adult mosquito control, J. Am. Mosq. Control Assoc. 22, 490-496.

22 Kline, D.L., G.C. Muller, A. Junnila, and R.D. Xue (2018),
Chapter 5: Attractive toxic sugar baits (ATSB): a novel vector management tool, Advances in the Biorational Control of Medical and Veterinary Pests. Ed. By E.J. Norris et al. ACS symposium Series, American Chemical Society, Washington, DC, 2018, P. 63-73.

23 Laurens, M.B. (2020),
RTS, S/AS01 vaccine (Mosquirix™): an overview. Hum Vaccin Immunother. 16,480-489.

24 Mains, J.W., P.H. Kelly, K.L. Dobson, W.D. Petrie, and S.L. Dobson (2019),
Localized control of *Aedes aegypti* (Diptera: Culicidae) in Miami, FL, via inundative releases of Wolbachia-infected male mosquitoes. J. Med. Entomol. 56,1296-1303.

25 Mains, J.W., C. L. Brelsfoard, and S.L. Dobson (2015),
Male mosquitoes as vehicles for insecticide, PLoS Negl. Trop. Dis. 9, e0003406, doi:10.1371/journal.pntd.0003406.

26 Mount, G.A. (1998),
https://pubmed.ncbi.nlm.nih.gov/9813829/, A critical review of ultralow-volume aerosols of insecticide applied with vehicle-mounted generators for adult mosquito control. J. Am. Mosq. Control Assoc. 14, 305-334.

27 Mount, G.A., T.L. Biery, and D.G. Haile (1996),
https://pubmed.ncbi.nlm.nih.gov/9046465/, A review of ultralow-volume aerial sprays of insecticide for mosquito control. J. Am. Mosq. Control Assoc. 12, 601-618.

28 Najera, J.A. and M. Zaim (2002),
Malaria vector control: Decision making criteria and procedures for judicious use of insecticides, WHO/CDS/WHOPES/2002.5 Rev.1., WHO Pesticide Evaluation Scheme, Geneva, P.1-106.

29 Pearson, M.A., K. Blore, C. Efstathion, V.S. Aryaprema, G.C. Muller, R.D. Xue, W.A. Qualls (2020),
Evaluation of boric acid as toxic sugar bait against resistant *Aedes aegypti* mosquitoes. J. Vector Ecology 45, 100-103.

30 Petersen, L.R., C.B. Beard, and S.N. Visser (2019),
Combatting the increasing threat of vector-borne disease in the United States with a national vector-borne disease prevention and control system, Am J. Trop. Med. Hyg. 100, 242-245.

31 Pluess, B., F.C. Taner, C. Lengeler, and B. L. Sharp (2010),
Indoor residual spraying for preventing malaria, Cochrane library 2010(4), CD006657, Doi:10.1002/14651858.CD006657.pub2.

32 Scott, J.M., K.E. Seeger, J. Gibson-Corrado, G.C. Muller, and R.D. Xue (2017)
Attractive toxic sugar bait (ATSB) mixed with pyriproxyfen for control of larval *Aedes albopictus* (Diptera: Culicidae) through fecal deposits by adult mosquitoes, J. Med. Entomol. 54, 236-238.

33 Sougoufara, S. E.C. Ottih, and F. Tripet (2020),
The need for new vector control approaches targeting outdoor biting *Anopheline* malaria vector communities, Parasite Vectors 13, 295.

34 Stoops, C.A., W.A. Qualls, T.V. T. Nguyen, and S.L. Richards (2018),
A review of studies evaluating insecticide barrier treatments for mosquito control from 1944 to 2018, Environ. Health Insights, 16, 26.

35 Talbalaghi, A., M. Farooq, W.A. Qualls, K. Blore, and R.D. Xue (2020)
Semi-field evaluation of a modified commercial My Mosquito Deleter larval trap with sticky paper against *Aedes aegypti*. J. Vector Ecol. 45.

36 Traore, M.M., A. Junnila, S.F. Traore, S. Doumbia, E.E. Revay, V.D. Kravchenko, Y. Schlein, K.L. Arheart, P. Gergely, R.D. Xue, A. Hausmann, R. Beck, A. Prozorov, R.A. Diarra, A. S. Kone, S. Majambere, J. Bradley, J. Vontas, J.C. Beier, and G.C. Muller (2020),
Large-scale field trial of attractive toxic sugar baits (ATSB) for control of malaria vector mosquitoes in Mali, West Africa. Malaria J. 19, 72, Doi:org/10.1186/s12936-020-3132-0.

37 World Health Organization (WHO) (2019),
Tenth meeting of the WHO vector control advisory group, WHO meeting report, 13-15, May 2019, Geneva, P. 1-32.

38 World Health Organization (WHO) (2006),
Global malaria programme: Indoor residual spraying, use of indoor residual spraying for scaling up global malaria control and elimination, WHO position statement, WHO/HTM/MAL/2006.1112, Geneva, P. 1-10.

39 World Health Organization (WHO) (2019),
Guidelines for malaria vector control, WHO, Geneva, P. 1-90.

40 World Health Organization (WHO) (2006),
Malaria vector control and personal protection, WHO Technical Report Series 936, Geneva, P. 1-61.

41 World Health Organization (WHO) (2008),
WHO position statement on integrated vector management, WHO, Geneva, WHO/HIM/NID/VEM/2008.2, P. 1-4.

42 Xue, R.D. and D.R. Barnard (2003),
Boric acid bait kills adult mosquitoes, J. Econ. Entomol. 96, 1559-1562.

43 Xue, R.D., G.C. Muller, W.A. Qualls, M.L. Smith, J.M. Scott, J. Lear, and S.E. Cope (2013),
Attractive target sugar baits: field evaluation and potential for use in mosquito control, Wing Beats 24, 13-18.

44 Xue, R.D., G.C. Muller, and J.F. Day (2015),
Chapter 19: Commercially available insect repellents and criteria for their use. In Insect Repellents Handbook, P. 339-350. ed. By M. Debboun, S.P. Frances, and D. Strickman. CRC Press, Boca Raton, FL, USA.

45 Zhu, D., E. Khater, S. Chao, D. Dixon, C.S. Bibbs, and R.D. Xue (2019),
Modifying the autocidal gravid ovitraps (AGO) with a powered suction fan and additional lures to increase the collection of released *Aedes aegypti* and a natural populations of *Aedes albopictus* (Diptera: Culicidae), J. Vector Ecol. 44, 282-284.

Chapter 3:

Concepts of the Best Management Practices, for Intergrated Pest Mosquito, and Vector Management

1 American Mosquito Control Association (AMCA), (2017)
Best practices for integrated mosquito mangement: a focused update, AMCA, www.mosquito.org.

2 Center for Disease Control and Prevention (CDC), (2020)
A national public health framework for the prevention and control of vector-borne diseases in humans, www.cdc.gov/ncezid/dvdb/framework.

3 CDC, 2020a
Integrated mosquito management, www.cdc.gov/mosquitoes.

4 Entomological Society of America (ESA), (2020)
Integrated pest management: Safe, economical, sustainable, and effective. ESA position statement on integrated Pest Management approved on September 20. 3 Park Place, Suite 307, Annapolis, MD, USA, www.entsoc.org.

5 Environmental Protection Agency (EPA), (2020)
Success in mosquito control: an integrated approach,Environmental Protection Agency, USA, www.epa.gov.

6 Florida Mosquito Control Associaiton (FMCA) and Florida Department of Agriculture and Consumer Services (FDACS), (2012)
Best management practices for integrated mosquito management, www.floridamosquito.org.

7 Fouet, C Kamdem, C., (2019)
Integrated mosquito management: Is precision control a luxury or necessity? Trends Parasitol, 35, 85-95.

8 IAEA & WHO/TDR, (2019)
Guidance framework for testing the sterile insect technique as a vector control tool against *Aedes*-borne diseases, Geneva, WHO.

9 Lloyd, AM, Connelly, CR, Carlson, DB, (2018)
Florida coordinating council on mosquito control, Florida mosquito control, http://fmel.ifas.ufl.edu.

10 Lu, Bao-Lin, (1984)
Integrated control of mosquitoes. Chinese Academy Press, Beijing, China, P.1-191.

11 Lu, Bao-Lin, (1999)
Integrated control of mosquitoes, 2nd edition, Chinese Academy Press, Beijing, China. P.1-277.

12 Najera, JA, Zaim, M., (2002)
Malaria vector control, decision making vriteria and procedures for judicious use of insecticides, WHO Pesticide Evaluation Scheme, Geneva, WHO/CDS/WHOPES/2002.5 Rev.1.

13 University of California San Francisco (UCSF), (2020)
Malaria elimination toolkit: Entomological surveillance planning too (ESPT), www.shrinkingthemalariamap.org.

14 World Health Organization (WHO), (2004)
Global strategic framework for integrated vector management, Geneva, Geneva, WHO/CDS/CPE/PVC/2004.10.

15 WHO, (2006)
Indoor residuel spraying. Geneva, WHO/HTM/MAL/2006.1112, www.who.int/malaria.

16 WHO (2006a)
Malaria vector control and personal protection, WHO, Geneva, WHO Technical Report Series 936.

17 WHO, (2008)
WHO position statemetn on integrated vector management, Geneva, WHO/HIM/NTD/VEM/2008.2, P.1-4.

18 WHO/TDR, (2016)
Global vector control response 2017-2030, WHO, Geneva.

19 WHO, (2019)
Tenth meeting of the WHO vector control advisory group, WHO meeting report, 13-15, May 2019, Geneva, P.1-32.

20 WHO, (2019a)
Guidelines for malaria vector control, WHO, Geneva, P. 1-90.

21 Xue, RD, Peper, S, Muller, GC, (2023)
Chapter "Practical control methods and new techniques for mosquito control", Bio-mathematics, Statistics and Nano-Technologies: Mosquito Control Strategies, Chapter 1. Editor: Peyman Ghaffari, CRC press Taylors & Francis Group.

Chapter 4:

Overview of Personal Protection Measures Through the Innovative Use of Repellent-Textiles

1 Arief, H., Saratian, E.T.P., Permana, D., Soelton, M., Rohman, F., & Mugiono, M., (2019)
Innovation of Natural Mosquito Repellent Products (Amuk Candle) as the Opportunity for Community Business, International Conference on Community Development, 2(1), 38-42, DOI: https://doi.org/10.33068/iccd.Vol2.Iss1.200.

2 The Barcelona Institute for Global Health (ISGlobal), https://www.isglobal.org/en_GB/nuestra-historia.

3 Barnard Donald Roy, Bernier Ulrich, Xue Rui-De and Debboun Mustapha, (2007),
Standard Methods for Testing Mosquito Repellents, DOI: 10.1201/9781420006650.ch5.

4 Brown, M., and Hebert, A. A., (1997)
Insect repellents: An Overview. Journal of the American Academy of Dermatology, 36(2), 243–249.

5 Debboun, M and Strickman, D., (2012)
Insect Repellents and Associated Personal Protection for a Reduction in Human Disease. Medical and Veterinary Entomology, 27(1), DOI:10.1111/j.1365-2915.2012.01020.x.

6 Diaz, J. H., (2016)
Chemical and Plant-Based Insect Repellents: Efficacy, Safety, and Toxicity. Wilderness and Environmental Medicine, 27(1),153-163.

7 European Centre for Disease Prevention and Control and European Food Safety Authority. The importance of vector abundance and seasonality – Results from an expert consultation, Stockholm and Parma: ECDC and EFSA, (2018).

8 Faulde M, Uedelhoven W., (2006)
A new clothing impregnation method for personal protection against ticks and biting insects. International Journal of Med Microbiology, 296(40), 225-9, DOI: 10.1016/j.ijmm.2006.01.008, PMID: 16524779.

9 Grancaric, A. M., Laird, K., Botteri, L., Shen, J. and Laatikainen, K., (2019)
Microencapsulation for Improved Mosquitoes Repellent Efficacy of Cotton Fabrics, Innovation Technology Management Consultancy Conference, Marrakech, Morocco.

10 Grancarić, A. M., Botteri, L. and Ghaffari, P., (2019)
Combating Invasive Mosquitoes by Textiles and Paints, AUTEX-2019-19th World Textile Conference on Textiles at the Crossroads.

11 Hebeish, A., Fouda, M.G., Hamdy, I.A., EL-Sawy, S.M., Abdel-Mohdy,F.A.,(2008)
Preparation of durable insect repellent cotton fabric: Limonene as insecticide Carbohydrate Polymers 74 (2), 268-273, https://doi.org/10.1016/j.carbpol.2008.02.013.

12 Maheshwari, V., and Ramya, K.,(2014)
Development of Eco-friendly Mosquito Repellent Fabric Finished with Andrographis paniculata plant extracts, International Journal of Pharmaceutical Sciences, 6(5), 115–117.

13 Maia, M.F., Moore, S.J., (2011)
Plant-based insect repellents: a review of their efficacy, development and testing, Malaria Journal 10(11), https://doi.org/10.1186/1475-2875-10-S1-S11.

14 Michaelakis A., V. Karras, Petric D, A. M. Grancaric, D. Papachristos, G. Balastos, L. Botteri, Department of Entomology and Agricultural Zoology, Benaki Phytopathological Institute, Athens – Greece , University of Novi Sad, Faculty of Agriculture, Novi Sad, Serbia University of Zagreb, Zagreb, Croatia.

15 Mok S., Ashley E.A., Ferreira P.E., Zhu L., Lin Z., Yeo T., Chotivanich K., Imwong M., Pukrittayakamee S., Dhorda M., Nguon C., Lim P., Amaratunga C., Suon S., Hien T.T., Htut Y., Faiz M.A., Onyamboko M.A., Mayxay M., Newton PN, Tripura R, Woodrow CJ, Miotto O, Kwiatkowski DP, Nosten F, Day N.P., Preiser P.R., White N.J., Dondorp A.M., Fairhurst R.M., Bozdech Z., (2015)
Drug resistance, Population Transcriptomics of Human Malaria Parasites Reveals the Mechanism of Artemisinin Resistance, Science, 347(6220), 431-5.

16 Morton F., Travis B. and Linduska J., (1947)
Results of Screening Tests with Materials Evaluated as Insecticides, Miticides, and Repellents at the Orlando Fla. Laboratory, United States Department of Agriculture, Agricultural Research Administration Bureau of Entomology and Plant Quarantine, Available online: http://ufdc.ufl.edu/AA00025211/00001.

17 Moutailler S, Yousfi L, Mousson L, Devillers E, Vazeille M, Vega-Rúa A, Perrin Y, Jourdain F, Chandre F, Cannet A, Chantilly S, Restrepo J, Guidez A, Dusfour I, Vieira Santos de Abreu F, Pereira dos Santos T, Jiolle D, Visser TM, Koenraadt CJM, Wongsokarijo M, Diallo M, Diallo D, Gaye A, Boyer S, Duong V, Piorkowski G, Paupy C, Lourenco de Oliveira R, de Lamballerie X, Failloux A-B., (2019)
A New High-Throughput Tool to Screen Mosquito-Borne Viruses in Zika Virus Endemic/Epidemic Areas, Viruses, 11(10), 904.

18 Norris, E. J. and Coats, J. R., (2017)
Current and Future Repellent Technologies: The Potential of Spatial Repellents and Their Place in Mosquito-Borne Disease Control, International Journal of Environmental Research and Public Health, 14 (2) 124.

19 Paluch G., Bartholomay L., Coats J., (2010)
Mosquito repellents: A Review of Chemical Structure Diversity and Olfaction, Pest Management Science, 66(9), 925–935, DOI: 10.1002/ps.1974.

20 Peter R.J., Bossche P., Van Den Penzhorn B.L., Sharp B., (2005)
Tick, Fly, and Mosquito Control—Lessons from the Past, Solutions for the Future, Veterinary Parasitology, 132(3-4), 205–215, DOI: 10.1016/j.vetpar.2005.07.004.

21 Peterson, C. and Coats, J., (2001)
Insect Repellents - Past, Present and Future, Pesticide Outlook, 12(4), 154-158, DOI:10.1039/b106296b.

22 Reynoso, M., Seccacini, E. A., Calcagno, J. A., Zerba, E. N., & Alzogaray, R. A., (2017)
Toxicity, repellency and flushing out in Triatoma infestans (Hemiptera: Reduviidae) exposed to the repellents DEET and IR3535. PeerJ, 5, e3292, https://doi.org/10.7717/peerj.3292.

23 Reisen, W.K., (2004)
University of California, Center for Vector-borne Diseases, Department of Pathology, Microbiology and Immunology, School of Veterinary -Vector Biology, Ecology and Control, 127-137.

24 Qualls Whitney A., Rui-De Xue, Muhammad Farooq, Steven Peper, Vindhya Aryaprema,Kai Blore, Richard Weaver, Dena Autry, Asghar Talbalaghi, James Kenar, Steven C. Cermak, and Junwei J. Zhu, (2020)
Evaluation of lotions of botanical-based repellents against Aedes aegypti Medical Entomology 2020, Journal of Medical Entomology, tjaa244 , https://doi.org/10.1093/jme/tjaa244.

25 Sritabutra, D., Soonwera, M., Waltanachanobon, S., and Poungjai, S., (2011)
Evaluation of Herbal Essential Oil as Repellents against Aedes aegypti (L.) and Anopheles dirus Peyton and Harrion, Asian Pacific Journal of Tropical Biomedicine, 1(1), 124–128.

26 Standards, A., (2006)
Standard Test Methods for Laboratory Testing of Non-Commercial Mosquito Repellent Formulations on the Skin, ASTM International, DOI:10.1520/E0951-94R06.

27 Talbalaghi, A., (2008),
Source PubMed from Parassitologia 50, 125-126, ISSN 0048-2951.

28 Talbalaghi, A., Ali, A. and Hassandoust S., (2018)
Evaluation of a Promising New Botanical Adult Mosquito Repellent on Horses, Journal of Translational Science, 5(2), 1-4 DOI:10.15761/JTS.1000250. ISSN:2059-268X.

29 Talbalaghi., A et al., (2010)
Are Aedes albopictus or other mosquito species from northern Italy competent to sustain new arbovi- ral outbreaks?, Medical and Veterinary Entomology 24, ed Vet Entomol 2010 Mar, 24(1), 83-7, DOI:10.1111/j.1365-2915.2009.00853.x.

30 Tawatsin, A., Wratten, S. D., Scott, R. R., Thavara, U., and Techadamrongsin, Y., (2001)
Repellency of Volatile Oils from Plants against Three Mosquito Vectors, Journal of Vector Ecology, 26, 76–82.

31 Tolle, M.A., (2009)
Mosquito-borne Diseases, Current Problems in Pediatric and Adolescent Health Care, 39(4) 97–140 DOI:10.1016/j.cppeds.2009.01.001.

32 WHO, World Health Organisation, (2020)
https://www.who.int/news-room/fact-sheets/detail/vector-borne-diseases, Vector-borne Diseases.

Chapter 5:

Biology, Surveillance and Control of Mosquito Vectors through the Innovative Use of Repellent-Textiles

1 The Ferguson College of Agriculture website: http://entoplp.okstate.edu/mosquito/lifecycle.html.

2 AFPM, (2002)
Armed Forces Pest Management Board: Technical Guide No 43, Guide to pest surveillance during contingency operations, Defense Pest Management Information Analysis Centre, Walter Reed Army Medical Centre, Washington, DC, 20307-50001.

3 Cameron Webb & Richard C. Russell, 2005
A comparison of four commercially available adult mosquito traps, Institute of Clinical pathology and Medical Research.

4 Centers for Disease Control and Prevention, (2005)
Mosquito Borne Disease, National Centre for Infectious Disease, Centers for Disease Control, Atlanta, Georgia, http://www.cdc.gov/ncidoc/diseases/list_mosquitoes.htm.

5 Cheong, W.H., Loong, K.P., Mahadevan, S., Mak, J.W. and Kan, S.K.P., (1984)
Mosquito fauna of the Bengkoka Peninsular, Sabah, Malaysia, Southeast Asian Journal of Tropical Medicine and Public Health 15, 19-25.

6 Cheong, W.H., Chiang, G.L., Loong, K.P., Mahadevan, S. and Samarawickrema, W.A., (1988)
Biting activities cycles of some mosquitoes in the Bengkoka Peninsula, Sabah state with notes on their importance, Tropical Biomedicine, 5, 27-21.

7 Colinvaux, Paul A. (1973)
Introduction to Ecology, Wiley, ISBN 0-471-16498-4.

8 Eliningaya, J., Kweka and Aneth, M., Mahande, (2009)
Comparative evaluation of four mosquitoes sampling methods in rice irrigation schemes of lower Moshi, northern Tanzania, Malar J. 2009, 8, 149, Published online 2009 July 6. DOI:10.1186/1475-2875-8-149.

9 Guimarães, A.E., C. Gentile, C.M. Lopes, and R. Pinto de Mello, (2000a)
Ecology of mosquitoes (Diptera: Culicidae) in areas of Serra do Mar State Park, State of São Paulo, Brazil, III. Daily biting rhythms and lunar cycle influence, Mem. Inst. Oswaldo Cruz, 95, 753-760.

10 Guimarães, A.E., R. Pinto de Mello, C.M. Lopes, and C. Gentile, (2000b)
Ecology of mosquitoes (Diptera: Culicidae) in areas of Serra do Mar State Park, State of São Paulo, Brazil, I. Monthly frequency and climatic factors, Mem. Inst. Oswaldo Cruz, 95, 1-16.

11 Harbach, R.E. and Kitching, I.J., (1998)
Phylogeny and classification of the Culicidae (Diptera), Systematic Entomology, 23, 327-370.

12 Harbach, R.E. and Kitching, I.J., 2005
Reconsideration of *Anopheline* mosquito phylogeny (Diptera: Culicidae, *Anophelinae*) based on morphological data, Systematics and Biodiversity, 3, 345-374.

13 Harbach, R.E. and Knight, K.L., (1980)
Taxonomists' Glossary of Mosquito Anatomy, Plexus Publishing, Inc. Marlton, NJ, 415 pp.

14 Harbach, R.E. and Kitching, I.J., (1998)
Phylogeny and classification of the Culicidae (Diptera), Systematic Entomology, 23, 327-370.

15 Hock, W., John, (2004)
CDC Miniature Light Trap - Model, 512, instr_512_cdcminiature.doc, Friday, December 03, 2004.

16 Jorge, R., (2001)
Rey. 2001. The Mosquito, HTTP://EDIS.IFAS.UFL.EDU/IN652.

17 Knight, K. and Stone, A., (1977)
A Catalog of the mosquito of the World (Diptera: Culicidae), Thomas Say Foundation, Vol. 6. College Park, Maryland, 611 pp.

18 Loong, K.P., Chiang, G.L., Yap, H.H., (1998)
Field study of the bionomics of *Anopheles maculatus* and it's in malaria transmission in Malaysia, Southeast Asian Journal of Tropical Medicine and Public Health, 19, 724-728.

19 Mosquito Larvae Anatomy - Florida Medical Entomology Laboratory,
fmel.ifas.ufl.edu/key/anatomy/larval.shtml.

20 Newson, H.D., (1977)
Arthropod problems in recreational areas, Annual Reviewers Entomology, 22, 333-353 pp.

21 Oli, K., Jeffery, J. and Vythilingam, I., (2005)
A comparative study of adult mosquito trapping using dry ice and yeast generated carbon dioxide, Tropical Biomedicine 22(2), 249–251.

22 Onyido, V., Ezike, N., Ozumba, E., Nwosu, O., Ikpeze, M., Obiukwu & E., Amadi, (2009)
Crepuscular Man-Biting Mosquitoes of a Tropical Zoological Garden in Enugu, South-Eastern Nigeria. The Internet Journal of Parasitic Diseases, 2009, Volume 4, No 1.

23 Reid, J.A., (1968)
Anophelinae mosquitoes in Malaya and Borneo, Stud. Inst. Med. Res. Malaysia, 520 pp.

24 Reiter, P. (2001)
Climate change and mosquito-borne disease. Envir. Hlth. Perspect, 109, 141-161.

25 Rancangan Kawalan Penyakit Bawaan Vektor, (1997)
Vector Borne Disease Control Programme, Ministry of Health, Malaysia.

26 Rogozi Elton, Enkelejda Velo, and Silva Bino, (2012a)
Mosquito species trappability during the summer season in some areas of Albania. A comparison between the techniques used for collecting adult mosquitoes, Journal of International Environmental Application & Science, Volume 7, Issue 5, pp 871-879.

27 Rogozi Elton, Rohani Bt. Ahmad and Zamree Ismail, (2012b)
Biting activity of some antopophilic mosquito species in Malaysia, Journal of International Environmental Application & Science, Volume 7, Issue 5, pp 894-900.

28 Rohani, A., Chan S.T., Abdullah, A.G., Tanrang, H. and Lee, H.L., (2008)
Species composition of mosquito fauna in Ranau, Sabah, Malaysia, Tropical Biomedicine, 25 (3), 232-236.

29 Rohani, A., Lokman Hakim, S., Hassan, A.R., Chan, S.T., Ong, Y.F., Abdullah, A.G. and Lee Han Lim, (1999)
Bionomic of *Anopheles balabacensis* baisas, the principal malaria vector, in Ranau, Sabah, Tropical Biomedicine, 16, 31-38.

30 Schaffner F., Angel G., Geoffroy B., Hervy J.-P., Rhaiem A. & Brunhes J.,Décembre, (2001)
The Mosquitoes of Europe / Les moustiques d'Europe, Logiciel d'identification et d'enseignement (CD-Rom), Montpellier, France, IRD, Editions & EID Méditerranée.

31 Service M.W., (1993a)
Mosquito ecology field sampling methods., 1. London, UK: Elsevier Applied Science.

32 Service M.W., (1993b)
Mosquito ecology field sampling methods, 2. London, UK: Elsevier Applied Science.

33 Simpson, E. H., (1951)
The Interpretation of Interaction in Contingency Tables, Journal of the Royal Statistical Society, Ser. B, 13, 238-241.

34 Sørensen, T., (1948)
A method of establishing groups of equal amplitude in plant sociology based on similarity of species and its application to analyses of the vegetation on Danish commons, Biologiske Skrifter/Kongelige Danske Videnskabernes Selskab, 5 (4), 1-34.

35 The Life Cycle of the Mosquito,
`www.mosquitoes.org/LifeCycle.html.`

36 World Health Organization, (1975)
Manual on practical entomology in malaria, Part II. Methods and Techniques. Geneva. WHO.

37 WHO, (2002)
Management of uncomplicated malaria and the use of antimalaria drugs for the protection of travelers, World Health Organization, Division of Control of Tropical Diseases, Geneva.

38 WHO, (1992)
Entomological field techniques for malaria control, Part 1, Learner's Guide, World Health Organization, Geneva.

Part (II):

Mathematical Modeling Immunity: An Overview Based on Malaria

Chapter 6:

Models of Acquired Immunity to Malaria: A Review

1 World Health Organization, (2018), World malaria report.

2 World Health Organization et al., (2016)
Eliminating malaria. World Health Organization, 2016.

3 Killen, Gerry F., et al., (2007)
Preventing childhood malaria in Africa by protecting adults from mosquitoes with insecticide-treated nets. PLoS Medicine, 2007, 4.7:e229.

4 Killen, Gerry F., Smith, Thomas, (2007)
A. Exploring the contributions of bed nets, cattle, insecticides and excitorepellency to malaria control: a deterministic model of mosquito host-seeking behaviour and mortality. Transactions of the Royal Society of Tropical Medicine and Hygiene, 2007, 101.9, 867-880.

5 White, Nicholas J., (2004)
Antimalarial drug resistance. The Journal of clinical investigation, 2004, 113.8, 1084-1092.

6 Pinkevych M, Petravic J, Chelimo K, Kazura JW, Moormann AM, Davenport MP, (2012)
The dynamics of naturally acquired immunity to Plasmodium falciparum infection, PLoS computational biology, 2012 Oct 18, 8(10):e1002729.

7 Port, G. R.; Boreham, P. F. L.; Bryan, Joan H., (1980)
The relationship of host size to feeding by mosquitoes of the *Anopheles gambiae* Giles complex(Diptera: Culicidae), Bulletin of Entomological Research, 1980, 70.1, 133-144.

8 World Health Organization, (WHO) and WHO Global Malaria Programme,
http://www.who.int/malaria/about_us/en/index.html, http://www.who.int/topics/malaria/en/.

9 Bathurst, Ian, Hentschel, Chris, (2006)
Medicines for Malaria Venture: sustaining antimalarial drug development, Trends in parasitology, 2006, 22.7: 301-307.

10 Duffy PE, Sahu T, Akue A, Milman N, Anderson C., (2012)
Pre-erythrocytic malaria vaccines: identifying the targets, Expert review of vaccines, 2012 Oct 1, 11(10), 1261-80.

11 J. David M. Edgar, (2011)
Clinical Immunology, The Ulster medical journal, 2011 Jan, 80(1), 5 14.

12 Mandal S, Sarkar RR, Sinha S., (2011), Mathematical models of malaria-a review, Malaria journal, 2011 Dec, 10(1), 202.

13 Govella, NJ, Okumu, FO, Killeen, GF, (2004)
Insecticide-treated nets can reduce malaria transmission by mosquitoes which feed outdoors. The American journal of tropical medicine and hygiene, 2010 Mar 1, 82(3), 415-9.

14 VAN ECK, Nees Jan, WALTMAN, Ludo, (2013)
VOSviewer manual. Leiden: Univeristeit Leiden, 2013, 1.1.

15 Covell G., (1960)
Relationship between malarial parasitaemia and symptoms of the disease: a review of the literature, Bulletin of the World Health Organization, 1960, 22(6), 605.

16 Geisse KV, Butler EJ, Cordovez JM., (2012)
Effects of Natural Acquired Immunity in an Age-Structured Malaria Model, Technical report, July; 2012 Jul 31.

17 Ataíde R, Ashley EA, Powell R, Chan JA, Malloy MJ, O'Flaherty K, Takashima E, Langer C, Tsuboi T, Dondorp AM, Day NP., (2017)
Host immunity to Plasmodium falciparum and the assessment of emerging artemisinin resistance in a multinational cohort, Proceedings of the National Academy of Sciences, 2017 Mar 28, 114(13), 3515-20.

18 Ataíde R, Powell R, Moore K, McLean A, Phyo AP, Nair S, White M, Anderson TJ, Beeson JG, Simpson JA, Nosten F., (2017)
Declining transmission and immunity to malaria and emerging artemisinin resistance in Thailand: A longitudinal study, The Journal of infectious diseases, 2017 Aug 3, 216(6), 723-31.

19 Bakary T, Boureima S, Sado T., (2018)
A mathematical model of malaria transmission in a periodic environment, Journal of biological dynamics, 2018 Jan 1, 12(1), 400-32.

20 Matuschewski K., (2017)
Vaccines against malaria—still a long way to go, The FEBS journal, 2017 Aug, 284(16), 2560-8.

21 Sherman IW, (2009)
The elusive malaria vaccine: miracle or mirage?, Washington, DC, USA, ASM Press, 2009.

22 Hviid L., (2005)
Naturally acquired immunity to Plasmodium falciparum malaria in Africa, Acta tropica, 2005 Sep 1, 95(3), 270-5.

23 Greenwood B., (2005)
Malaria vaccines: Evaluation and implementation, Acta tropica, 2005 Sep 1, 95(3), 298-304.

24 Rono J., (2013)
Naturally acquired immunity to plasmodium falciparum malaria: antibody responses and immunological memory, Inst för medicin, Solna/Dept of Medicine, Solna, 2013 Oct 11.

25 Scott N, Ataide R, Wilson DP, Hellard M, Price RN, Simpson JA, Fowkes FJ., (2018)
Implications of population-level immunity for the emergence of artemisinin-resistant malaria: a mathematical model, Malaria journal, 2018 Dec, 17(1), 279.

26 Yamana TK, Bomblies A, Laminou IM, Duchemin JB, Eltahir EA., (2013)
Linking environmental variability to village-scale malaria transmission using a simple immunity model. Parasites & vectors, 2013 Dec, 6(1), 226.

27 Yamana TK, Bomblies A, Eltahir EA., (2015)
Simulating malaria transmission in the current and future climate of West Africa, InAGU Fall Meeting Abstracts 2015 Dec.

28 Yamana,TK.
Mechanistic modelling of the links between environment, mosquitoes and malaria transmission in the current and future climates of West Africa (Doctoral dissertation, Massachusetts Institute of Technology).

29 Guinovart C, Navia MM, Tanner M, (2006)
oo PL. Malaria: burden of disease, Current molecular medicine, 2006 Mar 1, 6(2), 137-40.

30 Molineaux L, Träuble M, Collins WE, Jeffery GM, Dietz K., (2002)
Malaria therapy reinoculation data suggest individual variation of an innate immune response and independent acquisition of antiparasitic and antitoxic immunities, Transactions of the Royal Society of Tropical Medicine and Hygiene, 2002 Mar 1;96(2), 205-9.

31 Molineaux L, Diebner HH, Eichner M, Collins WE, Jeffery GM, Dietz K., (2001)
Plasmodium falciparum parasitaemia described by a new mathematical model, Parasitology, 2001 Apr, 122(4), 379-91.

32 Diebner HH, Eichner M, Molineaux L, Collins WE, Jeffery GM, Dietz K., (2000)
Modelling the transition of asexual blood stages of Plasmodium falciparum to gametocytes, Journal of Theoretical Biology, 2000 Jan 21, 202(2), 113-27.

33 Alonso PL, Smith T, Schellenberg JA, Masanja H, Mwankusye S, Urassa H, De Azevedo IB, Chongela J, Kobero S, Menendez C, Hurt N., (1994)
Randomised trial of efficacy of SPf66 vaccine against Plasmodium falciparum malaria in children in southern Tanzania, The Lancet, 1994 Oct 29, 344(8931), 1175-81.

34 Doolan DL, Dobaño C, Baird JK., (2009)
Acquired immunity to malaria, Clinical microbiology reviews, 2009 Jan 1, 22(1), 13-36.

35 Baird JK., (1995)
Host age as a determinant of naturally acquired immunity to Plasmodium falciparum, Parasitology today, 1995 Mar 1, 11(3), 105-11.

36 Langhorne J, Ndungu FM, Sponaas AM, Marsh K., (2008)
Immunity to malaria: more questions than answers, Nature immunology, 2008 Jul, 9(7), 725.

37 Yokley K, Lee JT, Brown A, Minor M, Mader G., (2013)
A simple agent-based model of malaria transmission investigating intervention methods and acquired immunity, Involve, a Journal of Mathematics, 2013 Oct 24, 7(1), 15-40.

38 Koella, JC., (1991)
On the use of mathematical models of malaria transmission, Acta tropica, 1991 Apr 1;49(1), 1-25.

39 Aguas R, White LJ, Snow RW, Gomes MG, (2008)
Prospects for malaria eradication in sub-Saharan Africa, PloS one, 2008 Mar 12, 3(3):e1767.

40 Dietz K, Molineaux L, Thomas A, (1974)
A malaria model tested in the African savannah, Bulletin of the World Health Organization, 1974, ,50(3-4), 347.

41 Bekessy, A., Molineaux, L., Storey, J., (1976)
Estimation of incidence and recovery rates of Plasmodium falciparum parasitaemia from longitudinal data, Bulletin of the World Health Organization, 1976, 54.6, 685.

42 Dietz K, Raddatz G, Molineaux L., (2006)
Mathematical model of the first wave of Plasmodium falciparum asexual parasitemia in non-immune and vaccinated individuals, The American journal of tropical medicine and hygiene, 2006 Aug 1, 75(2_suppl), 46-55.

43 Aron JL, (1988)
Mathematical modeling of immunity to malaria, Mathematical Biosciences, 1988 Jul 1, 90(1-2), 385-96.

44 Aron, J. L., May, R. M., (1982)
The population dynamics of malaria, Population Dynamics of Infectious Diseases, Theory and Applications, 1982.

45 Aron JL, (1983)
Dynamics of acquired immunity boosted by exposure to infection, Mathematical Biosciences. 1983 Jun 1, 64(2), 249-59.

46 Ngwa GA, Shu WS, (2000)
A mathematical model for endemic malaria with variable human and mosquito populations, Mathematical and Computer modeling, 2000 Oct 1, 32(7-8), 747-63.

47 Ngwa GA, (2004)
Modeling the dynamics of endemic malaria in growing populations, Discrete and Continuous Dynamical Systems Series B, 2004 Aug 1, 4, 1173-202.

48 Chitnis N, Cushing JM, Hyman JM, (2006)
Bifurcation analysis of a mathematical model for malaria transmission, SIAM Journal on Applied Mathematics, 2006 Nov 3, 67(1), 24-45.

49 Chitnis NR, (2005)
Using mathematical models in controlling the spread of malaria, PhD Dissertation, 2005.

50 Yang HM, (2000)
Malaria transmission model for different levels of acquired immunity and temperature-dependent parameters (vector), Revista de saude publica, 2000 Jun, 34(3), 223-31.

51 Yang HM, Ferreira MU, (2000)
Assessing the effects of global warming and local social and economic conditions on the malaria transmission, Revista de saude publica, 2000 Jun, 34(3), 214-22.

52 Filipe JA, Riley EM, Drakeley CJ, Sutherland CJ, Ghani AC, (2007)
Determination of the processes driving the acquisition of immunity to malaria using a mathematical transmission model, PLoS computational biology, 2007 Dec 28, 3(12):e255.

53 Okell LC, Drakeley CJ, Bousema T, Whitty CJ, Ghani AC, (2008)
Modeling the impact of artemisinin combination therapy and long-acting treatments on malaria transmission intensity, PLoS medicine, 2008 Nov 25, 5(11):e226.

54 Okell LC, Bousema T, Griffin JT, Ouédraogo AL, Ghani AC, Drakeley CJ, (2012)
Factors determining the occurrence of submicroscopic malaria infections and their relevance for control, Nature communications, 2012 Dec 4;3(1), 1-9.

55 Ghani AC, Sutherland CJ, Riley EM, Drakeley CJ, Griffin JT, Gosling RD, Filipe JA, (2009)
Loss of population levels of immunity to malaria as a result of exposure-reducing interventions: Consequences for interpretation of disease trends, PLoS One, 2009 Feb 9, 4(2):e4383.

56 Smith T, Maire N, Ross A, Penny M, Chitnis N, Schapira A, Studer A, Genton B, Lengeler C, Tediosi F, De Savigny D., (2008)
Towards a comprehensive simulation model of malaria epidemiology and control, Parasitology, 2008 Nov, 135(13), 1507-16.

57 Griffin JT, Hollingsworth TD, Okell LC, Churcher TS, White M, Hinsley W, Bousema T, Drakeley CJ, Ferguson NM, Basáñez MG, Ghani AC., (2010)
Reducing Plasmodium falciparum malaria transmission in Africa: a model-based evaluation of intervention strategies, PLoS medicine, 2010 Aug 10, 7(8):e1000324.

58 Cairns M, Ghani A, Okell L, Gosling R, Carneiro I, Anto F, Asoala V, Owusu-Agyei S, Greenwood B, Chandramohan D, Milligan P., (2011)
Modeling the protective efficacy of alternative delivery schedules for intermittent preventive treatment of malaria in infants and children, PLoS One, 2011 Apr 20, 6(4):e18947.

59 Anderson RM, May RM. Infectious diseases of humans: dynamics and control. Oxford university press; 1992 Aug 27.

60 Boyd, Mark F., (1949)
Epidemiology of malaria: factors related to the intermediate host, In: Malariology, WB Saunders Philadelphia, 1949, p. 551-607.

61 Boyd MF. Malariology, (1949)
A comprehensive Survey of all Aspects of this Group of Diseases from a global Standpoint, Malariology, A Comprehensive Survey of all Aspects of this Group of Diseases from a Global Standpoint, 1949, 2.

62 Labadin J, Kon M, Juan S., (2009)
Deterministic malaria transmission model with acquired immunity WCECS 2009, October 20–22, 2009, San Francisco, USA.

63 Molineaux L, Gramiccia G, (1980)
World Health Organization, The Garki project: research on the epidemiology and control of malaria in the Sudan savanna of West Africa, 1980.

64 Dutertre J., (1976)
Etude d'un modèle épidémiologique appliqué au paludisme, Ann Soc Belge Med Trop, 1976, 56, 127-41.

65 Hethcote HW, Stech HW, van den Driessche P., (1981)
Periodicity and stability in epidemic models: a survey, InDifferential equations and applications in ecology, epidemics, and population problems, 1981, (pp. 65-82).

66 Beier JC, Killeen GF, Githure JI., (1999)
Entomologic inoculation rates and Plasmodium falciparum malaria prevalence in Africa, The American journal of tropical medicine and hygiene, 1999 Jul 1, 61(1), 109-13.

67 Anderson RM, May RM., (1979)
Population biology of infectious diseases: Part I, Nature, 1979 Aug, 280(5721), 361.

68 Greenwood BM., (1990)
Immune responses to sporozoite antigens and their relationship to naturally acquired immunity to malaria, Bulletin of the World Health Organization, 1990, 68(Suppl), 184.

69 Kamuyu G., (2017)
Identifying Merozoite Targets of Protective Immunity Against Plasmodium falciparum Malaria (Doctoral dissertation, The Open University), 2017.

70 Milligan PJ, Downham DY, (1996)
Models of superinfection and acquired immunity to multiple parasite strains, Journal of applied probability, 1996 Dec, 33(4), 915-32.

71 Zwetyenga J, Rogier C, Tall A, Fontenille D, Snounou G, Trape JF, Mercereau-Puijalon O., (1998)
No influence of age on infection complexity and allelic distribution in Plasmodium falciparum infections in Ndiop, a Senegalese village with seasonal, mesoendemic malaria, The American journal of tropical medicine and hygiene, 1998 Nov 1, 59(5), 726-35.

72 Gu W, Killeen GF, Mbogo CM, Regens JL, Githure JI, Beier JC., (2003)
An individual-based model of Plasmodium falciparum malaria transmission on the coast of Kenya, Transactions of the Royal Society of Tropical Medicine and Hygiene, 2003 Jan 1, 97(1), 43-50.

73 Gurarie D, Karl S, Zimmerman PA, King CH, Pierre TG, Davis TM, (2012)
Mathematical modeling of malaria infection with innate and adaptive immunity in individuals and agent-based communities, PloS one, 2012 Mar 28, 7(3):e34040.

74 Kassim OO, Ako-Anai KA, Torimiro SE, Hollowell GP, Okoye VC, Martin SK, (2000)
Inhibitory factors in breastmilk, maternal and infant sera against in vitro growth of Plasmodium falciparum malaria parasite, Journal of Tropical Pediatrics, 2000 Apr 1, 46(2), 92-6.

75 Tumwiine J, Mugisha JY, Luboobi LS, (2007)
A mathematical model for the dynamics of malaria in a human host and mosquito vector with temporary immunity, Applied Mathematics and Computation, 2007 Jun 15, 189(2), 1953-65.

76 Maire N, Smith T, Ross A, Owusu-Agyei S, Dietz K, Molineaux L, (2006)
A model for natural immunity to asexual blood-stages of Plasmodium falciparum malaria in endemic areas, The American journal of tropical medicine and hygiene, 2006 Aug 1, 75(2_suppl), 19-31.

77 Eckhoff PA, (2012)
Malaria parasite diversity and transmission intensity affect development of parasitological immunity in a mathematical model, Malaria journal, 2012 Dec, 11(1), 419.

78 Chiyaka C, Garira W, Dube S, (2008)
Modeling immune response and drug therapy in human malaria infection, Computational and Mathematical Methods in Medicine, 2008 Jun 1, 9(2), 143-63.

79 Bosomprah S, (2014)
A mathematical model of seropositivity to malaria antigen, allowing seropositivity to be prolonged by exposure, Malaria journal, 2014 Dec, 13(1), 12.

80 Nasell I., (1986)
On superinfection in malaria, Mathematical Medicine and Biology: A Journal of the IMA, 1986 Jan 1, 3(3), 211-27.

81 Portugal S, Drakesmith H, Mota MM, (2011)
Superinfection in malaria: Plasmodium shows its iron will, EMBO reports, 2011 Dec 1, 12(12), 1233-42.

82 Portugal S, Carret C, Recker M, Armitage AE, Gonçalves LA, Epiphanio S, Sullivan D, Roy C, Newbold CI, Drakesmith H, Mota MM, (2011)
Host-mediated regulation of superinfection in malaria, Nature medicine, 2011 Jun, 17(6), 732.

83 Wohlin C., (2014)
Guidelines for snowballing in systematic literature studies and a replication in software engineering, InProceedings of the 18th international conference on evaluation and assessment in software engineering 2014 May 13 (pp. 1-10).

84 Richie TL., (1988)
Interactions between malaria parasites infecting the same vertebrate host, Parasitology, 1988 Jun, 96(3), 607-39.

85 Boyd MF, Kitchen SF, Matthews CB, (1939)
Consecutive Inoculations with Plasmodium Vivax and Plasmodium Falciparum, The American Journal of Tropical Medicine and Hygiene, 1939 Mar 1, 1(2), 141-50.

86 Garnham PC, (1966)
Malaria parasites and other haemosporidia,1966.

87 Hackett, L. W., (1941)
Malaria and the community. In "A Symposium on Human Malaria" (F. R. Moulton, ed.), pp. 148–156, American Association for the Advancement of Science, Washington DC.

88 McKenzie FE, Smith DL, O'Meara WP, Riley EM, (2008)
Strain theory of malaria: the first 50 years, Advances in parasitology, 2008 Jan 1, 66, 1-46.

89 Hackett LW. (1937)
Malaria in Europe, An Ecological Study, 1937.

90 Gatton ML, Cheng Q., (2004)
Modeling the development of acquired clinical immunity to Plasmodium falciparum malaria, Infection and immunity, 2004 Nov 1, 72(11), 6538-45.

91 Gelband H, Panosian CB, Arrow KJ, editors, (2004)
Saving lives, buying time: economics of malaria drugs in an age of resistance, National Academies Press, 2004 Oct 9.

92 Schofield L, Mueller I., (2006)
Clinical immunity to malaria, Current molecular medicine, 2006 Mar 1, 6(2), 205-21.

93 Cai LM, Lashari AA, Jung IH, Okosun KO, Seo YI, (2013)
Mathematical analysis of a malaria model with partial immunity to reinfection, InAbstract and applied analysis 2013 (Vol. 2013), Hindawi.

94 Niger AM, Gumel AB, (2008)
Mathematical analysis of the role of repeated exposure on malaria transmission dynamics, Differential Equations and Dynamical Systems, 2008 Jul 1, 16(3), 251-87.

95 Ross R., (1911)
The prevention of malaria, John Murray, London, 1911.

96 Macdonald G., (1950)
The analysis of infection rates in diseases in which super infection occurs, Tropical diseases bulletin, 1950, 47, 907-15.

97 Macdonald G., (1956)
Theory of the eradication of malaria, Bulletin of the World Health Organization, 1956, 15(3-5), 369.

98 Gupta S, Snow RW, Donnelly CA, Marsh K, Newbold C, (1999)
Immunity to non-cerebral severe malaria is acquired after one or two infections, Nature medicine, 1999 Mar, 5(3), 340.

99 Aponte JJ, Menendez C, Schellenberg D, Kahigwa E, Mshinda H, Vountasou P, Tanner M, Alonso PL, (2007)
Age interactions in the development of naturally acquired immunity to Plasmodium falciparum and its clinical presentation, PLoS medicine, 2007 Jul 31, 4(7):e242.

100 Griffin JT, Hollingsworth TD, Reyburn H, Drakeley CJ, Riley EM, Ghani AC, (2015)
Gradual acquisition of immunity to severe malaria with increasing exposure, Proceedings of the Royal Society of London B: Biological Sciences, 2015 Feb 22, 282(1801):20142657.

101 Barry A, Hansen D., (2016)
Naturally acquired immunity to malaria, Parasitology, 2016 143(2), 125-128.

102 Gurarie D, McKenzie FE, (2007)
A stochastic model of immune-modulated malaria infection and disease in children, Mathematical biosciences, 2007 Dec 1, 210(2), 576-97.

103 Laneri K, Paul RE, Tall A, Faye J, Diene-Sarr F, Sokhna C, Trape JF, Rodó X., (2015)
Dynamical malaria models reveal how immunity buffers effect of climate variability, Proceedings of the National Academy of Sciences, 2015 Jul 14, 112(28), 8786-91.

104 Peyerl-Hoffmann G, Jelinek T, Kilian A, Kabagambe G, Metzger WG, Von Sonnenburg F., (2001)
Genetic diversity of Plasmodium falciparum and its relationship to parasite density in an area with different malaria endemicities in West Uganda, Tropical Medicine & International Health, 2001 Aug, 6(8), 607-13.

105 Deitsch, Kirk W.; DEL PINAL, Amy; Wellems, Thomas E., (1999)
Intra-cluster recombination and var transcription switches in the antigenic variation of Plasmodium falciparum, Molecular and biochemical parasitology, 1999, 101.1-2: 107-116.

106 Mwanga GG, Haario H, Nannyonga BK., (2012)
Spread of Antimalarial Drug Resistance in a Population with Superinfection, Applied Mathematical Sciences, 2012, 6(118):5877-900.

107 Klein EY, (2013)
Antimalarial drug resistance: a review of the biology and strategies to delay emergence and spread, International journal of antimicrobial agents, 2013 Apr 1, 41(4), 311-7.

108 Klein EY, Smith DL, Boni MF, Laxminarayan R., (2008)
Clinically immune hosts as a refuge for drug-sensitive malaria parasites, Malaria Journal, 2008 Dec, 7(1), 67.

109 de Vries P., (2001)
An Individual Oriented Approach to Modelling Demography, Malaria and Illness, InProceedings of the Workshop on Spatial Aspects of Demography 2001 (Vol. 200).

110 de Vries P, Martens P., (2000)
A Camera focus on local eco-epidemiological malaria risk assessment-a model in development, ICIS Workingpaper serie, 2000.

111 McKenzie FE, Bossert WH, (1998)
A target for intervention in Plasmodium falciparum infections, The American journal of tropical medicine and hygiene, 1998 Jun 1, 58(6):763-7.

112 Molineaux L, Dietz K., (1999)
Review of intra-host models of malaria, Parassitologia, 1999 Sep, 41(1/3):221-32.

113 Maire N, Tediosi F, Ross A, Smith T., (2006)
Predictions of the epidemiologic impact of introducing a pre-erythrocytic vaccine into the expanded program on immunization in sub-Saharan Africa, The American journal of tropical medicine and hygiene, 2006 Aug 1, 75(2_suppl):111-8.

114 Ross A, Killeen G, Smith T, (2006)
Relationships between host infectivity to mosquitoes and asexual parasite density in Plasmodium falciparum, The American journal of tropical medicine and hygiene, 2006 Aug 1, 75(2_suppl):32-7.

115 Ross A, Maire N, Molineaux L, (2006)
T. An epidemiologic model of severe morbidity and mortality caused by Plasmodium falciparum, The American journal of tropical medicine and hygiene, 2006 Aug 1, 75(2_suppl):63-73.

116 Tediosi F, Hutton GU, Maire N, Smith TA, Ross A, (2006)
Tanner M. Predicting the cost-effectiveness of introducing a pre-erythrocytic malaria vaccine into the expanded program on immunization in Tanzania, The American journal of tropical medicine and hygiene, 2006 Aug 1, 75(2_suppl):131-43.

117 Chen I, Clarke SE, Gosling R, Hamainza B, Killeen G, Magill A, O'Meara W, Price RN, Riley EM., (2016)
"Asymptomatic" malaria: a chronic and debilitating infection that should be treated, PLoS medicine, 2016 Jan 19, 13(1):e1001942.

118 Smith DL, Dushoff J, Snow RW, Hay SI., (2005)
The entomological inoculation rate and Plasmodium falciparum infection in African children, Nature, 2005 Nov, 438(7067):492.

119 Saul A. (1996)
Transmission dynamics of Plasmodium falciparum, Parasitology today, 1996 Feb 1, 12(2):74-9.

120 S, Swinton J, Anderson RM., (1994)
Theoretical studies of the effects of heterogeneity in the parasite population on the transmission dynamics of malaria, Proceedings of the Royal Society of London, Series B: Biological Sciences, 1994 Jun 22, 256(1347):231-8.

121 Gupta S, Trenholme K, Anderson RM, Day KP, (1994)
Antigenic diversity and the transmission dynamics of Plasmodium falciparum, Science, 1994 Feb 18, 263(5149):961-3.

122 Gupta S, P. Day KA, (1994)
A theoretical framework for the immunoepidemiology of Plasmodium falciparum malaria, Parasite immunology, 1994 Jul, 16(7):361-70.

123 Gupta, S.; Day, K. P., (1994)
A strain theory of malaria transmission, Parasitology Today, 1994, 10.12: 476-481.

124 Bretscher MT, Maire N, Felger I, Owusu-Agyei S, Smith T., (2015)
Asymptomatic Plasmodium falciparum infections may not be shortened by acquired immunity, Malaria journal, 2015 Dec, 14(1):294.

125 Bretscher MT, Maire N, Chitnis N, Felger I, Owusu-Agyei S, Smith T., (2011)
The distribution of Plasmodium falciparum infection durations. Epidemics, 2011 Jun 1, 3(2):109-18.

126 Collins WE, Jeffery GM, (1999)
A retrospective examination of secondary sporozoite-and trophozoite-induced infections with Plasmodium falciparum: development of parasitologic and clinical immunity following secondary infection, The American journal of tropical medicine and hygiene, 1999 Jul 1, 61(1_Supplement):20-35.

127 Collins WE, Jeffery GM., (1999)
A retrospective examination of sporozoite-and trophozoite-induced infections with Plasmodium falciparum in patients previously infected with heterologous species of Plasmodium: effect on development of parasitologic and clinical immunity, The American journal of tropical medicine and hygiene, 1999 Jul 1, 61(1_Supplement):36-43.

128 Collins WE, Jeffery GM, (1999)
A retrospective examination of the patterns of recrudescence in patients infected with Plasmodium falciparum, The American journal of tropical medicine and hygiene, 1999 Jul 1, 61(1_Supplement):44-8.

129 Duffy, P. E., Fried, M., (1999)
Malaria during pregnancy: parasites, antibodies and chondroitin sulphate A, Biochemical Society Transactions, 1999, 27.4: 478-482.

130 Struik, Siske S., Riley, Eleanor M., (2004)
Does malaria suffer from lack of memory?, Immunological reviews, 2004, 201.1: 268-290.

131 Bouchaud, Olivier, et al., (2005)
Do African immigrants living in France have long-term malarial immunity?, The American journal of tropical medicine and hygiene, 2005, 72.1: 21-25.

132 Bonner P., et al., (2014)
Parasite burden and severity of malaria in Tanzanian children, New England Journal of Medicine, 2014, 370.19: 1799-1808.

133 Crompton, Peter D., et al., Malaria immunity in man and mosquito: insights into unsolved mysteries of a deadly infectious disease, Annual review of immunology, 2014, 32: 157-187.

134 Smith, Thomas, et al., (2006)
An epidemiologic model of the incidence of acute illness in Plasmodium falciparum malaria, The American journal of tropical medicine and hygiene, 2006, 75.2_suppl: 56-62.

135 Thomas L. Richie, Falgunee K. Parekh, (2009)
Vaccines for Biodefense and Emerging and Neglected Diseases, 2009.

136 Good, Michael F.; Yanow, Stephanie K., (2017)
A whole parasite transmission-blocking vaccine for malaria: an ignored strategy, Emerging Topics in Life Sciences, 2017, 1.6: 547-552.

137 Yazdani, S. S., et al., (2006)
Immune responses to asexual blood-stages of malaria parasites, Current molecular medicine, 2006, 6.2: 187-203.

138 Dzikowski, Ron; Templeton, Thomas J.; Deitsch, Kirk, (2006)
Variant antigen gene expression in malaria, Cellular microbiology, 2006, 8.9: 1371-1381.

139 De Mendonca, Vitor RR; Goncalves, Marilda Souza; Barral-Netto, Manoel, (2012)
The host genetic diversity in malaria infection, Journal of tropical medicine, 2012.

140 Bachmann, Anna, et al., (2019)
Controlled human malaria infection with Plasmodium falciparum demonstrates impact of naturally acquired immunity on virulence gene expression, PLoS pathogens, 2019, 15.7: e1007906.

141 Davey, D. G.; Robertson, G., (1957)
I. Experiments with antimalarial drugs in man: II. A description of methods. Transactions of the Royal Society of Tropical Medicine and Hygiene, 1957, 51.5: 450-456.

142 Beeson, J. G.; Duffy, P. E., (2005)
The immunology and pathogenesis of malaria during pregnancy, In: Immunology and Immunopathogenesis of Malaria, Springer, Berlin, Heidelberg, 2005. p. 187-227.

143 MacDonald, George, et al., (1957)
The epidemiology and control of malaria. The Epidemiology and Control of Malaria, 1957.

144 Bailey, Norman TJ, et al., (1975)
The mathematical theory of infectious diseases and its applications, Charles Griffin & Company Ltd, 5a Crendon Street, High Wycombe, Bucks HP13 6LE., 1975.

145 Molineaux, L.; Dietz, K.; Thomas, A., (1978)
Further epidemiological evaluation of a malaria model, Bulletin of the World Health Organization, 1978, 56.4: 565.

146 Elderkin, R. H., et al., (1977)
On the steady state of an age dependent model for malaria, In: Nonlinear systems and applications, Academic Press, 1977, p. 491-512.

147 Bejon P, Williams TN, Liljander A, Noor AM, Wambua J, Ogada E, Olotu A, Osier FH, Hay SI, Färnert A, Marsh K., (2010)
Stable and unstable malaria hotspots in longitudinal cohort studies in Kenya, PLoS medicine, 2010 Jul 6, 7(7):e1000304.

148 Colbourne M., (1966)
Malaria in Africa, 1966.

149 Lee, Sulggi A., et al., (2006)
Complexity of Plasmodium falciparum infections and antimalarial drug efficacy at 7 sites in Uganda, The Journal of infectious diseases, 2006, 193.8: 1160-1163.

150 Chiyaka, C.; Garira, W.; Dube, S., (2007)
Transmission model of endemic human malaria in a partially immune population, Mathematical and computer modelling, 2007, 46.5-6: 806-822.

151 Chiyaka, C., et al., (2008)
A mathematical analysis of the effects of control strategies on the transmission dynamics of malaria, Applied Mathematics and Computation, 2008, 195.2: 641-662.

152 Chiyaka, Christinah; Garira, Winston; Dube, Shadreck, (2009)
Effects of treatment and drug resistance on the transmission dynamics of malaria in endemic areas, Theoretical population biology, 2009, 75.1: 14-29.

153 Chiyaka C, Tatem AJ, Cohen JM, Gething PW, Johnston G, Gosling R, Laxminarayan R, Hay SI, Smith DL, (2013)
The stability of malaria elimination. Science. 2013 Feb 22;339(6122):909-10.

154 Smith, David L., et al., (2013)
A sticky situation: the unexpected stability of malaria elimination, Philosophical Transactions of the Royal Society B: Biological Sciences, 2013, 368.1623: 20120145.

155 McKenzie, F. Ellis; Bossert, William H., (2005)
An integrated model of Plasmodium falciparum dynamics, Journal of theoretical biology, 2005, 232.3: 411-426.

156 Brown, K. N., et al., (1966)
Immunity to malaria: antigenic variation in chronic infections of Plasmodium knowlesi, Geneva, World Health Organization, 1966.

157 Griffin, Jamie T., (2016)
Is a reproduction number of one a threshold for Plasmodium falciparum malaria elimination?, Malaria journal, 2016, 15.1: 389.

158 Killeen, Gerry F., et al., (2018)
Entomological surveillance as a cornerstone of malaria elimination: a critical appraisal, Towards malaria elimination—a leap forward, London, InTech, 2018, 403-29.

159 Smith, Thomas, et al., (2006)
Mathematical modeling of the impact of malaria vaccines on the clinical epidemiology and natural history of Plasmodium falciparum malaria: Overview, The American journal of tropical medicine and hygiene, 2006, 75.2_suppl: 1-10.

160 Killeen, Gerry F.; Ross, Amanda; Smith, Thomas, (2006)
Infectiousness of malaria-endemic human populations to vectors, The American journal of tropical medicine and hygiene, 2006, 75.2_suppl: 38-45.

161 Tediosi, Fabrizio, et al., (2006)
An approach to model the costs and effects of case management of Plasmodium falciparum malaria in sub-Saharan Africa, The American journal of tropical medicine and hygiene, 2006, 75.2_suppl: 90-103.

162 Hviid L, Staalsoe T., (2004)
Malaria immunity in infants: a special case of a general phenomenon?, Trends in parasitology, 2004 Feb 1, 20(2):66-72.

163 Ashley EA, White NJ, (2014)
The duration of Plasmodium falciparum infections, Malaria journal, 2014 Dec 1, 13(1):500.

164 Pilosof S, He Q, Tiedje KE, Ruybal-Pesantez S, Day KP, Pascual M., (2019)
Competition for hosts modulates vast antigenic diversity to generate persistent strain structure in Plasmodium falciparum, PLoS biology, 2019 Jun 24, 17(6):e3000336.

165 Smith T, Felger I, Tanner M, Beck HP, (1999)
11. Premunition in Plasmodium falciparum infection: insights from the epidemiology of multiple infections, Transactions of the Royal Society of Tropical Medicine and Hygiene, 1999 Feb 1, 93(Supplement_1):59-64.

166 Beck, H.P., et al., (1997)
Analysis of multiple Plasmodium falciparum infections in Tanzanian children during the phase III trial of the malaria vaccine SPf66, Journal of Infectious Diseases, 1997, 175.4: 921-926.

167 Sondo, Paul, et al., (2019)
Genetically diverse Plasmodium falciparum infections, within-host competition and symptomatic malaria in humans, Scientific reports, 2019, 9.1: 127.

168 Sergent E, Parrot L., (1935)
L'immunité, la prémunition et la résistance innée, Archives de l'institut Pasteur d'Algérie, 1935;13:279-319.

169 Cohen S, Deans JA., (1988)
Specific acquired immunity in experimental malaria, Malaria: principles and practice of malariology, 1988;1:515-57.

170 Baird JK, Jones TR, Danudirgo EW, Annis BA, Bangs MJ, Basri PH, Masbar S., (1991)
Age-dependent acquired protection against Plasmodium falciparum in people having two years exposure to hyperendemic malaria, The American journal of tropical medicine and hygiene, 1991 Jul 1;45(1):65-76.

171 Druilhe, P.; Perignon, J. L., (1997)
A hypothesis about the chronicity of malaria infection, Parasitology Today, 1997, 13.9: 353-357.

172 Kwiatkowski, D., (1991)
Cytokines and anti-disease immunity to malaria, Research in immunology, 1991, 142.8: 707-712.

173 Recker M, Nee S, Bull PC, Kinyanjui S, Marsh K, Newbold C, Gupta S., (2004)
Transient cross-reactive immune responses can orchestrate antigenic variation in malaria, Nature, 2004 Jun;429(6991):555.

174 BOUDIN, Christian, et al. Plasmodium falciparum transmission blocking immunity under conditions of low and high endemicity in Cameroon. Parasite immunology, 2004, 26.2: 105-110.

175 Lindsay, S. W., et al., (1989)
Impact of permethrin-treated bednets on malaria transmission by the *Anopheles gambiae* complex in The Gambia, Medical and veterinary entomology, 1989, 3.3: 263-271.

176 Babiker HA, Ranford-Cartwright LC, Walliker D., (1999)
3. Genetic structure and dynamics of Plasmodium falciparum infections in the Kilombero region of Tanzania, Transactions of the Royal Society of Tropical Medicine and Hygiene, 1999 Feb 1, 93:11-4.

177 Ranford-Cartwright LC, Balfe P, Carter R, Walliker D., (1993)
Frequency of cross-fertilization in the human malaria parasite Plasmodium falciparum, Parasitology, 1993 Jul, 107(1).11-8.

178 Walliker D, (1989)
Genetic recombination in malaria parasites, Exp Parasitol, 69: 303–309.

179 Reeder JC, Davern KM, Baird JK, Rogerson SJ, Brown GV, (1997)
The age-specific prevalence of Plasmodium falciparum in migrants to Irian Jaya is not attributable to agglutinating antibody repertoire, Acta tropica, 1997 May 30, 65(3):163-73.

180 Bull PC, Marsh K., (2002)
The role of antibodies to Plasmodium falciparum-infected-erythrocyte surface antigens in naturally acquired immunity to malaria, Trends in microbiology, 2002 Feb 1, 10(2):55-8.

181 Aron, Joan L., (1982)
Malaria epidemiology and detectability, Transactions of the Royal Society of Tropical Medicine and Hygiene, 1982, 76.5: 595-601.

182 Nedelman, Jerry, (1989)
Gametocytemia and infectiousness in falciparum malaria: observations and models, In: Advances in Disease Vector Research, Springer, New York, NY, 1989, p. 59-89.

183 Drakeley, Chris, et al., (2006)
The epidemiology of Plasmodium falciparum gametocytes: weapons of mass dispersion, Trends in parasitology, 2006, 22.9: 424-430.

184 Muirhead-Thomson, R. C., (1957)
The malarial infectivity of an African village population to mosquitoes (*Anopheles gambiae*), The American journal of tropical medicine and hygiene, 1957, 6.6: 971-979.

185 MacDonald, George., (1951)
Community Aspects of Immunity to Malaria, British medical bulletin, 1951, 8.1: 33-36.

186 Giha HA, Staalsoe T, Dodoo D, Elhassan IM, Roper C, Satti GM, Arnot DE, Theander TG, Hviid, L., (1999)
Nine-year longitudinal study of antibodies to variant antigens on the surface of Plasmodium falciparum-infected erythrocytes, Infection and immunity. 1999 Aug 1, 67(8):4092-8.

187 Eckhoff PA., (2011)
A malaria transmission-directed model of mosquito life cycle and ecology, Malaria journal, 2011 Dec 1, 10(1):303.

188 Smith, T., et al., (1999)
7. Dynamics of multiple Plasmodium falciparum infections in infants in a highly endemic area of Tanzania, Transactions of the Royal Society of Tropical Medicine and Hygiene, 1999, 93.Supplement_1 : 35-39.

189 Genton, B., et al., (1995)
The epidemiology of malaria in the Wosera area, East Sepik Province, Papua New Guinea, in preparation for vaccine trials I. Malariometric indices and immunity, Annals of Tropical Medicine & Parasitology, 1995, 89.4: 359-376.

190 Al-Yaman, F., et al., (1997)
Reduced risk of clinical malaria in children infected with multiple clones of Plasmodium falciparum in a highly endemic area: a prospective community study, Transactions of the Royal Society of Tropical Medicine and Hygiene, 1997, 91.5: 602-605.

191 Smith, Tom; Vounatsou, Penelope, (2003)
Estimation of infection and recovery rates for highly polymorphic parasites when detectability is imperfect, using hidden Markov models, Statistics in medicine, 2003, 22.10: 1709-1724.

192 Eckhoff, Philip, (2012)
P. falciparum infection durations and infectiousness are shaped by antigenic variation and innate and adaptive host immunity in a mathematical model, PloS one, 2012, 7.9: e44950.

193 Smith T, Beck HP, Kitua A, Mwankusye S, Felger I, Fraser-Hurt N, Irion A, Alonso P, Teuscher T, Tanner M., (1999)
4. Age dependence of the multiplicity of Plasmodium falciparum infections and of other malariological indices in an area of high endemicity, Transactions of the Royal Society of Tropical Medicine and Hygiene, 1999 Feb 1, 93:15-20.

194 Smith T, Ross A, Maire N, Chitnis N, Studer A, Hardy D, Brooks A, Penny M, Tanner M., (2012)
Ensemble modeling of the likely public health impact of a pre-erythrocytic malaria vaccine, PLoS Med., 2012 Jan 17, 9(1):e1001157.

195 Hafalla JC, Silvie O, Matuschewski K., (2011)
Cell biology and immunology of malaria, Immunological reviews, 2011 Mar, 240(1):297-316.

196 Amadi M, Shcherbacheva A, Haario H., (2021)
Agent-based modelling of complex factors impacting malaria prevalence, Malaria journal, 2021 Dec, 20(1):1-5.

197 Nahrendorf W, Scholzen A, Sauerwein RW, Langhorne J., (2015)
Cross-stage immunity for malaria vaccine development, Vaccine, 2015 Dec 22, 33(52):7513-7.

198 Ross A, Smith T, (2010)
Interpreting malaria age-prevalence and incidence curves: a simulation study of the effects of different types of heterogeneity, Malaria journal, 2010 Dec, 9(1):1-9.

199 Cushing JE, Campbell DH, (1957)
Principles Of Immunology, Principles of Immunology, 1957.

200 Rodriguez-Barraquer I, Arinaitwe E, Jagannathan P, Kamya MR, Rosenthal PJ, Rek J, Dorsey G, Nankabirwa J, Staedke SG, Kilama M, Drakeley C., (2018)
Quantification of anti-parasite and anti-disease immunity to malaria as a function of age and exposure, Elife, 2018 Jul 25, 7:e35832.

201 Trieu A, Kayala MA, Burk C, Molina DM, Freilich DA, Richie TL, Baldi P, Felgner PL, Doolan DL, (2011)
Sterile protective immunity to malaria is associated with a panel of novel *P. falciparum* antigens, Molecular & Cellular Proteomics, 2011 May 31, mcp-M111.

202 Bousema T, Okell L, Felger I, Drakeley C., (2014)
Asymptomatic malaria infections: detectability, transmissibility and public health relevance, Nature reviews Microbiology, 2014 Dec, 12(12):833.

203 Macdonald G., (1952)
The analysis of equilibrium in malaria, Tropical diseases bulletin, 1952 Sep, 49(9):813.

204 Dye C., (1986)
Vectorial capacity: must we measure all its components?, Parasitology Today, 1986 Aug 1, 2(8):203-9.

205 Smith T, Maire N, Dietz K, Killeen GF, Vounatsou P, Molineaux L, Tanner M., (2006)
Relationship between the entomologic inoculation rate and the force of infection for Plasmodium falciparum malaria, The American journal of tropical medicine and hygiene, 2006 Aug 1, 75(2_suppl):11-8.

206 Gumel AB, (2012)
Causes of backward bifurcations in some epidemiological models, Journal of Mathematical Analysis and Applications, 2012 Nov 1, 395(1):355-65.

207 Sachs J, Malaney P, (2002)
The economic and social burden of malaria, Nature, 2002 Feb, 415(6872):680-5.

208 Gallup JL, Sachs JD, (2001)
The economic burden of malaria, The American journal of tropical medicine and hygiene, 2001 Jan 1, 64(1_suppl):85-96.

209 Baird, J. Kevin, et al., (2002)
Epidemiological measures of risk of malaria, In: Malaria methods and protocols, Humana Press, 2002, p. 13-22.

210 Drakeley, C., et al., (2003)
An estimation of the entomological inoculation rate for Ifakara: A semi-urban area in a region of intense malaria transmission in Tanzania, Tropical Medicine & International Health, 2003, 8.9: 767-774.

211 Ademolue TW, Awandare GA, (2018)
Evaluating antidisease immunity to malaria and implications for vaccine design, Immunology, 2018 Apr, 153(4):423-34.

212 Smith, David L., et al., (2007)
Revisiting the basic reproductive number for malaria and its implications for malaria control, PLoS Biol, 2007, 5.3: e42.

213 Sama W, Killeen G, Smith T, (2004)
Estimating the duration of Plasmodium falciparum infection from trials of indoor residual spraying, The American journal of tropical medicine and hygiene, 2004 Jun 1, 70(6):625-34.

214 Ross A, Smith T., (2006)
The effect of malaria transmission intensity on neonatal mortality in endemic areas, The American journal of tropical medicine and hygiene, 2006 Aug 1, 75(2_suppl):74-81.

215 Deloron P, Chougnet C., (1992)
Is immunity to malaria really short-lived?, Parasitology today, 1992 Nov 1, 8(11):375-8.

216 Chaplin DD, (2010)
Overview of the immune response, Journal of Allergy and Clinical Immunology, 2010 Feb 1, 125(2):S3-23.

217 Indrayan A., (2019)
Research Methods for Medical Graduates, CRC Press, 2019 Oct 16.

Part (III):
Mathematical Epidemiology including Mosquito Dynamics and Control Theory

Chapter 7:
Multi-Strain Host-Vector Dengue Modeling: Dynamics and Control

1 M. Aguiar, S. Ballesteros, B. W. Kooi, and N. Stollenwerk, (2011)
The role of seasonality and import in a minimalistic multi-strain dengue model capturing differences between primary and secondary infections: complex dynamics and its implications for data analysis. *J Theor Biol*, 289:181-196, 2011.

2 M. Aguiar, B. W. Kooi, and N. Stollenwerk, (2008)
Epidemiology of dengue fever: a model with temporary cross-immunity and possible secondary infection shows bifurcations and chaotic behaviour in wide parameter regions. *Math Model Nat Phenom*, 3:48-70, 2008.

3 M. Aguiar, N. Stollenwerk, and S. B. Halstead, (2016)
The impact of the newly licensed dengue vaccine in endemic countries. *PLoS Negl Trop Dis*, 10:e5179, 2016.

4 B. M. Althouse, J. Lessler, A. A. Sall, M. Diallo, K. A. Hanley, D. M. Watts, S. C. Weaver, and D. A. T. Cummings, (2012)
Synchrony of sylvatic dengue isolations: A multi-host, multi-vector SIR model of dengue virus transmission in Senegal. *PLoS Negl Trop Dis*, 6(11):e1928, 2012.

5 R. M. Anderson and R. M. May, (1991)
Infectious Diseases of Humans: Dynamics and Optimal Control. Oxford University Press, Oxford, 1991.

6 H. Andersson and T. Britton, (2000)
Stochastic Epidemic Models and Their Statistical Analysis. Springer, 2000.

7 M. Andraud, N. Hens, C. Marais, and P. Beutels, (2012)
Dynamic epidemiological models for dengue transmission: A systematic review of structural approaches. *PLoS One*, 7:e349085, 2012.

8 J. Antonovics, (2017)
Transmission dynamics: critical questions and challenges, *Phil. Trans. R. Soc. B*, 372:20160087, 2017.

9 M. Bardi and I. Capuzzo-Dolcetta, (2008)
Optimal Control and Viscosity Solutions of Hamilton-Jacobi-Bellman Equations. Birkhäuser, Basel, 2008.

10 D. Bichara and C. Castillo-Chavez, (2016)
Vector-borne diseases models with residence times - A Lagrangian perspective, *Math Biosci*, 281:128-138, 2016.

11 D. Bichara and A. Iggidr, (2018)
Multi-patch and multi-group epidemic models: a new framework, *J Math Biol*, 77:107-134, 2018.

12 L. Billings, I. B. Schwartz, L. B. Shaw, M. McCrary, D. S. Burke, and D. A. T., Cummings, (2007)
Instabilities in multiserotype disease models with antibody-dependent enhancement. *J Theor Biol*, 246:18-27, 2007.

13 B. Buonomo, N. Chitnis, and A. d'Onofrio, (2018)
Seasonality in epidemic models: a literature review. *Ricerche mat*, 67:7-25, 2018.

14 B. Buonomo and R. Della Marca, (2018)
Optimal bed net use for a dengue disease model with mosquito seasonal pattern. *Math Meth Appl Sci*, 41(2):573-592, 2018.

15 V. Capasso and G. Serio, (1978)
A generalization of the Kermack-McKendrick deterministic epidemic model. *Math Biosci*, 42, 43-61, 1978.

16 P. Chanprasopchai, I. Ming Tang, and P. Pongsumpun, (2018)
SIR Model for Dengue Disease with Effect of Dengue Vaccination. *Comput Math Meth Medicine*, 9861572, 2018.

17 M. De Lara and L. S. Sepulveda Salcedo, (2016)
Viable control of an epidemiological model. *Math Biosci*, 280:24-37, 2016.

18 O. Diekmann and J. A. P. Heesterbeek, (2000)
Mathematical epidemiology of infectious diseases. Wiley series in mathematical and computional biology. Wiley, Chichester, 2000.

19 O. Diekmann, J. A. P. Heesterbeek, and J. A. J. Metz, (1990)
On the definition and the computation of the basic reproduction ratio R_0 in models for infectious diseases in heterogeneous populations. *J Math Biol*, 28:365-382, 1990.

20 O. Diekmann, M. de Jong, A. de Koeijer, and P. Reijnders, (1995)
The force of infection in populations of varying size: a modelling problem. *J Biol Systems*, 3(2):519-529, 1995.

21 K. Dietz, (1982)
Overall population patterns in the transmission cycle of infectious disease agents, in *Population Biology of Infectious Diseases* (R. M. Anderson and R. M. May, eds.), Springer, Berlin, Heidelberg, 1982, 87-102.

22 L. Esteva and C. Vargas, (1998)
Analysis of a dengue disease transmission model. *Math Biosci*, 150(2):131-151, 1998.

23 L. Esteva and C. Vargas, (2000)
Influence of vertical and mechanical transmission on the dynamics of dengue disease. *Math Biosci*, 167:51-64, 2000.

24 L. Esteva and C. Vargas, (2003)
Coexistence of different serotypes of dengue virus. *J Math Biol*, 46:31-47, 2003.

25 Z. Feng and J. X. Velasco-Hernandez, (1997)
Competitive exclusion in a vector-host model for the dengue fever. *J Math Biol*, 35:523-544, 1997.

26 N. Ferguson, R. Anderson, and S. Gupta, (1999)
The effect of antibody-dependent enhancement on the transmission dynamics and persistence of multiple-strain pathogens. *Proc Natl Acad Sci USA*, 96(9):790-794, 1999.

27 S. M. Garba, A. B. Gumel, and M. R. Abu Bakar, (2008)
Backward bifurcations in dengue transmission dynamics. *Math Biosci*, 215:11-25, 2008.

28 M. G. Guzman, M. Alvarez, and S. B. Halstead, (2013)
Secondary infection as a risk factor for dengue hemorrhagic fever/dengue shock syndrome: an historical perspective and role of antibody-dependent enhancement of infection. *Arch Virol*, 158:1445-59, 2013.

29 K. P. Hadeler and P. van den Driessche, (1997)
Backward bifurcation in epidemic control. *Math Biosci*, 146:15-35, 1997.

30 S. B. Halstead, (2003)
Neutralization and antibody-dependent enhancement of dengue viruses. *Adv Virus Res*, 60:421-467, 2003.

31 G. Hek, (2010)
Geometric singular perturbation theory in biological practice. *J Math Biol*, 60:347-386, 2010.

32 M. A. Johansson, J. Hombach, and D. A. T. Cummings, (2011)
Models of the impact of dengue vaccines: A review of current research and potential approaches. *Vaccine*, 29:5860-5868, 2011.

33 I. Z. Kiss, J. Miller, and P. L. Simon, (2017)
Mathematics of Epidemics on Networks. Springer, 2017.

34 B. W. Kooi, M. Aguiar, and N. Stollenwerk, (2013)
Bifurcation analysis of a family of multi-strain epidemiology models. *J Comput Appl Math*, 252:148-158, 2013.

35 B. W. Kooi, M. Aguiar, and N. Stollenwerk, (2014)
Analysis of an asymmetric two-strain dengue model. *Math Biosci*, 248:128-139, 2014.

36 B. W. Kooi, G. A. K. van Voorn and K. P. Das, (2011)
Stabilization and complex dynamics in a predator-prey model with predator suffering from an infectious disease, *Ecol Complex*, 8: 113-122, 2011.

37 A. A. Momoh and A. Fügenschuh, (2018)
Optimal control of intervention strategies and cost effectiveness analysis for a Zika virus model. *Oper Res Health Care*, 18:99-111, 2018.

38 G. G. Mwanga, H. Haario, and V. Capasso, (2015)
Optimal control problems of epidemic systems with parameter uncertainties: Application to a malaria two-age-classes transmission model with asymptomatic carriers. *Math Biosci*, 261:1-12, 2015.

39 H. Nishiura, (2006)
Mathematical and statistical analyses of the spread of dengue.

Dengue Bulletin, 30(51):67, 2006.

40 P. Rashkov, (2021)
A model for a vector-borne disease with control based on mosquito repellents: a viability analysis. *J Math Anal Appl*, 498: 124958, 2021.

41 P. Rashkov and B. W. Kooi, (2021)
Complexity of host-vector dynamics in a two-strain dengue model. *J Biol Dynam*, 15: 35-72, 2021.

42 P. Rashkov, E. Venturino, M. Aguiar, N. Stollenwerk, and B. W. Kooi, (2019)
On the role of vector modeling in a minimalistic epidemic model. *Math Biosci Eng*, 16(5):4314-4338, 2019.

43 M. Recker, K. B. Blyuss, C. P. Simmons, T. T. Hien, B. Wills, J. Farrar, and S. Gupta, (2009)
Immunological serotype interactions and their effect on the epidemiological pattern of dengue. *Proc Royal Soc B*, 276(1667):2541-2548, 2009.

44 F. Rocha, M. Aguiar, M. Souza, and N. Stollenwerk, (2013)
Time-scale separation and centre manifold analysis describing vector-borne disease dynamics. *Int J Comput Math*, 90(10):2105-2125, 2013.

45 H. S. Rodrigues, M. T. T. Monteiro, D. F. M. Torres and A. Zinober, (2012)
Dengue disease, basic reproduction number and control, *Int J Comp Math*, 89(3):334-346, 2012.

46 H. S. Rodrigues, M. T. T. Monteiro, and D. F. M. Torres, (2016)
Seasonality effects on dengue: basic reproduction number, sensitivity analysis and optimal control. *Math Meth Appl Sci*, 39(16):4671-4679, 2016.

47 H. S. Rodrigues, M. T. T. Monteiro, D. F. M. Torres, A. C. Silva, C. Sousa, and C. Conceição, (2015)
Dengue in Madeira island. In *Dynamics, Games and Science - International Conference and Advanced School Planet Earth, DGS II, Portugal, August 28-September 6, 2013* (J-P. Bourguignon, R. Jeltsch, A. A. Pinto, and M. Viana, eds.), Springer International, 2015, pages 593-605.

48 H. S. Rodrigues, M. T. T. Monteiro, and D. F. M. Torres, (2014)
Vaccination models and optimal control strategies to dengue. *Math Biosci*, 247:1-12, 2014.

49 I. B. Schwartz, L. B. Shaw, D. A. T. Cummings, L. Billings, M. McCrary, and D. S. Burke, (2005)
Chaotic desynchronization of multistrain diseases. *Phys Rev E*, 27:066201, 2005.

50 M. O. Souza, (2014)
Multiscale analysis for a vector-borne epidemic model. *J Math Biol*, 68(5):1269-1293, 2014.

51 Y. A. McLennan-Smith and G. N. Mercer, (2014)
Complex behaviour in a dengue model with a seasonally varying vector population. *Math Biosci*, 248, 22-30, 2014.

52 N. Stollenwerk and P. F. Sommer, B. W. Kooi, L. Mateus, P. Ghaffari, M. Aguiar, (2017)
Hopf and torus bifurcations, torus destruction and chaos in population biology *Ecol. Compl.*, 30, 91-99, 2017.

53 P. van den Driessche and J. Watmough, (2002)
Reproduction numbers and sub-threshold endemic equilibria for compartmental models of disease transmission. *Math Biosci*, 180:29-48, 2002.

54 T-T. Zheng and L-F. Nie, (2018)
Modelling the transmission dynamics of two-strain Dengue in the presence awareness and vector control. *J Theor Biol*, 443:82-91, 2018.

Chapter 8:

Mathematical Models and Optimal Control in Mosquito Transmitted Diseases

1 Bamgboye M. Afolabi, Olayemi T. Sofola, Bayo S. Fatunmbi, William Komakech, Festus Okoh, Oladele Saliu, Peju Otsemobor, Olusola B. Oresanya, Chioma N. Amajoh, David Fasiku, and Inuwa Jalingo, (2009)
Household possession, use and non-use of treated or untreated mosquito nets in two ecologically diverse regions of Nigeria – Niger Delta and Sahel Savannah. *Malaria Journal*, 8(1), 2009.

2 Folashade B. Agusto, Sara Y. Del Valle, Kbenesh W. Blayneh, Calistus N. Ngonghala, Maria J. Goncalves, Nianpeng Li, Ruijun Zhao, and Hongfei Gong, (2013)
The impact of bed-net use on malaria prevalance. *J. Theoret. Biol.*, 320:58-65, 2013.

3 Folashade B. Agusto and Jean M. Tchuenche, (2013)
Control strategies for the spread of malaria in humans with variable attractiveness. *Math. Popul. Stud.*, 20(2):82-100, 2013.

4 Nauman Ahmed, Muhammad Rafiq, Dumitru Baleanu, Ali Saleh Alshomrani, and Muhammad Aziz-ur Rehman, (2020)
Positive explicit and implicit computational techniques for reaction-diffusion epidemic model of dengue disease dynamics. *Adv. Difference Equ.*, pages Paper No. 202, 22, 2020.

5 Karam Allali, Sanaa Harroudi, and Delfim F. M. Torres, (2018)
Analysis and optimal control of an intracellular delayed HIV model with CTL immune response. *Math. Comput. Sci.*, 12(2):111-127, 2018.

6 Ebraheem O. Alzahrani, Wisal Ahmad, Muhammad Altaf Khan, and Sharaf J. Malebary, (2021)
Optimal Control Strategies of Zika Virus Model with Mutant. *Commun. Nonlinear Sci. Numer. Simul.*, 93:105532, 2021.

7 AMPL
AMPL streamlined modeling for real optimization.

8 Iván Area, Faïçal Ndaïrou, Juan J. Nieto, Cristiana J. Silva, and Delfim F. M. Torres, (2018)
Ebola model and optimal control with vaccination constraints. *J. Ind. Manag. Optim.*, 14(2):427-446, 2018.

9 Martin Bohner, Sabrina Streipert, and Delfim F. M. Torres, (2019)
Exact solution to a dynamic SIR model. *Nonlinear Anal. Hybrid Syst.*, 32:228-238, 2019.

10 Carlos Campos, Cristiana J. Silva, and Delfim F. M. Torres, (2020)
Numerical optimal control of HIV transmission in Octave/MATLAB. *Math. Comput. Appl.*, 25(1):25010001-25010000, 2020.

11 Lamberto Cesari, (1983)
Optimization–theory and applications, volume 17 of *Applications of Mathematics (New York)*. Springer-Verlag, New York, 1983.

12 Iboi Enahoro, Steffen Eikenberry, Abba B. Gumel, Silvie Huijben, and Krijn Paaijmans, (2020)
Long-lasting insecticidal nets and the quest for malaria eradication: a mathematical modeling approach. *J. Math. Biol.*, 81(1):113-158, 2020.

13 Wendell H. Fleming and Raymond W. Rishel, (1975)
Deterministic and stochastic optimal control. Springer-Verlag, Berlin-New York, 1975.

14 Bushra Hasan, Manmohan Singh, David Richards, and Aaron Blicblau, (2019)
Mathematical modelling of Zika virus as a mosquito-borne and sexually transmitted disease with diffusion effects. *Math. Comput. Simulation*, 166:56-75, 2019.

15 Doracelly Hincapié-Palacio, Juan Ospina, and Delfim F. M. Torres, (2016)
Approximated analytical solution to an Ebola optimal control problem. *Int. J. Comput. Methods Eng. Sci. Mech.*, 17(5-6):382-390, 2016.

16 Rashid Jan, Muhammad Altaf Khan, Poom Kumam, and Phatiphat Thounthong, (2019)
Modeling the transmission of dengue infection through fractional derivatives. *Chaos Solitons Fractals*, 127:189-216, 2019.

17 E. Jung, S. Lenhart, and Z. Feng, (2002)
Optimal control of treatments in a two-strain tuberculosis model. *Discrete Contin. Dyn. Syst. Ser. B*, 2(4):473-482, 2002.

18 Gerry F. Killeen and Thomas A. Smith, (2007)
Exploring the contributions of bed nets, cattle, insecticides and excitorepellency to malaria control: a deterministic model of mosquito host-seeking behaviour and mortality. *Transactions of the Royal Society of Tropical Medicine and Hygiene*, 101(9):867-880, 2007.

19 Olena Kostylenko, Helena Sofia Rodrigues, and Delfim F. M. Torres, (2019)
The risk of contagion spreading and its optimal control in the economy. *Stat. Optim. Inf. Comput.*, 7(3):578-587, 2019.

20 Ana P. Lemos-Paião, Cristiana J. Silva, and Delfim F. M. Torres, (2017)
An epidemic model for cholera with optimal control treatment. *J. Comput. Appl. Math.*, 318:168-180, 2017.

21 Ana P. Lemos-Paião, Cristiana J. Silva, Delfim F. M. Torres, and Ezio Venturino, (2020)
Optimal control of aquatic diseases: a case study of Yemen's cholera outbreak. *J. Optim. Theory Appl.*, 185(3):1008-1030, 2020.

22 Christian Lengeler and R. W. Snow, (1996)
From efficacy to effectiveness: insecticide-treated bednets in Africa. *Bulletin of the World Health Organization*, 74(3):325-332, 1996.

23 John Leventides and Iraklis Kollias, (2014)
Optimal control indicators for the assessment of the influence of government policy to business cycle shocks. *J. Dyn. Games*, 1(1):79-104, 2014.

24 Yijie Li, Zhiming Guo, and Yanyuan Xing, (2020)
Modeling *wolbachia* diffusion in mosquito populations by discrete competition model. *Discrete Dyn. Nat. Soc.*, pages Art. ID 8987490, 11, 2020.

25 Kate Macintyre, Joseph Keating, Yohannes B. Okbaldt, Mehari Zerom, Stephen Sosler, Tewolde Ghebremeskel, and Thomas P. Eisele, (2006)
Rolling out insecticide treated nets in Eritrea: examining the determinants of possession and use in malarious zones during the rainy season. *Tropical Medicine and International Health*, 11(6):824-833, 2006.

26 Joseph Malinzi, Rachid Ouifki, Amina Eladdadi, Delfim F. M. Torres, and K. A. Jane White, (2018)
Enhancement of chemotherapy using oncolytic virotherapy: mathematical and optimal control analysis. *Math. Biosci. Eng.*, 15(6):1435-1463, 2018.

27 Carrie A. Manore, Kyle S. Hickmann, James M. Hyman, Ivo M. Foppa, Justin K. Davis, Dawn M. Wesson, and Christopher N. Mores, (2015)
A network-patch methodology for adapting agent-based models for directly transmitted disease to mosquito-borne disease. *J. Biol. Dyn.*, 9(1):52-72, 2015.

28 Joaquim P. Mateus, Paulo Rebelo, Silvério Rosa, César M. Silva, and Delfim F. M. Torres, (2018)
Optimal control of non-autonomous SEIRS models with vaccination and treatment. *Discrete Contin. Dyn. Syst. Ser. S*, 11(6):1179-1199, 2018.

29 Radu Miron, (2002)
Lagrange and Hamilton spaces: geometrical models in mechanics, new theoretical physics, variational calculus and optimal control. *Cubo Mat. Educ.*, 4(2):227-251, 2002.

30 Sk Shahid Nadim, Indrajit Ghosh, Maia Martcheva, and Joydev Chattopadhyay, (2020)
Impact of venereal transmission on the dynamics of vertically transmitted viral diseases among mosquitoes. *Math. Biosci.*, 325:108366, 10, 2020.

31 Faïçal Ndaïrou, Iván Area, Juan J. Nieto, Cristiana J. Silva, and Delfim F. M. Torres, (2018)
Mathematical modeling of Zika disease in pregnant women and newborns with microcephaly in Brazil. *Math. Methods Appl. Sci.*, 41(18):8929-8941, 2018.

32 Calistus N. Ngonghala, Josephine Wairimu, Jesse Adamski, and Hardik Desai, (2020)
Impact of adaptive mosquito behavior and insecticide-treated nets on malaria prevalence. *J. Biol. Systems*, 28(2):515-542, 2020.

33 S. Olaniyi, K. O. Okosun, S. O. Adesanya, and R. S. Lebelo, (2020)
Modelling malaria dynamics with partial immunity and protected travellers: optimal control and cost-effectiveness analysis. *J. Biol. Dyn.*, 14(1):90-115, 2020.

34 L. S. Pontryagin, V. G. Boltyanskii, R. V. Gamkrelidze, and E. F. Mishchenko, (1962)
The mathematical theory of optimal processes. Translated from the Russian by K. N. Trirogoff; edited by L. W. Neustadt. Interscience Publishers John Wiley & Sons, Inc. New York-London, 1962.

35 B. G. Sampath Aruna Pradeep and Wanbiao Ma, (2015)
Global stability of a delayed mosquito-transmitted disease model with stage structure. *Electron. J. Differential Equations*, pages No. 10, 19, 2015.

36 Amira Rachah and Delfim F. M. Torres, (2018)
Analysis, simulation and optimal control of a SEIR model for Ebola virus with demographic effects. *Commun. Fac. Sci. Univ. Ank. Sér. A1 Math. Stat.*, 67(1):179-197, 2018.

37 Diana Rocha, Cristiana J. Silva, and Delfim F. M. Torres, (2018)
Stability and optimal control of a delayed HIV model. *Math. Methods Appl. Sci.*, 41(6):2251-2260, 2018.

38 Filipe Rodrigues, Cristiana J. Silva, Delfim F. M. Torres, and Helmut Maurer, (2018)
Optimal control of a delayed HIV model. *Discrete Contin. Dyn. Syst. Ser. B*, 23(1):443-458, 2018.

39 Helena Sofia Rodrigues, M. Teresa T. Monteiro, and Delfim F. M. Torres, (2010)
Dynamics of dengue epidemics when using optimal control. *Math. Comput. Modelling*, 52(9-10):1667-1673, 2010.

40 Helena Sofia Rodrigues, M. Teresa T. Monteiro, and Delfim F. M. Torres, (2016)
Seasonality effects on dengue: basic reproduction number, sensitivity analysis and optimal control. *Math. Methods Appl. Sci.*, 39(16):4671-4679, 2016.

41 Helena Sofia Rodrigues, M. Teresa T. Monteiro, Delfim F. M. Torres, and Alan Zinober, (2012)
Dengue disease, basic reproduction number and control. *Int. J. Comput. Math.*, 89(3):334-346, 2012.

42 Silvério Rosa and Delfim F. M. Torres, (2018)
Optimal control of a fractional order epidemic model with application to human respiratory syncytial virus infection. *Chaos Solitons Fractals*, 117:142-149, 2018.

43 Tridip Sardar, Sourav Rana, Sabyasachi Bhattacharya, Kamel Al-Khaled, and Joydev Chattopadhyay, (2015)
A generic model for a single strain mosquito-transmitted disease with memory on the host and the vector. *Math. Biosci.*, 263:18-36, 2015.

44 Cristiana J. Silva and Delfim F. M. Torres, (2012)
Optimal control strategies for tuberculosis treatment: a case study in Angola. *Numer. Algebra Control Optim.*, 2(3):601-617, 2012.

45 Cristiana J. Silva and Delfim F. M. Torres, (2013)
An optimal control approach to malaria prevention via insecticide-treated nets. *Conference Papers in Mathematics*, 2013:1-8, 2013.

46 Cristiana J. Silva and Delfim F. M. Torres, (2013)
Optimal control for a tuberculosis model with reinfection and post-exposure interventions. *Math. Biosci.*, 244(2):154-164, 2013.

47 T. Smith, N. Maire, A. Ross, M. Penny, N. Chitnis, A. Schapira, A. Studer, B. Genton, C. Lengeler, F. Tediosi, D. de Savigny, and M. Tanner, (2008)
Towards a comprehensive simulation model of malaria epidemiology and control, *Parasitology*, 135(13):1507-1516, 2008.

48 Akhil Kumar Srivastav, Naba Kumar Goswami, Mini Ghosh, and Xue-Zhi Li, (2018)
Modeling and optimal control analysis of Zika virus with media impact. *Int. J. Dyn. Control*, 6(4):1673-1689, 2018.

49 Akhil Kumar Srivastav, Junyuan Yang, XiaoFeng Luo, and Mini Ghosh, (2019)
Spread of Zika virus disease on complex network–a mathematical study. *Math. Comput. Simulation*, 157:15-38, 2019.

50 Maria Strazzullo, Francesco Ballarin, Renzo Mosetti, and Gianluigi Rozza, (2018)
Model reduction for parametrized optimal control problems in environmental marine sciences and engineering. *SIAM J. Sci. Comput.*, 40(4):B1055-B1079, 2018.

51 Miranda I. Teboh-Ewungkem, Gideon A. Ngwa, and Calistus N. Ngonghala, (2013)
Models and proposals for malaria: a review. *Math. Popul. Stud.*, 20(2):57-81, 2013.

52 Tomlab,
PROPT – Matlab Optimal Control Software (DAE, ODE).

53 Andreas Wächter and Lorenz T. Biegler, (2006)
On the implementation of an interior-point filter line-search algorithm for large-scale nonlinear programming. *Math. Program.*, 106(1, Ser. A):25-57, 2006.

54 WHO, (2007)
Insecticide-treated mosquito nets: a who position statement.

55 WHO, (2019)
World malaria report 2019.

56 Liang Zhang and Shuang-Ming Wang, (2020)
A time-periodic and reaction-diffusion Dengue fever model with extrinsic incubation period and crowding effects. *Nonlinear Anal. Real World Appl.*, 51:102988, 24, 2020.

Part (IV):

Topological Studies:

Topology Meets Mosquito Control

Chapter 9:

On the Shape and Design of Mosquito Abatement Districts

1 Bozeman JR, Pilling M., (2013)
The convexity ratio and applications, *Math Jap*, 76(1):47-53; 2013.

2 Bozeman JR, Davey M, Hutchins S, et al., (2018)
Redistricting without gerrymandering, utilizing the convexity ratio, and other applications to business and industry, *Appl Stochastic Models Bus Ind.*, 1-17; 2018, https://doi.org/10.1002/asmb.2396.

3 Programs agriculture mosquito control,
http://dem.ri.gov/programs/agriculture/mosquito-control.php.

4 Mosquitoes nuisance schedule,
https://winnipeg.ca/publicworks/insectcontrol/mosquitoes/nuisanceschedule.stm.

5 https://www.uaex.edu/publications/pdf/FSA-7060.pdf

6 American Mosquito Control Association (AMCA) – FAQ

7 Delaware Mosquito Control Section,
https://www.arcgis.com/apps/webappviewer/index.htmlid=91e67ef755914218af05429242174d62

8 Introduction to mosquito treatments,
https://doc.arcgis.com/en/arcgis-solutions/reference/introduction-to-mosquito-treatments.htm.

9 West-nile virus interactive map,
http://access.tarrantcounty.com/en/public-health/disease-control---prevention/west-nile-virus/west-nile-virus-interactive-map.html

Part (V):
Chemometric and Mathematical Approach for Modeling and Designing Mosquito Repellents

Chapter 10:
A Multiplatform Chemometric Approach to Molecular and Mathematical Modeling of Mosquito Repellents

1 Abushouk, A. I., Negida, A., Ahmed, H., (2016)
An updated review of Zika virus, Journal of Clinical Virology, 84:53-58.

2 Aguiar, M., Stollenwerk, N., Halstead, S. B., (2016)
The impact of the newly licensed dengue vaccine in endemic countries, PLOS Neglected Tropical Diseases, 16: e0005179.

3 Aungtikun, J., Soonwera, M., (2021)
Improved adulticidal activity against Aedes aegypti (L.) and Aedes albopictus (Skuse) from synergy between Cinnamomum spp. essential oils, Scientific Reports 11:4685.

4 Balachandran, C., Anbalagan, S., Kandeepan, C., et al. (2021)
Molecular docking studies of natural alkaloids as acetylcholinesterase (AChE1) inhibitors in *Aedes aegypti*. Journal of Asia-Pacific Entomology In Press, DOI: 10.1016/j.aspen.2021.05.011.

5 Benelli, G., Pavela, R., Rakotosaona, R., et al., (2020)
Insecticidal and mosquito repellent efficacy of the essential oils from stem bark and wood of Hazomalania voyronii. Journal of Ethnopharmacology 248:112333.

6 Bohbot, J., Strickman, D., Zwiebel, L., (2014)
The future of insect repellent discovery and development, Outlooks on Pest Managements - August 2014.

7 Chiro, N., Gramatica, P., (2011)
Real external predictivity of QSAR models: How to evaluate it? Comparison of different validation criteria and proposal of using the concordance correlation coefficient, Journal of Chemical Information and Modeling, 51:2320-2335.

8 Chiro, N., Gramatica, P., (2012)
Real external predictivity of QSAR models, Part 2. New intercomparable thresholds for different validation criteria and the need for scatter plot inspection, Journal of Chemical Information and Modeling 52:2044-2058.

9 Costa, A. A., Naspi, C. V., Lucia, A., Masuh, H. M., (2017)
Repellent and larvicidal activity of the essential oil from Eucalyptus nitens against Aedes aegypti and Aedes albopictus (Diptera: Culicidae), Journal of Medical Entomology, 54:670-676.

10 Das, N. G., Dhiman, S., Talukdar, P. K., Rabha, B., Goswami, D., Veer, V., (2015)
Synergistic mosquito-repellent activity of Curcuma longa, Pogostemon heyneanus and Zanthoxylum limonella essential oils, Journal of Infection and Public Health, 8:323-328.

11 Datoo, M. S., Natama, M. H., Somé, A., (2021)
Efficacy of a low-dose candidate malaria vaccine, R21 in adjuvant Matrix-M, with seasonal administration to children in Burkina Faso: a randomised controlled trial, The Lancet, 397:1809-1818.

12 de Oliveira, A. A., França, L. P., Ramos, A. de S., et al., (2021)
Larvicidal, adulticidal and repellent activities against *Aedes aegypti* L. of two commonly used spices, Origanum vulgare L. and Thymus vulgaris L. South African Journal of Botany, 140:17-24.

13 De, P., Aher, R. B., Roy, K., (2018)
Chemometric modeling of larvicidal activity of plant derived compounds against zika virus vector *Aedes aegypti*: application of ETA indices, RSC Advances, 8:4662-4670, development. Outlooks on Pest Management 25:265-270.

14 Dhimal, M., Ahrens, B., Kuch, U., (2015)
Climate change and spatiotemporal distributions of vector borne diseases in Nepal – A systematic synthesis of literature, Plos One 10:e0129869.

15 Doucet, J. P., Doucet-Panaye, A., Papa, E., (2019)
Topological QSAR Modelling of Carboxamides Repellent Activity to *Aedes Aegypti*, Molecular Information 38:e1900029

16 Fouque, F., Reeder, J. C., (2019)
Impact of past and on-going changes on climate and weather on vector-borne diseases transmission: a look at the evidence, Infectious Diseases of Poverty 8:51.

17 Gaddaguti, V., Rao, T. V., Rao, A. P., (2016)
Potential mosquito repellent compounds of Ocimum species against 3N7H and 3Q8I of *Anopheles gambiae*, Biotech 6:26.

18 Ghosh, S., Mali, S. N., Bhowmick, D. N., Pratap, A. P., (2021)
Neem oil as natural pesticide: Pseudo ternary diagram and computational study, Journal of the Indian Chemical Society 98:100088.

19 Githeko, A. K., Lindsay, S. W., Confalonieri, U. E., Patz, J. A., (2000)
Climate change and vector-borne diseases: a regional analysis, Bulletin of the World Health Organization 78:1136-1147.

20 Gramatica, P., Sangion, A., (2016)
A historical excursus on the statistical validation parameters for QSAR models: A clarification concerning metrics and terminology, Journal of Chemical Information and Modeling 56:1127-1131.

21 Gurunathan, A., Senguttuvan, J., Paulsamy, S., (2016)
Evaluation of mosquito repellent activity of isolated oleic acid, eicosyl ester from Thalictrum javanicum, Indian Journal of Pharmaceutical Sciences 78:103-110.

22 Héberger, K., (2010)
Sum of ranking differences compares methods or models fairly, Trends in Analytical Chemistry 29: 101-109.

23 Heberger, K., Kollar-Hunek, K., (2011)
Sum of ranking differences for method discrimination and its validation: comparison of ranks with random numbers, Journal of Chemometrics 25:151-158.

24 Jevrić, L. R., Karadžić, M. Ž., Mandić, A. I., et al., (2017)
Lipophilicity estimation and characterization of selected steroid derivatives of biomedical importance applying RP HPLC, Journal of Pharmaceutical and Biomedical Analysis 134:27-35.

25 Jiang, S., Tsikolia, M., Bernier, U. R., Bloomquist, J. R., (2017)
Mosquitocidal activity and mode of action of the isoxazoline fluralaner, International Journal of Environmental Research and Public Health 14:154.

26 Kajla, M. K., (2020)
Symbiotic bacteria as potential agents for mosquito control, Trends in Parasitology 36:4-7.

27 Kajla, M. K., Barrett-Wilt, G. A., Paskewitz, S. M., (2019)
Bacteria: A novel source for potent mosquito feeding-deterrents, Science Advances 5:eaau6141.

28 Karadžić Banjac, M. Ž., Kovačević, S. Z., Jevrić, L. R., Podunavac-Kuzmanović, S. O., Mandić, A. I., (2019)
On the characterization of novel biologically active steroids: Selection of lipophilicity models of newly synthesized steroidal derivatives by classical and non-parametric ranking approaches, Computational Biology and Chemistry 80:23-30.

29 Karadžić, M. Ž., Jevrić, L. R., Mandić, A. I., et al., (2017b)
Chemometrics approach based on chromatographic behavior, in silico characterization and molecular docking study of steroid analogs with biomedical importance, European Journal of Pharmaceutical Sciences 105:71-81.

30 Karadžić, M. Ž., Jevrić, L. R., Podunavac Kuzmanović, S. O., Lončar, E. S., Kovačević, S. Z., (2015b)
Structure-retention relationship study of 2,4-dioxotetrahydro-1,3-thiazole derivatives, Journal of Liquid Chromatography and Related Technologies 38:1247-1253.

31 Karadžić, M. Ž., Lončar, D. M., Benedeković, G., et al., (2017a)
A comparative study of chromatographic behavior and lipophilicity of selected natural styryl lactones, their derivatives and analogues, European Journal of Pharmaceutical Sciences 105:99-107.

32 Karadžić, M., Podunavac-Kuzmanović, S., Jevrić, L., Kovačević, S., (2015a)
QSRR analysis in characterization of some benzimidazole derivatives, Acta Chimica Slovenica 62:747-753.

33 Katritzky A. R., Wang Z., Slavov S., et al., (2008)
Synthesis and Bioassay of Improved Mosquito Repellents Predicted from Chemical Structure, Proceedings of the National Academy of Sciences of the United States of America 105: 7359-7364.

34 Khater, H. F., Selim, A. M., Abouelella, G. A., et al., (2020)
Commercial mosquito repellents and their safety concerns, In Malaria, ed. F. Kasenga, 1-27, IntechOpen.

35 Kollár-Hunek, K., Héberger, K., (2013)
Method and model comparison by sum of ranking differences in cases of repeated observations (ties), Chemometrics and Intelligent Laboratory Systems 127:139-146.

36 Kovačević, S. Z., Karadžić, M. Ž., Vukić, D. V., et al., (2019)
Toward steroidal anticancer drugs: Non-parametric and 3D-QSAR modeling of 17-picolyl and 17-picolinylidene androstanes with antiproliferative activity on breast adenocarcinoma cells, Journal of Molecular Graphics and Modelling 87:240-249.

37 Kovačević, S. Z., Podunavac-Kuzmanović, S. O., Jevrić, L. R., Jovanov, P. T., Djurendić, E. A., Ajduković, J. J., (2016b)
Comprehensive QSRR modeling as a starting point in characterization and further development of anticancer drugs based on 17α-picolyl and 17(E)-picolinylidene androstane structures, European Journal of Pharmaceutical Sciences 93:1-10.

38 Kovačević, S. Z., Podunavac-Kuzmanović, S. O., Jevrić, L. R., Vukić, V. R., Savić, M. P., Djurendić, E. A., (2016a)
Preselection of A- and B- modified D-homo lactone and D-seco androstane derivatives as potent compounds with antiproliferative activity against breast and prostate cancer cells – QSAR approach and molecular docking analysis, European Journal of Pharmaceutical Sciences 93:107-113.

39 Kovačević, S., Karadžić Banjac, M., Milošević, N., et al., (2020b)
Comparative chemometric and quantitative structure-retention relationship analysis of anisotropic lipophilicity of 1-arylsuccinimide derivatives determined in high-performance thin-layer chromatography system with aprotic solvents, Journal of Chromatography A 1628:461439.

40 Kovačević, S., Karadžić Banjac, M., Podunavac-Kuzmanović, S., et al., (2020a)
Chromatographic and computational screening of anisotropic lipophilicity and pharmacokinetics of newly synthesized 1-aryl-3-ethyl-3-methylsuccinimides, Computational Biology and Chemistry 84:107161.

41 Kovačević, S., Karadžić, M., Podunavac-Kuzmanović, S., Jevrić, L., Ivanović, E., Vojnović, M., (2018a)
Electrostatic and topological features as predictors of antifungal potential of oxazolo derivatives as promising compounds in treatment of infections caused by Candida albicans, Acta Chimica Slovenica 65:483-491.

42 Kovačević, S., Karadžić, M., Podunavac-Kuzmanović, S., Lidija Jevrić, L., (2018b)
Binding affinity toward human prion protein of some anti-prion compounds – Assessment based on QSAR modeling, molecular docking and non-parametric ranking, European Journal of Pharmaceutical Sciences 111: 215-225.

43 Kröber, T., Koussis, K., Bourquin, M., et al., (2018)
Odorant-binding protein-based identification of natural spatial repellents for the African malaria mosquito *Anopheles gambiae*, Insect Biochemistry and Molecular Biology 96:36-50.

44 Legeay, S., Clere, N., Apaire-Marchais, V., Faure, S., Lapied, B., (2018)
Unusual modes of action of the repellent DEET in insects highlight some human side effects, European Journal of Pharmacology 825:92-98.

45 Ming-Xiang, L., Yong-Peng, M., Hong-Xia, Z., et al., (2020)
Repellent, larvicidal and adulticidal activities of essential oil from Dai medicinal plant Zingiber cassumunar against *Aedes albopictus*, Plant Diversity In Press, DOI: 10.1016/j.pld.2020.11.008.

46 Moreira, A. S. N., Fernandes, R. O. S., Lemos, F. J. A., Braz-Filho, R., Vieira, I. J. C., (2016)
Larvicidal activity of Ramalina usnea lichen against *Aedes aegypti*, Brasilian Journal of Pharmacognosy 26:530-532.

47 Mourão, E. D. S., de Carvalho, T. G. C., de Lima, S. Y. E. M., de Alencar Filho, E. B., (2021)
Identification of molecular scaffolds from Caatinga Brazilian biome with potential against *Aedes aegypti* by molecular docking and molecular dynamics simulations, Journal of Molecular Structure 1229:129621.

48 Natarajan, R., Basak, S. C., Mills, D., et al., (2008)
Quantitative Structure-Activity Relationship Modeling of Mosquito repellents Using Calculated Descriptors, Croatica Chemica Acta 81:333-340.

49 Parham, P. E., Waldock, J., Christophides, G. K., et al., (2015)
Climate, environmental and socio-economic change: weighing up the balance in vector-borne disease transmission, Philosophical Transactions of the Royal Society B: Biological Sciences 370:20130551.

50 Poland, G. A., Ovsyannikova, I. G., Kennedy. R. B., (2019)
Zika vaccine development: Current status, Thematic Review on Vaccines 94:2572-2586.

51 Rashkov, P., (2021)
A model for a vector-borne disease with control based on mosquito repellents: A viability analysis, Journal of Mathematical Analysis and Applications 498:124958.

52 Rashkov, P. Venturino, E., Aguiar, M., Stollenwerk, N., Kooi, B. W., (2019)
On the role of vector modeling in a minimalistic epidemic model, Mathematical Biosciences and Engineering 16:4314-4338.

53 Rocklöv, J., Dubrow, R., (2020)
Climate change: an enduring challenge for vector-borne disease prevention and control, Nature Immunology 21:479-483.

54 Roy, D. N., Goswami, R., Pal, A., (2017)
The insect repellents: A silent environmental chemical toxicant to the health, Environmental Toxicology and Pharmacology 50:91-102.

55 Sharma, M., Alexander, A., Saraf, S., et al., (2021)
Mosquito repellent and larvicidal perspective of weeds Lantana camara L. and Ocimum gratissimum L. found in central India, Biocatalysis and Agriculture Biotechnology 34:102040.

56 Singh, A., Sheikhj J., (2021)
Development of multifunctional polyester using disperse dyes based through a combination of mosquito repellents, Journal of Molecular Structure 1232:129988.

57 Thireou, T., Kythreoti, G., Tsitsanou, K. E., et al., (2018)
Identification of novel bioinspired synthetic mosquito repellents by combined ligand-based screening and OBP-structure-based molecular docking, Insect Biochemistry and Molecular Biology 98: 48-61.

58 Tsikolia, M., Bernier, U. R., Agramonte, et al., (2018)
Insecticidal and repellent properties of novel trifluoromethylphenyl amides II. Pesticide Biochemistry and Physiology, 151:40-46.

59 Ulbert, S., (2019)
West Nile virus vaccines – current situation and future directions, Human Vaccines & Immunotherapeutics 15:2337-2342.

60 Vukic, V. R., Loncar, D. M., Vukic, D. V., et al., (2019)
In vitro antitumor activity, ADME-Tox and 3D-QSAR of synthesized and selected natural styryl lactones, Computational Biology and Chemistry 83:107-112.

61 Wang, P., Xu, X., Liao, S., et al., (2017)
Quantitative structure–activity relationship study of amide mosquito repellents, SAR and QSAR in Environmental Research, 28:341-353.

62 Wendimu, A., Tekalign, W., (2021)
Field efficacy of ethnomedicinal plant smoke repellency against Anopheles arabiensis and *Aedes aegypti*, Heliyon 7:e07373.

63 World Health Organization (WHO), (2021)
https://www.who.int/news-room/fact-sheets/detail/vector-borne-diseases.

64 Wu, H., Zhang, M., Zang, Z., (2019)
Repellent activity screening of 12 essential oils against *Aedes albopictus Skuse*: Repellent liquid preparation of Mentha arvensis and Litsea cubeba oils and bioassay on hand skin, Industrial Crops & Products 128:464-470.

65 Zhu, J. J., Cermak, S. C., Kenar, J. A., et al., (2018)
Better than DEET repellent compounds derived from coconut oil, Scientific Reports 8:14053.

Part (VI):

Pharmacy Meets Mosquito Control: Using Pharmacological Tools Combating Mosquito Transmitted VBDs

Chapter 11:

Pharmacological Approach to Combat Mosquito Transmitted Malaria

1 Madhav H, Hoda N., (2021)
An insight into the recent development of the clinical candidates for the treatment of malaria and their target proteins, *Eur J Med Chem*, 15; 201:112955, 2021.

2 Varo R, Chaccour C, Bassat Q. Update on malaria, (2020)
Med Clin (Barc), 155(9): 395-402, 2020.

3 Yang CY, Qian D, Lu DL, Liu Y, Zhou RM, Li SH, Zhang HW, Zhao YL, (2020)
Epidemic status of malaria and progress of malaria elimination in Henan Province, 2018. *Zhongguo Xue Xi Chong Bing Fang Zhi Za Zhi*, 32(3):298-300, 2020.

4 Beavogui AH, Delamou A, Camara BS, Camara D, Kourouma K, Camara R, Sagara I, Lama EK, Djimde A., (2020)
Prevalence of malaria and factors associated with infection in children aged 6 months to 9 years in Guinea: Results from a national cross-sectional study. Parasite *Epidemiol Control.* 11:e00162, 2020.

5 Kabaghe AN, Chipeta MG, Terlouw DJ, McCann RS, van Vugt M, Grobusch MP, Takken W, Phiri KS, (2017)
Short-Term Changes in Anemia and Malaria Parasite Prevalence in Children under 5 Years during One Year of Repeated Cross-Sectional Surveys in Rural Malawi. *Am J Trop Med Hyg.* 97(5):1568-1575, 2017.

6 Park GS, John CC, (2014)
Cerebral malaria. In: Peterson P., Toborek M. (eds) *Neuroinflammation and Neurodegeneration* pp 405-428. Springer, New York, NY, 2014.

7 Ashley EA, Poespoprodjo JR, (2020)
Treatment and prevention of malaria in children. *Lancet Child Adolesc Health.* 4(10):775-789, 2020.

8 Mathanga DP, Walker ED, Wilson ML, Ali D, Taylor TE, Laufer MK, (2012)
Malaria control in Malawi: current status and directions for the future. *Acta Trop.* 121(3):212-217, 2012.

9 Melody D, Bauleni A, Chimuna T, Nsona HK, Kaunda-Khangamwa BN, Kalengamaliro H, Sande JH, Phiri TB, Mathanga DP, (2016)
Feasibility, acceptability and impact of integrating malaria rapid diagnostic tests and pre-referral rectal artesunate into the integrated community case management programme. A pilot study in Mchinji district, Malawi. *Malar. J.* 15, 1–8, 2016.

10 D'Alessandro U, Hill J, Tarning J, Pell C, Webster J, Gutman J, Sevene E., (2018)
Treatment of uncomplicated and severe malaria during pregnancy. *The Lancet Infect. Dis.* 18 (4) e133-146, 2018.

11 Desai M, Hill J, Fernandes S, Walker P, Pell C, Gutman J, Kayentao K, Gonzalez R, Webster J, Greenwood B, Cot M, Ter Kuile FO, (2018)
Prevention of malaria in pregnancy. *Lancet Infect Dis.* 18(4):e119-e132, 2018.

12 Nkoka O, Chuang TW, Chen YH, (2020)
Effects of Malaria Interventions During Pregnancy on Low Birth Weight in Malawi, *Am J Prev Med*, 59(6):904-913, 2020.

13 Saito M, Briand V, Min AM, McGready R, (2020)
Deleterious effects of malaria in pregnancy on the developing fetus: a review on prevention and treatment with antimalarial drugs, *Lancet Child Adolesc Health*, 4(10):761-774, 2020.

14 Bassat Q, Ogutu B, Djimde A, Stricker K, Hamed K., (2015)
Tailoring a pediatric formulation of artemether-lumefantrine for treatment of Plasmodium falciparum malaria. *Antimicrobial agents and chemotherapy*, 59(8), 4366-4374, 2015.

15 WHO, (2015)
Guidelines for the treatment of malaria, 3rd Edition. World Health Organization, 2015.

16 Nasir B, Shah SN, Murtaza G, Shahid N, Akhtar M, Khan BA, Azhar S, Mumtaz A, Waseem A, Khan SA, Ubaid M., (2012)
New HPLC method for the determination of artemether in injections. *Scientific Research and Essays*. 7(10):1165-1168, 2012.

17 Byakika-Kibwika P, Lamorde M, Mayanja-Kizza H, Khoo S, Merry C., (2011)
Artemether-lumefantrine combination therapy for treatment of uncomplicated malaria: the potential for complex interactions with antiretroviral drugs in HIV-infected individuals. *Malaria research and Treatment.*, 2011.

18 Cui L, Su XZ, (2009)
Discovery, mechanisms of action and combination therapy of artemisinin. *Expert Review of Anti-Infective Therapy*, 7(8):999-1013, 2009.

19 White NJ, (2004)
Antimalarial drug resistance, *J Clin Invest*, 113:1084–1092, 2004.

20 WHO, (2015)
Global action plan on antimicrobial resistance, Geneva, 2015. `https://www.who.int/publications-detail-redirect/global-action-plan-on-antimicrobial-resistance`

21 Staehli Hodel EM, Guidi M, Zanolari B, Mercier T, Duong S, Kabanywanyi AM, Ariey F, Buclin T, Beck HP, Decosterd LA, Olliaro P, Genton B, Csajka C, (2013)
Population pharmacokinetics of mefloquine, piperaquine and artemether-lumefantrine in Cambodian and Tanzanian malaria patients, *Malar J*, 10;12:235, 2013.

22 Maganda BA, Ngaimisi E, Kamuhabwa AA, Aklillu E, Minzi OM, (2015)
The influence of nevirapine and efavirenz-based anti-retroviral therapy on the pharmacokinetics of lumefantrine and anti-malarial dose recommendation in HIV-malaria co-treatment. *Malar J*. 25;14:179, 2015.

23 Borrmann S, Sallas WM, Machevo S, González R, Björkman A, Mårtensson A, Hamel M, Juma E, Peshu J, Ogutu B, Djimdé A, D'Alessandro U, Marrast A-M, Lefèvre G, Kern SE, (2010)
The effect of food consumption on lumefantrine bioavailability in African children receiving artemether–lumefantrine crushed or dispersible tablets (Coartem®) for acute uncomplicated Plasmodium falciparum malaria. *Eur J Trop Med Int Health*. 15:434-441, 2010.

24 Hietala SF, Mårtensson A, Ngasala B, Dahlström S, Lindegårdh N, Annerberg A, Premji Z, Färnert A, Gil P, Björkman A, Ashton M., (2010)
Population pharmacokinetics and pharmacodynamics of artemether and lumefantrine during combination treatment in children with uncomplicated falciparum malaria in Tanzania. *Antimicrobial agents and chemotherapy*, 54(11), 4780-4788, 2010.

25 White NJ, van Vugt M, Ezzet F., (1999)
Clinical Pharmacokinetics and Pharmacodynamics of Artemether Lumefantrine. *Clin. Pharmacokin*. 37:105-125, 1999.

26 Bonica JJ, McDonald JS, (1995)
Principles and Practice of Obstetric Analgesia and Anesthesia. 2nd. Vol. 1995. Baltimore, MD: Williams & Wilkins, 1995.

27 Nakai A, Sekiya I, Oya A, Koshino T, Araki T., (2002)
Assessment of the hepatic arterial and portal venous blood flows during pregnancy with Doppler ultrasonography. *Arch Gynecol Obstet.*, **266**:25-29, 2002.

28 Feghali M, Venkataramanan R, Caritis S., (2016)
Pharmacokinetics of drugs in pregnancy. *Semin Perinatol*, **39**:512-519, 2016.

29 George B, Lumen A, Nguyen C, Wesley B, Wang J, Beitz J, Crentsil V., (2020)
Application of physiologically based pharmacokinetic modeling for sertraline dosing recommendations in pregnancy. *NPJ Syst Biol Appl.*, **6**:36, 2020.

30 Dellicour S, Sevene E, McGready R, Tinto H, Mosha D, Manyando C, Rulisa S, Desai M, Ouma P, Oneko M, Vala A., (2017)
First-trimester artemisinin derivatives and quinine treatments and the risk of adverse pregnancy outcomes in Africa and Asia: A meta-analysis of observational studies, *PLoS Med* 14(5): e1002290, 2017.

31 Abduljalil K, Furness P, Johnson TN, Rostami-Hodjegan A, Soltani H., (2012)
Physiological, anatomical, and metabolic changes with gestational age during normal pregnancy: creating a database and analysing trends for parameters required in physiologically based pharmacokinetic modelling. *Clin Pharmacokinet*. **51**:365–96, 2012.

32 Gaohua L, Abduljalil K, Jamei M, Johnson TN, Rostami-Hodjegan A, (2012)
A pregnancy physiologically based pharmacokinetic (p-PBPK) model for disposition of drugs metabolized by CYP1A2, CYP2D6 and CYP3A4. *Br J Clin Pharmacol*, **74**:873-885, 2012.

33 Baselt RC, (2015)
Disposition of Toxic Drugs and Chemicals in Man. 10th Edition. Biomedical Publications, California, p. 162-162 and 1177, 2015.

34 Desai M, ter Kuile FO, Nosten F, McGready R, Asamoa K, Brabin B, Newman RD, (2007)
Epidemiology and burden of malaria in pregnancy, *Lancet Infect Dis* **7**:93–104, 2007.

35 Bonate PL, Wang T, Passier P, Bagchus W, Burt H, Lüpfert C, Abla N, Kovac J, Keiser J, (2018)
Extrapolation of praziquantel pharmacokinetics to a pediatric population: a cautionary tale. *J. Pharmacokin Pharmacodyn* 45:747-762, 2018.

36 Accorsi R, Karp JS, Surti S, (2010)
Improved dose regimen in pediatric PET. *J Nucl Med.* **51**:293-300, 2010.

37 Rowland M, Tozer TN, (2011)
Age, weight, and gender (Chapter 14) in *Clinical Pharmacokinetics and Pharmacodynamics*, 4th Edition. Lippencott Williams & Wilkins, p.373-402, 2011.

38 Lefèvre G, Carpenter P, Souppart C, Schmidli H, McClean M, Stypinski D, (2002)
Pharmacokinetics and electrocardiographic pharmacodynamics of artemether-lumefantrine (Riamet) with concomitant administration of ketoconazole in healthy subjects. *Br J Clin Pharmacol*,**54**:485-92, 2002.

39 Ezzet F, van Vugt M, Nosten F, Looareesuwan S, White NJ, (2000)
Pharmacokinetics and Pharmacodynamics of Lumefantrine (Benflumetol) in Acute Falciparum Malaria. *Antimicrob Agents Chemother*, **44**:697-704, 2000.

40 Kabwang J. Na-Bangchang K, Congpuong K, Molunto P, Thanavibul A, (1997)
Pharmacokinetics and bioavailability of oral and intramuscular artemether. *Eur J Clin Pharmacol.* **52**:307–310, 1997.

41 Salman S, Page-Sharp M, Griffin S, Kose K, Siba PM, Ilett KF, Mueller I, Davis TME, (2011)
Population Pharmacokinetics of Artemether, Lumefantrine, and Their Respective Metabolites in Papua New Guinean Children with Uncomplicated Malaria. *Antimicrob. Agents Chemother*, **55**:5306–5313, 2011.

42 Mwesigwa J, Parikh S, McGee B, German P, Drysdale T, Kalyango JN, Clark TD, Dorsey G, Lindegardh N, Annerberg A, Rosenthal PJ, Kamya MR, Aweeka F, (2010)
Pharmacokinetics of Artemether-Lumefantrine and Artesunate-Amodiaquine in Children in Kampala, Uganda, *Antimicrob. Agents Chemother*, **54**:52–59, 2010

43 Tchaparian E, Sambol NC, Arinaitwe E, McCormack SA, Bigira V, Wanzira H, Muhindo M, Creek DJ, Sukumar N, Blessborn D, Tappero JW, Kakuru A, Bergqvist Y, Aweeka FT, Parikh S, (2016)
Population Pharmacokinetics and Pharmacodynamics of Lumefantrine in Young Ugandan Children Treated With Artemether-Lumefantrine for Uncomplicated Malaria. *J Infect Dis*, **214**:1243-51, 2016.

44 Kloprogge F, Workman L, Borrmann S, Tékété M, Lefèvre G, Hamed K, Piola P, Ursing J, Kofoed PE, Mårtensson A, Ngasala B, Björkman A, Ashton M, Hietala SF, Aweeka F, Parikh S, Mwai L, Davis TME, Karunajeewa H, Salman S, Checchi F, Fogg C, Newton PN, Mayxay M, Deloron P, Faucher JF, Nosten F, Ashley EA, McGready R, van Vugt M, Proux S, Price RN, Karbwang J, Ezzet F, Bakshi R, Stepniewska K, White NJ, Guerin PJ, Barnes KI, Tarning J, (2018)
Artemether-lumefantrine dosing for malaria treatment in young children and pregnant women: A pharmacokinetic-pharmacodynamic meta-analysis, *Plos Med.*, **15**:e1002579, 2018.

45 Francis J, Barnes KI, Workman L, Kredo T, Vestergaard LS, Hoglund RM, Byakika-Kibwika P, Lamorde M, Walimbwa SI, Chijioke-Nwauche I, Sutherland CJ, Merry C, Scarsi KK, Nyagonde N, Lemnge MM, Khoo SH, Bygbjerg IC, Parikh S, Aweeka FT, Tarning J, Denti P, (2020)
An individual participant data population pharmacokinetic meta-analysis of drug-drug interactions between lumefantrine and commonly used antiretroviral treatment. *Antimicrob Agents Chemother*, 64, 2020.

46 Gordi T, Xie R, Huong N V, Huong DX, Karlsson MO, Ashton M, Toufigh Gordi C, Hall H, (2005)
British Journal of Clinical Pharmacology A semiphysiological pharmacokinetic model for artemisinin in healthy subjects incorporating autoinduction of metabolism and saturable first-pass hepatic extraction. *Br J Clin Pharmacol* 2005, 59:189.

Part (VII):

Using Natural Oils and Micro-encapsulation Combatting Mosquitoes: An Overview

Chapter 12:

Plant Based Repellents - Green Mosquito Control

1 Braack, L., Gouveia De Almeida, A.P., Cornel, A.J., Swanepoel, R. and De Jager, C., (2018)
Mosquito - borne arboviruses of African origin: Review of key viruses and vectors, Parasites and Vectors, 11(1).

2 Reiter, P, (2008)
Global warming and malaria: Knowing the horse before hitching the cart. Malaria Journal, 7(1),S3.

3 Khanikor, B., Parida, P., Yadav, R.N.S. and Bora, D, (2013)
Comparative mode of action of some terpene compounds against octopamine receptor and acetyl cholinesterase of mosquito and human system by the help of homology modeling and docking studies. Journal of Applied Pharmaceutical Science, 3(2), 6-12.

4 Khater, H., (2013)
Bioactivity of essential oils as green biopesticides: Recent global scenario. In: Essentials Oils. II, Recent Progress in Medicinal Plants, 37 151-218. USA: Studium Press LLC; 2013.

5 Islam, J., Zaman, K., Duarah, S., Raju, P.S. and Chattopadhyay, P., (2017)
Mosquito repellents: An insight into the chronological perspectives and novel discoveries. Acta Tropica, 167, 216-230.

6 Pavela, R. and Benelli, G., (2016)
Essential oils as ecofriendly biopesticides. Challenges and constraints, Trends in Plant Science, 21(12), 1000-1007.

7 Sharifi-Rad, J., Sureda, A., Tenore, G.C. et al., (2017)
Biological activities of essential oils : From plant chemoecology to traditional healing systems, Molecules, 22(1), 70.

8 Lee, M.Y., (2018)
Essential oils as repellents against arthropods. BioMed Research International, 2018(1), 1-9.

9 Maia, M.F. and Moore, S.J., (2011)
Plant-based insect repellents: A review of their efficacy, development and testing, Malaria Journal, 10(1), S11.

10 Khater, H.F. (2012)
Ecosmart biorational insecticides: Alternative insect control strategies, In: Insecticides—Advances in Integrated Pest Management, Rijeka, Croatia: InTech; 2012.

11 Bakkali, F., Averbeck, S., Averbeck, D. and Idaomar, M., (2008)
Biological effects of essential oils -A review. Food and Chemical Toxicology ,46, 446-475.

12 Sangwan, N.S., Farooqi, A.H.A., Shabih, F. and Sangwan, R.S., (2001)
Regulation of essential oil production in plants. Plant Growth Regulation, 34(1), 3-21.

13 Tripathi, A.K., Upadhyay, S., Bhuiyan, M. and Bhattacharya,P.R., (2009)
A review on prospects of essential oils as biopesticide in insect-pest management, Journal of Pharmacognosy and Phytotherapy, 1(5), 052-063.

14 Amer, A.M., (2005)
Evaluation of various essential oils as repellents and insecticides against mosquitoes (Diptera : Culicidae), Inaugural dissertation for obtaining the doctoral degree of Faculty of Mathematics and Natural Sciences, Heinrich - Heine University, Düsseldorf.

15 Isman, M.B., (2006)
Botanical insecticides, deterrents, and repellents in modern agriculture and an increasingly regulated world, *Annual Review* of *Entomology, 51*, 45-66.

16 Kuvendziev, S., Lisichkov, K., Zeković, Z., Marinkovski, M. and Musliu, Z.H., (2018)
Supercritical fluid extraction of fish oil from common carp (Cyprinus carpio) L. tissues, Journal of Supercritical Fluids, 2018 (133), 528-534.

17 Loza-Tavera, H., (1999)
Monoterpenes in Essential Oils, In: Shahidi F., Kolodziejczyk P., Whitaker J.R., Munguia A.L., Fuller G. (eds) Chemicals via Higher Plant Bioengineering. Advances in Experimental Medicine and Biology, 464. Springer, Boston, MA.

18 Barasa, S.S., Ndiege, I.O., Lwande, W. and Hassanali, A., (2002)
Repellent activities of stereoisomers of p-menthane-3,8-diols against Anopheles gambiae (Diptera: Culicidae). *Journal of Medical Entomology*, 39,736-741.

19 Emily Zielinski-Gutierrez, R.A.W. and Roger, S.N., (2010)
Protection against mosquitoes, ticks and other insects and arthropods. CDC Health Information for International Travel ("The Yellow Book") Atlanta: Centers for Disease Control and Prevention.

20 EPA: p-Menthane-3,8-diol (011550) Fact Sheet, http://www.epa.gov/oppbppd1/biopesticides/ingredients/factsheets/factsheet_011550.htm

21 Rodriguez, S.D., Drake, L.L., Price, D.P. and Hammond, J.I. (2015),
The efficacy of some commercially available insect repellents for Aedes aegypti (Diptera: Culicidae) and Aedes albopictus (Diptera: Culicidae). Journal of Insect Science, 15(1), 140.

22 Rodriguez, S.D., Chung, H.N., Gonzales, K.K., Vulcan, J., Li, Y., Ahumada, J.A., Romero, H.M., De La Torre, M., Shu, F. and Hansen, I.A. (2017). Efficacy of some wearable devices compared with spry-on insect repellents for the Yellow fever mosquito, Aedes aegypti (L.) (Diptera: Culicidae). Journal of Insect Science, 17(1), 24, 1–6.

23 Trongtokit, Y., Curtis, C.F. and Rongsriyam, Y., (2005)
Efficacy of repellent products against caged and free flying Anopheles stephensi mosquitoes. Southeast Asian Journal of Tropical Medicine and Public Health, 36, 1423-1431.

24 Fradin, M.S. and Day, J.F., (2002)
Comparative efficacy of insect repellents against mosquito bites, New England Journal of Medicine, 347, 13-18.

25 Frances,S.P., Rigby, L.M. and Chow, W.K., (2014)
Comparative Laboratory and Field Evaluation of Repellent Formulations Containing Deet and Lemon Eucalyptus Oil Against Mosquitoes in Queensland, Australia, Journal of the American Mosquito Control Association, 30(1), 65-67.

26 Conti B., Canale A., Bertoli A., Gozzini F. & Pistelli L., (2010)
Essential oil composition and larvicidal activity of six Mediterranean aromatic plants against the mosquito *Aedes albopictus* (Diptera: Culicidae), Parasitology Research, 107, 1455-1461.

27 Zainulabeuddin S., Leal W.S., (2008)
Mosquitoes smell and avoid the insect repellent DEET, Proceedings of the National Academy of Sciences of the United States of America, 105(36), 13598-13603.

28 Günter C.M., Junnila, A., Butler, J., Kravchenko, V.D., Revay, E.E., Weiss, R.W. and Schlein, Y., (2009)
Efficacy of the botanical repellents geraniol, linalool, and citronella against mosquitoes, Journal of Vector Ecology, 34(1),2-8.

29 Moore, S.J., Hill, N., Ruiz, C. and Cameron, M.M., (2007)
Field evaluation of traditionally used plant-based insect repellents and fumigants against the malaria vector Anopheles darling in Riberalta, Bolivian Amazon. *Journal of Medical Entomology*, 44, 624-630.

30 Trongtokit, Y., Rongsriyam, Y., Komalamisra, N. and Apiwathnasorn, C., (2005)
Comparative repellency of 38 essential oils against mosquito bites, Phytotherapy Research, 19, 303-309.

31 Tawatsin, A., Wratten, S.D., Scott, R.R., Thavara, U. and Techadamrongsin, Y., (2001)
Repellency of volatile oils from plants against three mosquito vectors, Journal of Vector Ecology, 26, 76-82.

32 Amer, A. and Mehlhorn, H., (2006)
Repellency effect of forty-one essential oils against Aedes, Anopheles, and Culex mosquitoes, Parasitology Research, 99,478.

33 Phasomkusolsil, S. and Soonwera, M., (2011)
Comparative mosquito repellency of essential oils against *Aedes aegypti* (Linn.), *Anopheles dirus* (Peyton and Harrison) and *Culex quinquefasciatus* (Say) Asian Pacific Journal of Tropical Biomedicine, 1, S113-S118.

34 Adam, A.A., Ahmed, S.A., Mohamed, T.A., Azrag, R.A., Mustafa, S.E. and Hamdi, O.A., (2019)
Evaluation of repellent activities of the essential oil of Ocimum basilicum against *Anopheles* mosquito and formulation of mosquito repellent cream. Biomedical Research and Clinical Practice, 4, 1-5.

35 Won-Sik C., Byeoung-Soo P., Sae-Kwang K. and Sung-Eun L., (2002)
Repellent activities of essential oils and monoterpenes against *Culex pipiens pallens*, Journal of American Mosquito Control Association, 18(4), 348-351.

36 Sharma, S.K., Dua, V.K. and Sharma, V.P., (1995)
Field studies on the mosquito repellent action of neem oil, *Southeast Asian Journal of Tropical Medicine and Public Health*, 26(1),180-2.

37 Govindarajan, M., (2011)
Larvicidal and repellent properties of some essential oils against *Culex tritaeniorhynchus* Giles and *Anopheles subpictus* Grassi (Diptera: Culicidae), Asian Pacific Journal of Tropical Medicine, 4, 106-111.

38 Das, N.G., Dhiman, S., Talukdar, P.K., Rabha, B., Goswami, D. and Veer, V., (2015)
Synergistic mosquito-repellent activity of Curcuma longa, Pogostemon heyneanus and Zanthoxylum limonella essential oils, Journal of Infection and Public Health, 8(4), 323-328.

39 Muturi, E.J., Ramirez, J.L., Doll, K.M. and Bowman, M.J., (2017)
Combined toxicity of three essential oils against *Aedes aegypti* (Diptera: Culicidae) Larvae, *Journal of Medical Entomology*, 54(6), 1684-1691.

40 Chung, S.K., Seo, J.Y., Lim, J.H., Park, H., Yea, M.J. and Park, H.J., (2013)
Microencapsulation of essential oil for insect repellent in food packaging system, Journal of Food Science, 78(5),709-714.

41 Chattopadhyay P., Dhiman S., Borah S., Rabha B., Chaurasia A. K. and Veer V., (2015)
Essential oil based polymeric patch development and evaluating its repellent activity against mosquitoes, *Acta Tropica*, 147,45-53.

42 Yadav, N.P., Rai, V.K., Mishra, N., Sinha, P., Bawankule, D.U., Anirban, P., Tripathi, A.K. and Chanotiya, C.S., (2014)
A novel approach for development and characterization of effective mosquito repellent cream formulation containing citronella oil, BioMed Research International, 2014, 11 pages.

43 Murugan, K., Dinesh, D., Paulpandi, M., et al., (2015)
Nanoparticles in the fight against mosquito-borne diseases: bioactivity of Bruguiera cylindrica-synthesized nanoparticles against dengue virus DEN-2 (in vitro) and its mosquito vector *Aedes aegypti* (Diptera: Culicidae) *Parasitology Research*, 114(12), 4349-4361.

44 Govindarajan, M. and Benelli G., (2017)
A facile one-pot synthesis of eco-friendly nanoparticles using Carissa carandas: Ovicidal and larvicidal potential on malaria, dengue and filariasis mosquito vectors, *Journal of Cluster Science*, 28(1), 15-36.

Chapter 13:

Microencapsulation of Essential Oils for Antimicrobial Function and Mosquito Repellency

1 Abang, S. et al., (2012)
Effects of process variables on the encapsulation of oil in ca-alginate capsules using an inverse gelation technique. *Journal of Microencapsulation,* 29 (5), pp. 417-428.

2 Ali, S.W., Purwar, R., Joshi, M. and Rajendran, S., (2014)
Antibacterial properties of Aloe vera gel-finished cotton fabric. *Cellulose*, **21**, 2063-2072.

3 Anuar A A and Yusof N, (2016)
Methods of imparting mosquitoes repellents agents and the assessing mosquito repellency on textiles, *Fashion and Textiles*, **3**, 12, DOI:10.1186/s40691-016-0064-y.

4 Azeem, M., Zaman, T., Tahir, M., Haris, A., Iqbal, Z., Binyameen, M., Nazir, A., Shad, S.A., Majeed, S. and Mozūraitis, R., (2019)
Chemical composition and repellent activity of native plants essential oils against dengue mosquito, *Aedes aegypti*, *Ind Crops Prod*, **140**, 111609. DOI: 10.1016/j.indcrop.2019.111609.

5 Aziz, S. et al., (2014)
Microencapsulation of krill oil using complex coacervation, *Journal of Microencapsulation*, 31 (8), pp. 774-784.

6 Bakry, A.M. et al., (2016)
Microencapsulation of Oils: A Comprehensive Review of Benefits, Techniques, and Applications, *Comprehensive Reviews in Food Science and Food Safety*, 15 (1), pp. 143-182.

7 Berendsen, R. et al., (2015)
Spray dried double emulsions containing procyanidin-rich extracts produced by premix membrane emulsification: Effect of interfacial composition *Food Chemistry*, 178 (0), pp. 251-258.

8 Buranasuksombat, U. et al., (2011)
Influence of emulsion droplet size on antimicrobial properties, *Food Science and Biotechnology*, 20 (3), pp. 793-800.

9 Butstraen, C. and Salaün, F., (2014)
Preparation of microcapsules by complex coacervation of gum Arabic and chitosan *Carbohydrate Polymers*, 99 (0), pp. 608-616.

10 Calvo, P. et al., (2012)
Influence of the microencapsulation on the quality parameters and shelf-life of extra-virgin olive oil encapsulated in the presence of BHT and different capsule wall components, *Food Research International*, 45 (1), pp. 256-261.

11 Chouhan, S., Sharma, K., Guleria, S., (2017)
Antimicrobial Activity of Some Essential Oils - Present Status and Future Perspectives, *Medicines*, 4, DOI: 10.3390/medicines4030058.

12 da Silva, P.T. et al., (2014)
Microencapsulation: concepts, mechanisms, methods and some applications in food technology, *Ciência Rural*, 44 (7), pp. 1304-1311.

13 Dima, C. et al., (2016)
The kinetics of the swelling process and the release mechanisms of Coriandrum sativum L. essential oil from chitosan/alginate/inulin microcapsules, *Food Chemistry*, 195, pp. 39-48.

14 Dong, Z. et al., (2011)
Morphology and release profile of microcapsules encapsulating peppermint oil by complex coacervation*Journal of Food Engineering*, 104 (3), pp. 4.

15 Dong, Y. et al., (2013)
Scalable ionic gelation synthesis of chitosan nanoparticles for drug delivery in static mixers *Carbohydrate Polymers*, 94 (2), pp. 940-945.

16 Dürrigl, M. et al. (2011) Spray dried microparticles for controlled delivery of mupirocin calcium: Process–tailored modulation of drug release , *Journal of Microencapsulation*, 28 (2), pp. 108-121.

17 Elcocks, E.R., Spencer-Phillips, P.T.N. and Adukwu, E.C., (2020)
Rapid bactericidal effect of cinnamon bark essential oil against Pseudomonas aeruginosa, *J Appl Microbiol*, **128**, 1025-1037

18 Fan, W. et al., (2012)
Formation mechanism of monodisperse, low molecular weight chitosan nanoparticles by ionic gelation technique, *Colloids and Surfaces B: Biointerfaces*, 90, pp. 21-27.

19 Fàbregas, A. et al., (2013)
Impact of physical parameters on particle size and reaction yield when using the ionic gelation method to obtain cationic polymeric chitosan–tripolyphosphate nanoparticles, *International Journal of Pharmaceutics*, 446 (1-2), pp. 199-204.

20 Georgiev, V., Ananga, A., Dincheva, I., Badjakov, I., Gochev, V. and Tsolova, V., (2019)
Chemical composition, in vitro antioxidant potential, and antimicrobial activities of essential oils and hydrosols from Native American muscadine grapes, *Molecules*, **24**, 3355, DOI:10.3390/molecules24183355.

21 Ghayempour, S. and Montazer, M., (2016)
Micro/nanoencapsulation of essential oils and fragrances: Focus on perfumed, antimicrobial, mosquito-repellent and medical textiles, *Journal of Microencapsulation*, 33 (6), pp. 497-510.

22 Gómez Gaete, C. et al., (2008)
Morphology, structure and supramolecular organization of hybrid 1,2-dipalmitoyl-sn-glycero-3-phosphatidylcholine–hyaluronic acid microparticles prepared by spray drying, *European Journal of Pharmaceutical Sciences*, 34 (1), pp. 12-21.

23 Gray, A. et al., (2016)
Determination of microcapsule physicochemical, structural, and mechanical properties, *Particuology*, 24, 32-43.

24 Haidong, L. et al., (2012)
Use of combinations of gum arabic, maltodextrin and soybean protein to microencapsulate ginkgo leaf extracts and its inhibitory effect on skeletal muscle injury, *Carbohydrate Polymers*, 88 (2), pp. 435-440.

25 Heinzelmann, K. et al., (2000)
Protection of fish oil from oxidation by microencapsulation using freeze-drying techniques, *European Journal of Lipid Science and Technology*, 102 (2), pp. 114-121.

26 Hosseini, S.F. et al., (2013)
Two-step method for encapsulation of oregano essential oil in chitosan nanoparticles: Preparation, characterization and in vitro release study, *Carbohydrate Polymers*, 95 (1), pp. 50-56.

27 Jaya, S. et al., (2009)
Effect of alginate-pectin composition on drug release characteristics of microcapsules, *Journal of Microencapsulation*, 26 (2), pp. 143-153.

28 Javid, A., Raza, Z.A., Hussain, T. and Rehman, A., (2014)
Chitosan microencapsulation of various essential oils to enhance the functional properties of cotton fabric, *J Microencapsulation*, 31, 461-468.

29 Keawchaoon, L. and Yoksan, R., (2011)
Preparation, characterization and in vitro release study of carvacrol-loaded chitosan nanoparticles, *Colloids and Surfaces B: Biointerfaces*, 84 (1), pp. 163-171.

30 Kesavan, K. et al., (2013)
Mucoadhesive chitosan-coated cationic microemulsion of dexamethasone for ocular delivery: in vitro and in vivo evaluation, *Current Eye Research*, 38 (3), pp. 342-352.

31 Krokida, M.K. and Philippopoulos, C., (2006)
Volatility of apples during air and freeze drying, *Journal of Food Engineering*, 73 (2), pp.135-141.

32 Lv, Y. et al., (2014)
Formation of heat-resistant nanocapsules of jasmine essential oil via gelatin/gum arabic based complex coacervation, *Food Hydrocolloids*, 35, pp. 305-314.

33 Madene, A., Jacquot, M., Scher, J., and Desobry, S., (2006)
Flavour encapsulation and controlled release – a review, Jou*rnal of Food Science and Technology*, 41 (1), pp.1-21.

34 Martins, E. et al., (2015)
Oil core microcapsules by inverse gelation technique, *Journal of Microencapsulation*, 32 (1), pp. 86-95.

35 Munoz-Ibanez, M. et al., (2016)
The microstructure and component distribution in spray-dried emulsion particles, *Food Structure*, 8, pp. 16-24.

36 Nakagawa, K. and Nagao, H., (2012)
Microencapsulation of oil droplets using freezing-induced gelatin–acacia complex coacervation, *Colloids and Surfaces A: Physicochemical and Engineering Aspects*, 411, pp. 129-139.

37 Najafi-Soulari, S. et al., (2016)
Encapsulation optimization of lemon balm antioxidants in calcium alginate hydrogels, *Journal of Biomaterials Science, Polymer Edition*, 27 (16), pp. 1631-1644.

38 Nuisin, R. et al., (2013)
Microencapsulation of menthol by crosslinked chitosan via porous glass membrane emulsification technique and their controlled release properties, *Journal of Microencapsulation*, 30 (5), pp. 498-509.

39 Pedro, A.S, Cabral-Albuquerque, E., Ferreira, D. and Sarmento, B., (2009)
Chitosan: An option for development of essential oil delivery systems for oral cavity care? *Carbohydr Pol*, 76, 501-508.

40 Pérez-Limiñana, M.Á et al., (2014)
Effect of the shell-forming polymer ratio on the encapsulation of tea tree oil by complex coacervation as a natural biocide, *Journal of Microencapsulation*, 31 (2), pp. 176-183.

41 Piacentini, E. et al., (2013)
Microencapsulation of oil droplets using cold water fish gelatine/gum arabic complex coacervation by membrane emulsification, *Food Research International*, 53 (1), pp. 362-372.

42 Sayed, U., Sharma, K. and Parte, S. (2017) Application of essential oils for finishing of textile substrates. *J Text Eng Fash Technol* 1, 42-47.

43 Shinde, U. and Nagarsenker, M., (2011)
Microencapsulation of eugenol by gelatin-sodium alginate complex coacervation, *Indian Journal of Pharmaceutical Sciences*, 73 (3), pp. 311-315.

44 Sinha, V. et al., (2007)
Influence of operational variables on properties of piroxicam pellets prepared by extrusion-spheronization: A technical note, *AAPS PharmSciTech*, 8 (1), pp. E13-E141.

45 Soliman, E.A. et al., (2013)
Microencapsulation of Essential Oils within Alginate: Formulation and in Vitro Evaluation of Antifungal Activity, *Journal of Encapsulation and Adsorption Sciences*, 3 (1), pp. 48-55.

46 Specos, M.M., García, J.J., Tornesello, J., Marino, P., Vecchia, M.D., Tesoriero, M.D. and Hermida, L.G., (2010)
Microencapsulated citronella oil for mosquito repellent finishing of cotton textiles, *Trans R Soc Trop Med Hyg*, 104, 653-658.

47 Sun, G. and Zhang, Z., (2002)
Mechanical strength of microcapsules made of different wall materials, *International Journal of Pharmaceutics*, 242 (1–2), pp. 307-311.

48 Tian, W. et al., (2016)
Physical Stability and Antimicrobial Activity of Encapsulated Cinnamaldehyde by Self-Emulsifying Nanoemulsion, *Journal of Food Process Engineering*, 39 (5), pp. 462-471.

49 Tariq, S., Wani, S., Rasool, W., Shafi, K., Bhat, M.A., Prabhakar, A., Shalla, A.H. and Rather, M.A., (2019)
A comprehensive review of the antibacterial, antifungal and antiviral potential of essential oils and their chemical constituents against drug-resistant microbial pathogens,*Microb Pathog*, 134, 103580, DOI:10.1016/j.micpath.2019.103580.

50 Teeka, P. et al., (2014)
Preparation of Poly (methyl methacrylate) Microcapsule with Encapsulated Jasmine Oil, *Energy Procedia*, 56, pp. 181-186.

51 Tomaro-Duchesneau, C. et al., (2013)
Microencapsulation for the therapeutic delivery of drugs, live mammalian and bacterial cells, and other biopharmaceutics: current status and future directions, *Journal of Pharmaceutics*, 2013, pp. 103527-19.

52 Velasco, J. et al., (2003)
Variables affecting lipid oxidation in dried microencapsulated oils, *Grasas Y Aceites*, 54 (3), pp. 304-314.

53 Wilson, B. et al., (2010)
Chitosan nanoparticles as a new delivery system for the anti-Alzheimer drug tacrine, Nanomedicine: *Nanotechnology, Biology and Medicine*, 6 (1), pp. 144-152.

54 Winska, K., Maczka, W., Lyczko, J., Grabarczyk, M., Czubaszek, A. and Szumny, A., (2019)
Essential oils as antimicrobial agents—myth or real alternative? *Molecules*, 24, 2130. DOI:10.3390/molecules24112130.

55 Xu, Y. and Du, Y., (2003)
Effect of molecular structure of chitosan on protein delivery properties of chitosan nanoparticles, *International Journal of Pharmaceutics*, 250 (1), pp. 215-226.

56 Yang, K. et al., (2014)
Bioactivity of essential oil of *Litsea cubeba* from China and its main compounds against two stored product insects, *Journal of Asia-Pacific Entomology*, 17 (3), pp. 459-466.

57 Yang, J. et al., (2015)
Preparation and application of micro/nanoparticles based on natural polysaccharides, *Carbohydrate Polymers*, 123, pp. 53-66.

58 Yang, X. et al., (2015)
Development and evaluation of novel microcapsules containing poppy-seed oil using complex coacervation, *Journal of Food Engineering*, 161, pp. 87-93.

59 Zhang, K. et al., (2012)
Synthesis and release studies of microalgal oil-containing microcapsules prepared by complex coacervation, *Colloids and Surfaces B: Biointerfaces*, 89, pp. 61-66.

Part (VIII):

Textiles and Paints as Mosquito Control Tools

Chapter 14:

Mosquito Repellent against *Anopheles Spp.* and *Aedes Aegypti* on Cotton Fabric

1 Grancaric, A. M., T. Pušić, A. Tarbuk, (2006)
Enzymatic Scouring for Better Textile Properties of Knitted Fabrics, *Journal of Natural Fibres*, Vol. 3 (2006) 2/3.

2 Grancaric, A.M., Tarbuk, A. Kovaček, I., (2009)
Nanoparticles of Activated Natural Zeolite on Textiles for Protection and Therapy, *Chemical Industry & Chemical Engineering Quarterly*, 15 (2009), 4, 203-210.

3 Devaux, C. A., (2012)
Emerging and re-emerging viruses: A global challenge illustrated by Chikungunya virus outbreaks, *World Journal of Virology*, **Vol.** 1 (2012), No.1, pp. 11-22, ISSN 2220-3249, https://dx.doi.org/10.5501/wjv.v1.i1.11.

4 Caraballo H,, King K., (2014)
Emergency department management of mosquito-borne illness: malaria, dengue, and West Nile virus, *Emergency medicine practice*, **Vol.**16, (2014), No.5, pp.1-23.

5 Vilibic-Cavlek T., et al., (2017)
First detection of Zika virus infection in Croatian traveler returning from Brazil, 2016, *Journal of Infection in Developing Countries*, **Vol.**1 (2017), No.8, pp. 662-667, ISSN, 1972-2680, DOI:https://doi.org/10.3855/Jidc.9410.

6 Valentbiosciences
https://www.valentbiosciences.com/publichealth/pests/mosquitoes/mosquitoes-anopheles/ , Accessed: 2020-03-25.

7 Sinkins, S, (2007)
Genome sequence of Aedes aegypti, a major arbovirus vector, Science, **Vol.** 316, (2007), No. 5832, pp. 1718–1723, https://doi.org/10.1126/science.1138878.

8 WHO, (2017)
Global vector control response 2017–2030, World Health Organization, ISBN 978-92-4-151297-8, Geneva, (2017).

9 Grancarić, A. M. et al., (2018)
Natural Based Textile Protection From The Invasive Mosquitoes, *Proceedings of 18th Autex World Textile Conference*, Kalaoglu F. (Ed), pp.314-318, ISSN: 15606074883, Istanbul, June 2018.

10 Coleman, R.E., et al., (1993)
Laboratory evaluation of repellents against four anopheline mosquitoes (Diptera: Culicidae) and two phlebotomine sand flies (Diptera: Psychodidae), *Journal of Medical Entomology*, **Vol.** 30. (1993) No.3., pp.499–502, ISSN:0022-2585, https://doi.org/10.1093/jmedent/30.3.499.

11 Govere, J. M. & Durrheim, D. V., (2006)
Techniques for evaluating repellents, In: *Insect repellents: principles methods, and use*, CRC Press, ISBN 9780429123382, Boca, (2006), pp. 147-160.

12 Giatropoulos A. et al., (2012)
Evaluation of bioefficacy of three Citrus essential oils against the dengue vector Aedes albopictus (Diptera: Culicidae) in correlation to their components enantiomeric distribution, Parasitology Research **Vol.** 111., (2012) No.6, pp. 2253–2263, ISSN 0932-0113, https://doi.org/10.1007/s00436-012-3074-8.

13 Grancaric, A. M. et al., (2020)
Microencapsulation for Improved Mosquitoes Repellent Efficacy of Cotton Fabrics, *7th International Conference on Intelligent Textiles & Mass Customisation (ITMC 2019) IOP Conf. Series: Materials Science and Engineering*, 827, (2020), 012056, https://doi.org/10.1088/1757-899X/827/1/012056.

Chapter 15:

Recent Progress in Silica-Based Organic/Inorganic Hybrid Treatments as Anti-Mosquito Textile Finishing

1 Abdelhameed RM, Kamel Omhm, Amr A, et al., (2017)
Antimosquito Activity of a Titanium–Organic Framework Supported on Fabrics, ACS Appl Mater Interfaces 9:22112–22120, https://doi.org/10.1021/acsami.7b03164

2 Amiri S, Rahimi A, (2016)
Hybrid nanocomposite coating by sol–gel method: a review. Iran Polym J 25:559–577, https://doi.org/10.1007/s13726-016-0440-x

3 Ardanuy M, Faccini M, Amantia D, et al., (2014)
Preparation of durable insecticide cotton fabrics through sol–gel treatment with permethrin, Surf Coatings Technol 239:132–137, https://doi.org/10.1016/j.surfcoat.2013.11.031.

4 Böttcher H, Kallies K-H, Haufe H, Seidel J, (1999)
Silica Sol-Gel Glasses with Embedded Organic Liquids, Adv Mater 11:138–141, https://doi.org/10.1002/(SICI)1521-4095(199902)11:2<138::AID-ADMA138>3.0.CO;2-3.

5 Danks AE, Hall SR, Schnepp Z, (2016)
The evolution of 'sol-gel' chemistry as a technique for materials synthesis, Mater Horizons 3:91-112, https://doi.org/10.1039/C5MH00260E.

6 El-Sayed AA, Amr A, Kamel OMHM, et al.,(2020)
Eco-friendly fabric modification based on AgNPs@Moringa for mosquito repellent applications, Cellulose 27:8429–8442,https://doi.org/10.1007/s10570-020-03355-8.

7 Ghayempour S, Montazer M, (2016)
Micro/nanoencapsulation of essential oils and fragrances: Focus on perfumed, antimicrobial, mosquito-repellent and medical textiles. J Microencapsul 33:497-510, https://doi.org10.1080/02652048.2016.1216187.

8 Gonzalez E, Vejar N, Solis R, et al., (2019)
Sol-Gel Films: Corrosion Protection Coating for Aluminium Alloy, In: Sol-Gel Method - Design and Synthesis of New Materials with Interesting Physical, Chemical and Biological Properties, IntechOpen.

9 Grancaric AM, Laird K, Botteri L, et al., (2020)
Microencapsulation for improved mosquitoes' repellent efficacy of cotton fabrics, IOP Conf Ser Mater Sci Eng 827:012056, https://doi.org/10.1088/1757-899X/827/1/012056.

10 Haufe H, Muschter K,Siegert J, Böttcher H, (2008)
Bioactive textiles by sol–gel immobilised natural active agents, J Sol-Gel Sci Technol 45:97–101, https://doi.org/10.1007/s10971-007-1636-5.

11 Kakihana M, (1996)
Invited review "sol-gel" preparation of high temperature superconducting oxides, J Sol-Gel Sci Technol 6:7-55,https://doi.org/10.1007/BF00402588.

12 Li F-Y, Xing Y-J, Ding X, (2007)
Immobilization of papain on cotton fabric by sol–gel method, Enzyme Microb Technol 40:1692-1697, https://doi.org/10.1016/j.enzmictec.2006.09.007.

13 Mahltig B, Haufe H,Bottcher H, (2005)
Functionalisation of textiles by inorganic sol-gel coatings, J Mater Chem 15:4385–4398, https://doi.org/10.1039/b505177k.

14 Mulyani WE, Sunendar B, (2013)
Synthesis and Characterization of Silica-Lavender Microencapsulation by Sol Gel-Emulsion Method for Anti Mosquito Textile, Adv Mater Res 789:215–218, https://doi.org/10.4028/www.scientific.net/AMR.789.215.

15 Plutino MR, Colleoni C, Donelli I, et al., (2017)
Sol-gel 3-glycidoxypropyltriethoxysilane finishing on different fabrics: The role of precursor concentration and catalyst on the textile performances and cytotoxic activity, J Colloid Interface Sci 506:504–517, https://doi.org/10.1016/j.jcis.2017.07.048

16 Puoci F, Saturnino C, Trovato V, et al., (2020)
Sol–Gel Treatment of Textiles for the Entrapping of an Antioxidant/Anti-Inflammatory Molecule: Functional Coating Morphological Characterization and Drug Release Evaluation, Appl Sci 10:2287, https://doi.org/10.3390/app10072287.

17 Raja, ASM; Kawlekar, Sujata; Saxena, Sujata; Arputharaj, A; Patil P, (2015)
Mosquito protective textiles - A review, Int J Mosq Res 2:49-53.

18 Schindler W.D.; Hauser P.J., (2004)
Chemical Finishing of Textiles, Woodhead Publishing, Cambridge.

19 Tseghai GB, (2016)
Mosquito Repellent Finish of Cotton Fabric by Extracting Castor Oil, Int J Sci Eng Res 7:873-878.

Chapter 16:

Cotton and Polyester Fabrics Plasma Coated with Hydrogenated Amorphous Carbon Films (A-C:H) as Platform for Further Refinement

1 J. Peran, (2020)
Application of atmospheric pressure plasma technology for textile surface modification, (2020), https://doi.org/10.1177/0040517519883954.

2 A. Zille, F. R. Oliveira, A. P. Souto, (2015)
Plasma Treatment in Textile Industry, Plasma Process. Polym. 12 (2015) 98-131, https://doi.org/10.1002/ppap.201400052.

3 R. A. Jelil, (2015)
A review of low-temperature plasma treatment of textile materials, Springer US, 2015, https://doi.org/10.1007/s10853-015-9152-4.

4 C. Tudoran, M. Corina, M. Coro, (2020)
A concise overview on plasma treatment for application on textile and leather materials, (2020), 1-15, https://doi.org/10.1002/ppap.202000046.

5 S. Shahidi, B. Moazzenchi, M. Ghoranneviss, (2015)
Physical Journal a review-application of physical vapor deposition (PVD), (2015), 1-13, https://doi.org/10.1051/epjap/2015140439.

6 D. Caschera, P. Cossari, F. Federici, S. Kaciulis, A. Mezzi, G. Padeletti, D.M. Trucchi, (2011)
In fluence of PECVD parameters on the properties of diamond-like carbon films, Thin Solid Films. 519 (2011), 4087-4091, https://doi.org/10.1016/j.tsf.2011.01.197.

7 G. Gigli, G.M. Ingo, G. Padeletti, D. Caschera, B. Cortese, A, (2013)
brief review of surface functionalized cotton fabrics, Surf. Innov. 1, (2013), 1-43, https://doi.org/10.1680/si.13.00008.

8 A. Haji, M. Naebe, (2020)
Cleaner dyeing of textiles using plasma treatment and natural dyes: A review, J. Clean. Prod. 265 (2020) 121866, https://doi.org/10.1016/j.jclepro.2020.121866.

9 N. V. Bhat, R. N. Bharati, A. V. Gore, a J. Patil, (2011)
Effect of atmospheric pressure air plasma treatment on desizing and wettability of cotton fabrics, Text. 36 (2011), 42-46.

10 J. Robertson, Diamond-like amorphous carbon, Mater. Sci. Eng., R 37 (2002), 129-281, https://doi.org/10.1016/S0927-796X(02)00005-0.

11 A. Grill, (1999)
Plasma-deposited diamondlike carbon and related materials, IBM J. Res. & Dev. 43 (1999) 147–162, https://doi.org/10.1147/rd.431.0147.

12 R.K. Roy, K.R. Lee, (2007)
Biomedical applications of diamond-like carbon coatings: A review, J. Biomed. Mater. Res. - Part B Appl. Biomater. 83 (2007) 72-84, https://doi.org/10.1002/jbm.b.30768.

13 T. Hubáček, J. Siegel, R. Khalili, N. Slepičková-Kasálková, V. Švorčík, (2013)
Carbon coatings on polymers and their biocompatibility, Appl. Surf. Sci. 275 (2013) 43-48, https://doi.org/10.1016/j.apsusc.2013.01.127.

14 L. Kleinen, U. Böde, K. Schenk, H. Busch, J. Bradenahl, S.C. Müller, B. Hillebrands, N. Laube, (2007)
Amorphous carbon coatings inhibit crystalline biofilm formation on urological implants, Plasma Process. Polym. 4 (2007) 386-391, https://doi.org/10.1002/ppap.200731005.

15 J. Wang, N. Huang, C.J. Pan, S.C.H. Kwok, P. Yang, Y.X. Leng, J.Y. Chen, H. Sun, G.J. Wan, Z.Y. Liu, P.K. Chu, (2004)
Bacterial repellence from polyethylene terephthalate surface modified by acetylene plasma immersion ion implantation-deposition, Surf. Coatings Technol. 186, (2004) 299-304, https://doi.org/10.1016/j.surfcoat.2004.02.046.

16 Z.A. Boeva, A. Catena, L. Höfler, S, Wehner, C.B. Fischer, T. Lindfors, (2017)
Improved water barrier properties of polylactic acid films with an amorphous hydrogenated carbon (a-C:H) coating, Carbon 120, (2017), 157-164, https://doi.org/10.1016/j.carbon.2017.05.005

17 C.B. Fischer, M. Rohrbeck, S. Wehner, M. Richter, D. Schmeißer, (2013)
Interlayer formation of diamond-like carbon coatings on industrial polyethylene: Thickness dependent surface characterization by SEM, AFM and NEXAFS, Applied Surface Science 271 (2013) 381-389, https://doi.org/10.1016/j.apsusc.2013.01.210.

18 T. Schlebrowski, W. Rouabeh, S. Wehner, C.B. Fischer, (2019)
Specifying the interlayer turning point and dehydrogenation in a-C:H layers plasma deposited on high-density polyethylene with X-ray synchrotron techniques, Thin Solid Films 691 (2019) 137617, https://doi.org/10.1016/j.tsf.2019.137617.

19 M. Rohrbeck, S. Körsten, C.B. Fischer, S. Wehner, B. Kessler, (2013)
Diamond-like carbon coating of a pure bioplastic foil, Thin Solid Films. 545 (2013) 558-563, https://doi.org/10.1016/j.tsf.2013.07.028.

20 A. Catena, S. Agnello, L.M. Rösken, H. Bergen, E. Recktenwald, F. Bernsmann, H. Busch, M. Cannas, F.M. Gelardi, B. Hahn, S. Wehner, C.B. Fischer, (2016)
Characteristics of industrially manufactured amorphous hydrogenated carbon (a-C:H) depositions on high-density polyethylene, Carbon 96 (2016) 661-671, https://doi.org/10.1016/j.carbon.2015.09.101.

21 A. Catena, Q. Guo, M.R. Kunze, S. Agnello, F.M. Gelardi, S. Wehner, C.B. Fischer, (2016)
Morphological and Chemical Evolution of Gradually Deposited Diamond-Like Carbon Films on Polyethylene Terephthalate: From Subplantation Processes to Structural Reorganization by Intrinsic Stress Release Phenomena, ACS Appl. Mater. Interfaces 8 (2016) 10636–10646, https://doi.org/10.1021/acsami.6b02113.

22 T. Schlebrowski, L. Beucher, H. Bazzi, B. Hahn, S. Wehner, C.B. Fischer, (2019)
Prediction of a-C:H layer failure on industrial relevant biopolymer polylactide acide (PLA) foils based on the sp2/sp3 ratio, Surface and Coatings Technology 368 (2019) 79–87, https://doi.org/10.1016/j.surfcoat.2019.03.069.

23 T. Schlebrowski, L. Beucher, H. Bazzi, B. Hahn, S. Wehner, C.B. Fischer, (2019)
Changing Contents of Carbon Hybridizations in Amorphous Hydrogenated Carbon Layers (a-C:H) on Sustainable Polyhydroxybutyrate (PHB) Exhibit a Significant Deterioration in Stability, Depending on Thickness, C 5 (2019) 52, https://doi.org/10.3390/c5030052.

24 L. Xu, J. Deng, Y. Guo, W. Wang, R. Zhang, J. Yu, (2019)
Fabrication of super-hydrophobic cotton fabric by low-pressure plasma-enhanced chemical vapor deposition, (2019), https://doi.org/10.1177/0040517518780000.

25 D. Kundu, D. Banerjee, S. Ghosh, N.S. Das, S. Thakur, B. Das, K.K. Chattopadhyay, (2019)
Plasma enhanced Chemical Vapour deposited amorphous carbon coating for hydrophobicity enhancement in commercial cotton fabrics, Physica E: Low-dimensional Systems and Nanostructures 114 (2019), 1-10, https://doi.org/10.1016/j.physe.2019.113594.

26 Q. Gao, Q. Zhu, Y. Guo, C.Q. Yang, (2009)
Formation of Highly Hydrophobic Surfaces on Cotton and Polyester Fabrics Using Silica Sol Nanoparticles and Nonfluorinated Alkylsilane, (2009), 9797-9803.

27 D. Caschera, B. Cortese, A. Mezzi, M. Brucale, G.M. Ingo, G. Gigli, G. Padeletti, (2013)
Ultra Hydrophobic/Superhydrophilic Modified Cotton Textiles through Functionalized Diamond-Like Carbon Coatings for Self- Cleaning Applications, Langmuir 29 (2013) 2775–2783, https://doi.org/10.1021/la305032k.

28 D. Caschera, R. G. Toro, F. Federici, C. Riccucci, G.M. Ingo, G. Gigli, B. Cortese, (2015)
Flame retardant properties of plasma pre-treated/diamond-like carbon (DLC) coated cotton fabrics, Cellulose 22 (2015) 2797–2809, https://doi.org/10.1007/s10570-015-0661-8.

29 N. Kitahara, T. Sato, H. Isogawa, Y. Ohgoe, S. Masuko, F. Shizuku, K.K. Hirakuri, (2010)
Antibacterial property of DLC film coated on textile material, Diam. Relat. Mater. 19 (2010) 690-694, https://doi.org/10.1016/j.diamond.2010.03.013.

30 H. Zhou, L. Xu, A. Ogino, M. Nagatsu, (2008)
Investigation into the antibacterial property of carbon films, Diam. Relat. Mater. 17, (2008), 1416-1419, https://doi.org/10.1016/j.diamond.2008.01.047.

31 S.K. Nema, P.B. Jhala, (2015)
Plasma Technologies for Textile and Apparel, 1st ed. New Delhi: Woodhead Publishing India in Textiles, 2015, p.36.

32 J. Friedrich, (2015)
The plasma chemistry of polymer surfaces: Advanced techniques for surface design, 1st ed. Weinheim: Wiley-VC, 2015, pp.3-4.

33 G. Buyle, (2009)
Nanoscale finishing of textiles via plasma treatment, Mater Technol 2009; 24: 46-51.

34 F. Rombaldoni, K. Mahmood, A.Varesano, et al., (2013)
Adhesion enhancement of electrospun nanofiber mats to polypropylene nonwoven fabric by low-temperature oxygen plasma treatment. Surf Coat Technol, 2013, 216: 178-184.

35 B. Cortese, C. Piliego, I. Viola, S. D'Amone, R. Cingolani, G. Gigli, (2009)
Engineering transfer of micro- and nanometer-scale features by surface energy modification, Langmuir, 25 (2009) 7025-7031, https://doi.org/10.1021/la900248j.

36 Mokbul M. Hossain, A.S. Herrmann, D. Hegemann, (2006)
Plasma Hydrophilization Effect on different textile structures, Plasma Processes and Polymers, DOI:10.1002/ppap.200500152.

37 H.-U. Poll, S. Schreiter, (1998)
Melliand Textilber. 1998, 6, 466.

38 A. M. Sarmadi, T. H. Ying, F. Denes, (1993)
Text. Res. J. 1993, 63, 697, https://doi.org/10.1177/004051759306301201.

39 A.M. Grancaric, L. Botteri, J. Alongi, G. Malucelli, (2015)
Synergistic effects occurring between water glasses and urea/ammonium dihydrogen phosphate pair for enhancing the flame retardancy of cotton, Cellulose (2015), 22:2825-2835. DOI:10.1007/s10570-015-0671-6.

40 International Organization for Standardization, (1995)
Textiles - Determination of the permeability of fabrics to air, EN ISO Standard No.9237:1995, https://www.iso.org/standard/16869.html.

41 International Organization for Standardization, (2013)
Textiles - Tensile properties of fabrics - Part 1: Determination of maximum force and elongation at maximum force using the strip method, ISO Standard No. 13934-1:2013, https://www.iso.org/standard/60676.html.

Part (IX): Testing Methods for Treated Textiles with Mosquito-Repellents: An Overview

Chapter 17:

Testing Methods for Mosquito-Repellent Treated Textiles

1 Anuar, A. A., and N. Yusof, (2016)
Methods of imparting mosquito repellent agents and the assessing mosquito repellency on textile, *Fashion and Textiles*, 3-12.

2 Barnard, D.R., U.R. Bernier, R.D. Xue, and M. Debboun, 2006
Chapter 5. Standard methods for testing mosquito repellents, P. 103-110, Insect Repellents, Principles, Methods, and Uses, ed. By M. Debboun, S.P. Frances, and D. Strickman, CRC Press, Boca Raton, FL, USA.

3 Barnard, D.R. and R.D. Xue, 2006
Chapter 6. Biometrics and behavior in mosquito repellent assays. P. 111-124, Insect Repellents, Principles, Methods, and Uses, ed. By M. Debboun, S.P. Frances, and D. Strickman, CRC Press, Boca Raton, FL, USA.

4 Brown, M., and A. A. Hebert, (1997)
Insect repellents: an overview, *Journal of American Academy of Dermatology*, 36, 243-249.

5 Carnevale, P. and F. Gay, (2019)
Insecticide-treated mosquito nets, Method Mol. Biol., 2013, 221-232.

6 Chareonviriyaphap, T., A. Prabaripai, and S. Sungvornyothrin, (2002)
An improved excito-repellency test chamber for mosquito behavioral tests, *Journal of Vector Ecology*, 27, 250-252.

7 Frances, S.P., (2015)
Chapter 17. Strategies for using personal protection products, In Insect Repellents Handbook. P.317-329. ed. By M. Debboun, S.P. Frances, and D. Strickman, CRC Press, Boca Raton, FL, USA.

8 Govere, J.M. and D.N. Durrheim, (2006)
Chapter 8. Techniques for evaluating repellents, In Insect Repellents Handbook, P.147-159. ed. By M. Debboun, S.P. Frances, and D. Strickman, CRC Press, Boca Raton, FL, USA.

9 Kawada, H., K. Ohashi, G. O. Dida, G. Sonye, S. M. Njenga, C. Mwandawiro, and N. Minakawa, (2014)
Insecticidal and repellent activities of pyrethroids to the three major pyrethroid-resistant malaria vectors in western Kenya, *Parasites and Vectors* 7, 208.

10 Kawada, H., K. Futami, Y. Higa, G. Rai, T. Suzuki, and S. K. Rai, (2020)
Distribution and pyrethroid resistance status of *Aedes aegypti* and *Aedes albopictus* populations and possible phylogenetic reasons for the recent invasion of *Aedes aegypti* in Nepal, *Parasites and Vectors* 13, 213.

11 Kuramoto, K., and H. Kawada, (2018)
Development of a bioassay device for evaluating mosquito repellency, *Pyrethrum Workshop 2018*, September 3-5, 2018, Cambridge, UK.

12 Kuramoto, K., T. Mitsuhashi, T. Saito, Y. Takahashi, A. Watanabe, S. Harada, C. Tsurukawa, Y. Morimoto, and H. Kawada, (2019)
Development of the bioassay device for evaluating mosquito repellency, *The 6th International Forum for Surveillance and Control of Mosquitoes and Vector-borne Diseases (IFSCMVD)*, May 27-31, 2019, Xia-men, China.

13 McCain W.C., and G. J. Leach, (2006)
Chapter 13. Repellents used in fabric: The experience of the U.S. military, P. 261-273. Insect Repellents, Principles, Methods, and Uses, ed. By M. Debboun, S.P. Frances, and D. Strickman. CRC Press, Boca Raton, FL, USA.

14 Obermayr U., (2015)
Chapter 6. Excitorepellency. In Insect Repellents Handbook, P. 91-115, ed. By M. Debboun, S.P. Frances, and D. Strickman, CRC Press, Boca Raton, FL, USA.

15 Rutledge, L.C., Z.A. Mehr, and M. Debboun, (2015)
Chapter 8. Testing methods for insect repellents, In Insect Repellents Handbook, P.159-178, ed. By M. Debboun, S.P. Frances, and D. Strickman, CRC Press, Boca Raton, FL, USA.

16 U.S. Department of Agriculture, (1967)
Materials evaluated as insecticides, repellents, and chemosterilants at Orlando and Gainesville, Fla. 1952-1964. Technical Handbook 340, U.S. Department of Agriculture, Washington DC.

17 World Health Organization, (2005)
Guidelines for laboratory and field testing of long-lasting insecticidal mosquito nets, WHO/CDS/WHOPES/GCDPP/2005.11, 1-18 pages.

Part (X):

Case Studies: Putting Knowledge into Action

Chapter 18:

A Case Study: How the Rephaiah Project Combats Malaria in Young Children

1 WHO, World Malaria Report, (2019)
World Health Organization, Geneva, 2019.

2 WHO, (2015)
Guidelines for the treatment of Malaria 3rd edition, World Health Organization, Geneva, 2015

3 NMCP and ICF, Malawi Malaria Indicator Survey (2017)
Lilongwe: National Malaria Control Programme, Malawi Ministry of Health; 2018.

4 U.S. President's Malaria Initiative Malawi Malaria Operational Plan FY, (2020)
https://www.pmi.gov/docs/default-source/default-document-library/malaria-operational-plans/fy20/fy-2020-malawi-malaria-operational-plan.pdf?sfvrsn=6.

5 National malaria control programme, (2019)
Guidelines for the treatment of Malaria in Malawi, 5th Edition, 2019.

6 Chilanga E, Collin-Vézina D, MacIntosh H, Mitchell C, Cherney K, (2020)
Prevalence and determinants of malaria infection among children of local farmers in Central Malawi, Malar J. 19: 308, 2020, DOI:10.1186/s12936-020-03382-7.

7 Klootwijk L, Chirwa AE, Kabaghe AN, van Vugt M., (2019)
Challenges affecting prompt access to uncomplicated malaria case management in children in rural primary health facilities in Chikhwawa Malawi, BMC Health Services Research, 19:735, 2019, DOI:10.1186/s12913-019-4544-9.

8 Whitty CJ, Chandler C, Ansah E, Leslie T, Staedke SG, (2008)
Deployment of ACT antimalarials for treatment of malaria: challenges and opportunities, Malar J , 11 (7 Suppl 1), S7, 2008.

9 Lowe R, Chirombo J, Tompkins AM, (2013)
Relative importance of climatic, geographic and socio-economic determinants of malaria in Malawi, Malar J. 12, 416, 2013.

10 Malawi National Statistical Office, (2018)
Population and Housing Census, Zomba: National Statistical Office of Malawi, 4, 2019.

11 Mpando, LRS, (2000)
Fertility Levels and Trends, Malawi Demographic and Health Survey, 2000.

12 Population Reference Bureau, (2020)
Why Population Matters to Malawi's Development: Managing Population Growth for Sustainable Development, https://www.prb.org/wp-content/uploads/2012/05/malawi-population-matters.pdf, Published May 7, 2012, Accessed December 17, 2020.

13 World Bank Group, (2020)
Malawi Systematic Country Diagnostic: Breaking the Cycle of Growth and Slow Poverty Reduction, https://openknowledge.worldbank.org/handle/10986/31131, Published December 2018, Accessed December 17, 2020.

14 Ferguson, H.M., Dornhaus, A., Beeche, A., Borgemeister, C., Gottlieb, M., Mulla, M.S., Gimnig JE, Fish D, Killeen GF., (2010)
Ecology: a prerequisite for malaria elimination and eradication, PLoS Med, 7(8), p.e1000303, 2010.

15 Okiro EA, Noor AM, Malinga J, Mitto B, Mundia CW, Mathanga D, Mzilahowa T, Snow RW, (2014)
An epidemiological profile of malaria and its control in Malawi, A report prepared for the Ministry of Health, the Roll Back Malaria partnership and the Department for International Development, UK, 2014.

16 Van den Berg H, van Vugt M, Kabaghe AN, Nkalapa M, Kaotcha R, Truwah Z, Malenga T, Kadama A, Banda S, Tizifa T, Gowelo S, (2018)
Community-based malaria control in southern Malawi: a description of experimental interventions of community workshops, house improvement and larval source management, Malaria Journal. 17(1):266, 2018.

17 Hunt RH, Edwardes M, Coetzee M, (2010)
Pyrethroid resistance in southern African Anopheles funestus extends to Likoma Island in Lake Malawi, Parasites & Vectors, 3(1):1-4, 2010.

18 Mzilahowa T, Ball AJ, Bass C, Morgan JC, Nyoni B, Steen K, Donnelly MJ, Wilding CS, (2008)
Reduced susceptibility to DDT in field populations of *Anopheles quadriannulatus* and *Anopheles arabiensis* in Malawi: evidence for larval selection, Medical and Veterinary Entomology. 22(3):258-63, 2008.

19 Idro R, Jenkins NE, Newton CR, (2005)
Pathogenesis, clinical features, and neurological outcome of cerebral malaria. The Lancet Neurology, 4(12), 827-840, 2005.

20 Idro R, Kakooza-Mwesige A, Balyejjussa S, Mirembe G, Mugasha C, Tugumisirize J, Byarugaba J, (2010)
Severe neurological sequelae and behaviour problems after cerebral malaria in Ugandan children, BMC research notes, 3(1), 104, 2010.

21 Birbeck GL, (2004)
Cerebral Malaria, Current Treatment Options in Neurology, 6(2), 125–137, 2004.

22 Birbeck GL, Molyneux ME, Kaplan PW, Seydel KB, Chimalizeni YF, Kawaza K, Taylor TE, (2010)
Blantyre Malaria Project Epilepsy Study (BMPES) of neurological outcomes in retinopathy-positive paediatric cerebral malaria survivors: a prospective cohort study, The Lancet Neurology, 9(12), 1173-1181, 2010.

23 Boivin MJ, Vokhiwa M, Sikorskii A, Magen JG, Beare NA, (2014)
Cerebral malaria retinopathy predictors of persisting neurocognitive outcomes in Malawian children, The Pediatric Infectious Disease Journal, 33(8), 821, 2014.

24 Boivin MJ, Gladstone MJ, Vokhiwa M, Birbeck GL, Magen JG, Page C, Semrud Clikeman M, Kauye F, Taylor TE, (2011)
Developmental outcomes in Malawian children with retinopathy-positive cerebral malaria, Tropical Medicine & International Health, 16(3), 263–271, 2011.

25 Boivin MJ, Bangirana P, Byarugaba J, Opoka RO, Idro R, Jurek AM, John CC, (2007)
Cognitive impairment after cerebral malaria in children: A prospective study, Pediatrics, 119(2), e360–366, 2007.

26 Grau GER, Craig AG, (2012)
Cerebral malaria pathogenesis: revisiting parasite and host contributions, Future microbiology, 7(2), 291-302, 2012.

27 Idro R, Kakooza-Mwesige A, Asea B, Ssebyala K, Bangirana P, Opoka RO, Lubowa SK, Semrud-Clikeman M, John CC, Nalugya J, (2016)
Cerebral malaria is associated with long-term mental health disorders: a cross sectional survey of a long-term cohort, Malaria Journal, 15(1), 184, 2016.

28 John CC, Bangirana P, Byarugaba J, Opoka RO, Idro R, Jurek AM, Wu B, Boivin MJ, (2008)
Cerebral malaria in children is associated with long-term cognitive impairment. Pediatrics, 122(1), e92–99, 2008.

29 Langfitt JT, McDermott MP, Brim R, Mboma S, Potchen MJ, Kampondeni SD, Seydel KB, Semrud-Clikeman M, Taylor TE, (2019)
Neurodevelopmental impairments 1 year after cerebral malaria, Pediatrics, 143(2), 2019.

30 Siddiqui AJ, Adnan M, Jahan S, Redman W, Saeed M, Patel M, (2020)
Neurological disorder and psychosocial aspects of cerebral malaria: what is new on its pathogenesis and complications? A minireview, Folia Parasitologica, 67, 015, 2020.

31 Ssenkusu JM, Hodges JS, Opoka RO, Idro R, Shapiro E, John CC, Bangirana P, (2016)
Long-term behavioral problems in children with severe malaria, Pediatrics, 138(5), 2016.

Chapter 19:

Strengthening the Control of Mosquito Vectors in Cabo Verde: New Approaches to Improve Intervention Strategies

1 Patterson KD., (1988)
Epidemics, Famines, and Population in the Cape Verde Islands, 1580-1900, Int J Afr His Stud. 1988; 21(2): 291-313.

2 Franco A, Menezes A, (1955)
A filaríase autóctone (W. bancrofti) na ilha de Santiago (Estudo preliminar), Ann. Inst. Med. Trop. 1955; 12: 369-393.

3 Ministério da Saúde (Cabo Verde), (2009)
Plano Estratégico de pré-eliminação do Paludismo 2009-2013. Praia, 2009 Mar; 1–64. Available from: http://www.insp.gov.cv/index.php/documentos/outors-documentos/8-programa-nacional-de-luta-contra-o-paludismo/file.

4 World Health Organisation. Dengue fever in Cape Verde. City of Praia; 2009 Nov 18. Available from: https://www.who.int/csr/don/2009_11_18/en/.

5 Ministério da Saúde e da Segurança Social (Cabo Verde), (2016)
Infeção por Vírus Zika (ZIKV) Ano 2016: (Semanas de 1 a 21), Praia, 2016, Available from: https://www.minsaude.gov.cv/index.php/documentosite/zika-1/341-boletim-informativo-semanal-da-infecao-por-virus-zika-semana-21-ano-2016/file.

6 Ministério da Saúde e da Segurança Social (Cabo Verde), (2018)
Manual de Luta integrada de vetores e engajamento comunitário, MSSS. Praia, 2018.

7 Ministério da Saúde e da Segurança Social (Cabo Verde), (2017)
Boletim Informativo da Evolução dos Casos de Paludismo, Cabo Verde, 2017 Nov 12: 1-8, Available from: https://www.minsaude.gov.cv/index.php/documentosite/paludismo/449-boletim-informativo-evolucao-dos-casos-do-paludismo-ate-12-de-novembro-2017/file.

8 Instituto Nacional da Estatística (Cabo Verde), (2013)
Projeção Demográficas de Cabo Verde, 2010-2030. INE. Cabo Verde; 2013.

9 Santos ME, Torrão MM; Soares MJ, (2007)
História Concisa de Cabo Verde, Instituto de Investigação Científica Tropical, Instituto Nacional de Investigação e Património Culturais de Cabo Verde, Lisboa-Praia, 2007, ISBN: 978-972-672-973-0.

10 Instituto Nacional da Estatística (Cabo Verde), (2018)
Dados Estatísticos sobre a Cidade da Praia; 2018: 1937–2017.

11 Braga IA, Gomes AC, Nelson Mello R, Bergamashi D, de souza JM, (2000)
Comparação entre pesquisa larvária e armadilha de oviposição, para detecção de Aedes aegypti, Revista da Sociedade Brasileira de Medicina Tropical, 2000; 33(4):347-353.

12 Braga IA, Valle, D, (2007)
- *Aedes aegypti*: vigilância, monitoramento da resistência e alternativas de controle no Brasil, Epidemiol, Serv. Saúde. Brasília, 2007; 16(4):295-302.

13 Santos, SRA, Melo-Santos, MAV, Regis, L & Albuquerque, CMR,(2003)
Field evaluation of ovitraps consociated with grass infusion and Bacillus thuringiensis var. israelensis to determine oviposition rates of *Aedes aegypti*, Dengue Bulletin. 2003,27.

14 Tilak R, Gupta V, Suryam V, Yadav JD, Gupta KD, (2011)
A Laboratory Investigation into Oviposition Responses of *Aedes aegypti* to Some Common Household Substances and Water from Conspecific Larvae, Med J Armed Forces India, 2005 Jul;61(3):227-9, DOI:10.1016/S0377-1237(05)80159-5.Epub, 2011 May 30, PMID: 27407765; PMCID: PMC4925447.

15 Stoops C. Influence of Bacillus thuringiensis var. israelensis on oviposition of Aedes albopictus (Skuse). Journal of Vector Ecology. Clemson: Departament of entomology, 2005, 30(1):41-44.

16 Araújo AP, Araujo Diniz DF, Helvecio E, de Barros RA, de Oliveira CM, Ayres CF, de Melo-Santos MA, Regis LN, Silva-Filha MH, (2013)
The susceptibility of *Aedes aegypti* populations displaying temephos resistance to Bacillus thuringiensis israelensis: a basis for management, Parasit Vectors, 2013;6(1):297, DOI:10.1186/1756-3305-6-297.

17 Aronson AI, Shai Y, (2001)
Why Bacillus thuringiensis insecticidal toxins are so effective: unique features of their mode of action, FEMS Microbiol Lett. 2001, 195(1):1-8, DOI:10.1111/j.1574-6968.2001.tb10489.x.

18 Gómez LF, Oliveira AL de, Moura AJF da, Rocha HDR, Miquel M, Ayres CF, (2015)
Spatio-temporal survey of *Aedes aegypti* population in Cape Verde throught geographic information systems, XIV Curso Internacional de Dengue, La Habana, Cuba, 2015.

19 Acioli, R., (2006)
O uso de armadilhas de Oviposição (ovitrampas) como ferramenta para monitoramento populacional do *Aedes spp* em bairros do Recife, Dissertação (Mestrado em Saúde Pública) – Centro de Pesquisa Aggeu Magalhães, Fundação Oswaldo Cruz, Recife, 2006.

20 Reiter P, Nathan M., (2001)
Guidelines for assessing the eficacy of insecticidal space sprays for control of the Dengue vector *Aedes aegypti*, WHO/CDS/CPE/PVC/2001, 2001.

21 Fay, R., Perry, A, (1965)
Laboratory studies of ovipositional preferences of *Aedes aegypti*, Mosquito News, 1965; 25(3):276-281.

22 Alves J, Gomes B, Rodrigues R, Silva J, Arez AP and Pinto J, (2010)
Mosquito fauna on the Cape Verde Islands (West Africa): an update on species distribution and a new finding, Journal of Vector Ecology 35: 307–312, DOI:10.1111/j.1948-7134.2010.00087.x.

23 Leal SDV, Fernandes Varela IB, Lopes Gonçalves AAL, Sousa Monteiro DD, Ramos de Sousa CM, Lima Mendonça MDL, De Pina AJ, Alves MJ, Osório HC, (2020)
Abundance and Updated Distribution of *Aedes aegypti* (Diptera: Culicidae) in Cabo Verde Archipelago: A Neglected Threat to Public Health, Int J Environ Res Public Health, 2020 Feb 17, 17(4):1291, DOI:10.3390/ijerph17041291.

24 Regis L, Monteiro AM, Melo-Santos MA, Silveira JC Jr, Furtado AF, Acioli RV, Santos GM, Nakazawa M, Carvalho MS, Ribeiro PJ Jr, Souza WV, (2008)
Developing new approaches for detecting and preventing *Aedes aegypti* population outbreaks: basis for surveillance, alert and control system, Mem Inst Oswaldo Cruz, 2008, 103(1):50-9, DOI:10.1590/s0074-02762008000100008.

25 Barbosa RM, Regis LN, (2011)
Monitoring temporal fluctuations of *Culex quinquefasciatus* using oviposition traps containing attractant and larvicide in an urban environment in Recife, Brazil, Mem Inst Oswaldo Cruz, 2011 Jun, 106(4):451-5, DOI:10.1590/s0074-02762011000400011.

26 Barbosa RM, Souto A, Eiras AE, Regis L, (2007)
Laboratory and field evaluation of an oviposition trap for *Culex quinquefasciatus* (Diptera: Culicidae), Mem Inst Oswaldo Cruz, 2007 Jun, 102(4):523-9, DOI:10.1590/s0074-02762007005000058.

27 Xavier MN, Santos EM, Silva AP, Gomes Júnior PP, Barbosa RM, Oliveira CM, (2018)
Field evaluation of sticky BR-OVT traps to collect culicids eggs and adult mosquitoes inside houses, Rev Soc Bras Med Trop, 2018, 51:297-303.

28 Alvarado-Castro V, Paredes-Solís S, Nava-Aguilera E, Morales-Pérez A, Alarcón-Morales L, Balderas-Vargas NA, Andersson N, (2017)
Assessing the effects of interventions for *Aedes aegypti* control: systematic review and meta-analysis of cluster randomised controlled trials, BMC Public Health, 2017 May 30, 17(Suppl 1):384, DOI:10.1186/s12889-017-4290-z.

29 Bouzid M, Brainard J, Hooper L, Hunter PR, (2016)
Public Health Interventions for *Aedes* Control in the Time of Zikavirus- A Meta-Review on Effectiveness of Vector Control Strategies, PLoS Negl Trop Dis, 2016 Dec 7, 10(12):e0005176, DOI:10.1371/journal.pntd.0005176.

30 Achee NL, Gould F, Perkins TA, Reiner RC Jr, Morrison AC, Ritchie SA, Gubler DJ, Teyssou R, Scott TW, (2015)
A critical assessment of vector control for dengue prevention, PLoS Negl Trop Dis, 2015 May 7, 9(5):e0003655, DOI:10.1371/journal.pntd.0003655.

31 Wilke ABB, Beier JC, Benelli G, (2019)
Complexity of the relationship between global warming and urbanization - an obscure future for predicting increases in vector-borne infectious diseases, Curr Opin Insect Sci, 2019 Oct;35, 1-9. DOI:10.1016/j.cois.2019.06.002.

32 Otmani Del Barrio M, Simard F, Caprara A, (2018)
Supporting and strengthening research on urban health interventions for the prevention and control of vector-borne and other infectious diseases of poverty: scoping reviews and research gap analysis, Infect Dis Poverty, 2018 Sep 3, 7(1):94, DOI:10.1186/s40249-018-0462-z.

33 Schiøler KL, Alifrangis M, Kitron U, Konradsen F, (2016)
Insecticidal Paints: A Realistic Approach to Vector Control?, PLoS Negl Trop Dis, 2016 Apr 21, 10(4):e0004518, DOI:10.1371/journal.pntd.0004518.

34 Mosqueira B, Duchon S, Chandre F, Hougard JM, Carnevale P, Mas-Coma S, (2010)
Efficacy of an insecticide paint against insecticide susceptible and resistant mosquitoes - part 1: laboratory evaluation, Malar J., 2010,25;9:340, DOI:10.1186/1475-2875-9-340.

35 World Health Organization, (2006)
Guidelines for testing mosquito *adulticides* for indoor residual spraying and treatment of mosquito nets, 2006, https://apps.who.int/iris/handle/10665/69296.